Eating Disorders in Children and Adolescents

Anorexia nervosa and other eating disorders are arguably the most complex mental health problems that a child or adolescent may experience. Numbers seeking help are on the increase, and the complexity of these disorders challenges even the most experienced clinician. In this timely book the experience of numerous practitioners with international reputations in the field is brought to bear on the broad range of issues a good clinician needs to know about, from the history of the disorder through to treatment, psychopharmacology, the psychotherapies, epidemiology, comorbidities, eating disorders in boys and neuroimaging. The book is divided into five parts detailing the scientific underpinnings, abnormal states, the evidence base for treatments, and finally public health issues, including service delivery models and perspectives on prognosis and outcomes. Clinicians encountering eating disorders will find this latest addition to the Cambridge Child and Adolescent Psychiatry series invaluable.

Tony Jaffa is Consultant Child and Adolescent Psychiatrist for Cambridgeshire and Peterborough NHS Mental Health Trust and Associate Lecturer of the University of Cambridge. He is also Clinical Director of the Cambridge Child and Adolescent Mental Health Service. He has worked in the area of child and adolescent anorexia nervosa and other eating disorders for nearly 15 years and in 1998 opened the first UK NHS inpatient unit solely for teenagers with anorexia nervosa. He has published widely in the professional literature with recent papers and chapters focusing mostly on issues of service delivery and on eating disorders. He has presented on these in national and international conferences.

Brett McDermott is a Consultant Child and Adolescent Psychiatrist, Director of the Mater Child and Youth Mental Health Service in Brisbane, Australia, and an Associate Professor at the University of Queensland. He has worked in the area of child and adolescent anorexia nervosa and other eating disorders for over 10 years and was the foundation Director of the Eating Disorders Team at the Princess Margaret Hospital for Children in Perth. He has presented at national and international conferences on eating disorders in children and adolescents and published on this topic, as well as on emotional trauma in children and children's responses to natural disasters.

Cambridge Child and Adolescent Psychiatry

Child and adolescent psychiatry is an important and growing area of clinical psychiatry. The last decade has seen a rapid expansion of scientific knowledge in this field and has provided a new understanding of the underlying pathology of mental disorders in these age groups. This series is aimed at practitioners and researchers both in child and adolescent mental health services and in developmental and clinical neuroscience. Focusing on psychopathology, it highlights those topics where the growth of knowledge has had the greatest impact on clinical practice and on the treatment and understanding of mental illness. Individual volumes benefit from both the international expertise of their contributors and a coherence generated through a uniform style and structure for the series. Each volume provides first an historical overview and a clear descriptive account of the psychopathology of a specific disorder or group of related disorders. These features then form the basis for a thorough critical review of the etiology, natural history and later adult adjustment. Whilst each volume is therefore complete in its own right, volumes also relate to each other to create a flexible and collectable series that should appeal to students as well as to experienced scientists and practitioners.

Editorial board

Already published in this series

Eating disorders in children and adolescents

Edited by
Tony Jaffa
and
Brett McDermott

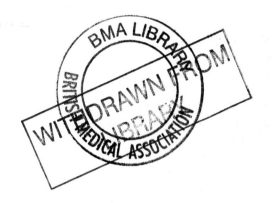

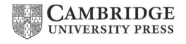

CAMBRIDGE
UNIVERSITY PRESS

CAMBRIDGE UNIVERSITY PRESS
Cambridge, New York, Melbourne, Madrid, Cape Town, Singapore, São Paulo

CAMBRIDGE UNIVERSITY PRESS
The Edinburgh Building, Cambridge CB2 2RU, UK

Published in the United States of America by Cambridge University Press, New York

www.cambridge.org
Information on this title: www.cambridge.org/9780521613125

© Cambridge University Press 2007

First published 2007

Printed in the United Kingdom at the University Press, Cambridge

A catalogue record for this publication is available from the British Library

ISBN-13 978-0-521-61312-5 paperback
ISBN-10 0-521-61312-4 paperback

Contents

Part III   Abnormal states

Part IV   Evidence-based care

Part V   Public health perspectives

Contributors

Alan Apter
Feinberg Child Study Centre,
Schneider Children's
Medical Centre
14 Kaplan Street
Petah Tikva 49202,
Israel

Lynne Green
University of Liverpool,
Section of Adolescent Psychiatry,
Academic Unit,
79 Liverpool Road,
Chester CH2 1AW, UK

C. Laird Birmingham
Department of Psychiatry,
University of British Columbia,
Saint Paul's Hospital,
1081 Burrard Street,
Vancouver, BC
Canada V6Z 1Y6

Caroline Braet,
Ghent University,
H-Dunantlaan 2,
B-900 Ghent, Belgium

Timothy Brewerton
Department of Psychiatry and
Behavioral Sciences,
Medical University of
South Carolina,
67 President Street,
Charleston, SC 29482, USA

Rachel Bryant-Waugh
Department of Child and
Adolescent Mental Health,
Great Ormond Street Hospital for
Children NHS Trust,
Great Ormond Street,
London WC1N 3JH, UK

Emily Burton
Department of Psychology,
The University of Texas at Austin,
1 University Station A8000
Austin, TX 78712, USA

Meghan Butryn
Department of Psychology,
Mail Stop 626,
Drexel University,
245 N. 15th Street,
Philadelphia, PA 19102, USA

Jennifer Couturier
Eating Disorders Program for
Children and Adolescents,
London Health Sciences Centre,
800 Commissioners Road East,
London, ON,
Canada N6C 2V5

Ida Dancyger
North Shore University Hospital,
NYU School of Medicine,
400 Community Drive,
Manhasset, NY 11030, USA

Gina Dimitropoulos
Division of Behavioural
Sciences and Health,
Toronto General Research Institute,
TGH, Room 8-219, Eaton N Wing,
200 Elizabeth Street,
Toronto, ON, Canada

Victor Fornari
North Shore University Hospital,
NYU School of Medicine,
400 Community Drive,
Manhasset, NY 11030, USA

Hans-Christoph Friederich
Department of Psychosomatic and
General Internal Medicine,
Heidelberg University,
Im Neuenheimer Feld 410,
69120 Heidelberg, Germany

Simon Gowers
University of Liverpool,
Section of Adolescent Psychiatry,

Academic Unit,
79 Liverpool Road,
Chester CH2 1AW, UK

Phillipa Hay
Discipline of Psychiatry,
School of Medicine,
James Cook University,
Townsville,
QLD 4811, Australia

Andrew Hill
Academic Unit of Psychiatry and
Behavioural Sciences,
Leeds University School
of Medicine,
15 Hyde Terrace,
Leeds LS2 9LT, UK

Tony Jaffa
The Phoenix Centre, Ida Darwin,
Fulbourn,
Cambridge CB1 5EE, UK

Debra K. Katzman
Division of Behavioural
Sciences and Health,
Toronto General Research Institute,
TGH, Room 8-219, Eaton N Wing,
200 Elizabeth Street,
Toronto, ON, Canada

Richard Kreipe
Golisano Children's Hospital at
Strong,
Division of Adolescent Medicine,
601 Elmwood Avenue, Box 690,
Rochester, NY 14642, USA

Orit Krispin
Feinberg Child Study Centre,
Schneider Children's Medical
Centre,
14 Kaplan Street,
Petah Tikva 49202, Israel

Shani Leor
Feinberg Child Study Centre,
Schneider Children's Medical Centre
14 Kaplan Street,
Petah Tikva 49202, Israel

James Lock
Lucile Salter Packard Children's
Hospital at Stanford,
401 Quarry Road,
Stanford, CA 94305, USA

Michael Lowe
Department of Psychology,
Mail Stop 626,
Drexel University,
245 N. 15th Street,
Philadelphia, PA 19102, USA

Brett McDermott
Mater Child & Youth Mental Health
Service,
Management Unit, Level 2,
Community Services Building,
Annerley Road,
South Brisbane, QLD 4101,
Australia

Julian Mercer
Division of Obesity and Metabolic
Health,

Rowett Research Institute,
Aberdeen AB21 0SB, Scotland

James E. Mitchell
Neuropsychiatric Research Institute,
P.O. Box 1415,
120 8th Street South,
Fargo, ND 58107, USA

Dasha Nicholls
Department of Child and
Adolescent Mental Health,
Great Ormond Street Hospital for
Children NHS Trust,
London WC1N 3JH, UK

Søren Nielsen
Storstrom County Psychiatric
Services,
Storstrom County Hospital in
Naestved,
Ringstedgade 61,
DK-4700, Naestved, Denmark

Greta Noordenbos,
Department of Clinical Psychology,
Leiden University,
Wassenaarseweg 52,
2333 AK Leiden, the Netherlands

Leora Pinhas
Division of Behavioural
Sciences and Health,
Toronto General Research Institute,
TGH, Room 8-219,
Eaton N Wing,
200 Elizabeth Street,
Toronto, ON, Canada

James Roerig
Neuropsychiatric Research Institute,
P.O. Box 1415,
120 8th Street South,
Fargo, ND 58107, USA

Kristine J. Steffen
Neuropsychiatric Research Institute,
P.O. Box 1415,
120 8th Street South,
Fargo, ND 58107, USA

Hans Steiner
Department of Psychiatry and
Behavioral Sciences,
Stanford University School of
Medicine,
401 Quarry Road,
Stanford, CA 94305-5719, USA

H.-C. Steinhausen
Department of Child and Adolescent
Psychiatry,
University of Zurich,
Neumensterallee 9,
Postfach CH-8032,
Zurich, Switzerland

Eric Stice
Psychology Department,
Seay Psychology Building,

University of Texas,
Austin, TX 78712, USA

Peter B. Sullivan
Department of Paediatrics,
John Radcliffe Hospital,
Headington,
Oxford OX3 9DU, UK

Janet Treasure
Department of Academic Psychiatry,
5th Floor Thomas Guy House,
Guy's Hospital,
London SE1 9RT, UK

Mytilee Vemuri
Department of Psychiatry and
Behavioral Sciences,
Stanford University School of
Medicine,
401 Quarry Road,
Stanford, CA 94305-5719, USA

D. Blake Woodside
Division of Behavioural
Sciences and Health,
Toronto General Research Institute,
TGH, Room 8-219,
Eaton N Wing,
200 Elizabeth Street,
Toronto, ON, Canada

Part I

Introduction

1

Historical and current conceptualizations of eating disorders: a developmental perspective

Mytilee Vemuri and Hans Steiner

Stanford University School of Medicine, Stanford, CA, USA

There is no human society that deals rationally with food in its environment, that eats according to the availability, edibility, and nutritional values alone.

(Hilde Bruch, 1973, p. 3)

Introduction

Eating disorders are complex, multi-faceted and acutely sensitive to societal and cultural pressures. They challenge clinicians to expand their understanding beyond the individual and consider external pressures that trigger and maintain the process of disordered eating. In this chapter, we review how conceptualizations of eating disorders have evolved, and highlight the power of social context in the development and maintenance of these 'diseases'. We shall also review current research into eating disorders, which spans numerous disciplines, including psychology, psychiatry, sociology, and more recently genetics and molecular biology. Multidisciplinary approaches are particularly helpful for conceptualizing eating disorders. As these disorders generally develop in childhood and adolescence, we pay particular attention to a developmental approach that also considers societal pressures, developmental norms, mutability of behaviours, and the individual's unique response to his or her environment.

History of anorexia nervosa

While the term 'anorexia nervosa' (AN) was first introduced into medical literature in 1874 by Dr William Gull, reports of self-starvation may date back to times of early Christianity (Keel & Klump, 2003). Cases of self-starvation

Eating Disorders in Children and Adolescents, ed. Tony Jaffa and Brett McDermott. Published by Cambridge University Press. © Cambridge University Press 2007.

attributed to demonic possession were documented in the fifth century (Keel & Klump, 2003). Saint Wilgefortis, thought to have lived between the eighth and twelfth centuries, reportedly engaged in self-starvation resulting in emaciation and (what has been speculated to be) lanugo – the fine downy hair that may result from anorexia and malnutrition (Keel & Klump, 2003). Detailed accounts of eating disorders prior to the twelfth century are limited, therefore it has been difficult to apply the diagnosis of AN or bulimia nervosa (BN) to such cases.

Holy starvation

Self-starvation in medieval times was often seen in the context of religious piety. The best known of the abstinent medieval religious figures was St Catherine of Siena who entered a pattern of self-starvation that ultimately resulted in her death in 1380 at age 32–33. Of note, starvation was only one of many austerities St Catherine partook in, including self-flagellation, scalding and sleeping on a bed of thorny substances (Brumberg, 1989), raising the question of whether starvation was a meaningful (or pathological) behaviour in its own right. The various accounts of self-starvation (primarily in women) in the Middle Ages were often interpreted as signs of extreme religious piety, or perhaps even miracles that they had continued to survive on so little nourishment. However, with the coming of the Christian reformation, self-starvation as a means of achieving holiness was viewed with greater suspicion, and perhaps even viewed as demoniacal (Brumberg, 1989; Keel & Klump, 2003).

Miraculous maids

By the seventeenth and eighteenth centuries, young women who abstained from food were termed 'miraculous maids' and were scrutinized with both scepticism and awe (Brumberg, 1989). During this period, prolonged abstinence from food was seen as a symptom of organic illness. Richard Morton's 1694 thesis on consumption is often cited as the first clinical description of what we currently call anorexia nervosa (Strober, 1986). He described a state of 'nervous atrophy' characterized by decreased appetite, amenorrhea, food aversion, emaciation, hyperactivity and indifference to the condition. He attributed the condition to a malfunction of the brain and nerves as well as observing a pathological emotional component contributing to a mind-body process (Strober, 1986). The eighteenth century, which saw advances in anatomy and reflex neurophysiology, also brought new conceptualizations of eating disorders. For example, in 1767, the English scientist Richard Whytt attributed food aversions and food cravings to the gastric nerves. Until the nineteenth century the term 'anorexia', or loss of appetite, was applied to the symptom associated with a variety of physical and emotional disorders such as hysteria, mania, melancholy, chlorosis and psychotic disorders.

Emergence of anorexia nervosa in the 20th century

Anorexia nervosa emerged as a distinctive syndrome in the latter part of the nineteenth century, as described by separate reports by William Gull and Charles Lasègue. Gull took note of onset during adolescence, preponderance in females and significant psychological component. Lasègue's report on 'l'anorexia hysterique' likewise underscores the psychological component to the disease in his case study,

A young girl . . . suffers from some emotion which she avows or conceals . . . At first she feels uneasiness after food. At the end of some weeks there is no longer a supposed temporary repugnance, but a refusal of food that may be indefinitely prolonged.

(Cited in Strober, 1986, p. 235.)

It also pointed out the role of the family in the disease form and process.

The family has but two methods at its service which it always exhausts – entreaties and menaces, and which both serve as a touchstone. The delicacies of the table are multiplied in the hope of stimulating the appetite; but the more the solicitude increases, the more the appetite diminishes. (Cited in Strober, 1986, p. 235.)

The debate over fasting girls existed against the backdrop of the Victorian debate between science and religion. The existence of these young women, despite their abstinence from nourishment, seemed to defy science, and aroused suspicion particularly from scientists and medical doctors. As fame and fortune were potential outcomes of the publicity surrounding such girls, scrutiny of their means and motivation was not uncommon.

While Gull and Lasègue's work clearly defined the clinical features of AN, conceptualizations of the disease and treatments remained controversial. The beginning of the twentieth century saw a trend towards medicalization of diseases. In 1914, Simmond published a case report about cachexia due to pituitary dysfunction. For several years following this publication, the notion of hypophyseal insufficiency and a largely biological/medical conceptualization of the disease dominated popular conceptualizations (Vandereycken, 2002).

Psychoanalytic theories

The 1940s and 1950s saw the rise of psychoanalysis in psychiatry, and so followed a dominance of psychoanalytic perspectives on anorexia and obesity.

Hunger was seen as an innate drive, and food viewed as an unconscious symbol of desires (e.g. love, hatred, sexual gratification, pregnancy). The fear of food intake seen in anorexia was linked with unconscious fears of oral impregnation, or fears of adulthood and sexuality (Bruch, 1973; Brumberg, 1989).

Psychodynamic theories

Hilde Bruch's prolific studies of eating disorders in the latter half of the twentieth century brought a broader, deeper perspective to eating disorders. She supported the notion of early developmental problems resulting in a disruption of an individual's emotional and physiological experience of food and satiation (Bruch, 1973). She argued that inappropriate reciprocal feedback patterns between mother and child around feeding may result in disturbances in hunger awareness, particularly if feeding occurred to gratify the mother's needs over the child's (e.g. in order to keep the child quiet, or timing feeds to suit mother's needs). Such disruptions may affect a child's development of autonomy or inner-directedness (Bruch, 1973). She noted in both obese and anorexic patients: a misperception of their body size, misperceptions of satiety, misperceptions or resistance to their sexual role, and misperceptions of their affective states. She speculated that anorexic and obese patients alike experience their bodies as not being truly their own, but under the influence of others. She viewed the behaviours associated with anorexia as a means of undoing feelings of passivity, ineffectiveness and control by outside forces.

History of bulimia

The term bulimia nervosa (BN) was first introduced into the medical literature by Gerald Russell in 1979 and, it should be noted, was first introduced as a sub-type of AN. While historical examination shows evidence of behaviours similar to AN, it is difficult to find the same pattern for bulimia. Bingeing behaviours and purging behaviours have certainly existed prior to the twentieth century. Vomitoriums existed in ancient roman times, and bingeing/purging may have been common behaviours. Excessive appetites have also been described historically. However, a consistent pattern of behaviours, or afflicted populations, has not been elucidated. Many of the historical descriptions cited in literature seem more consistent with other disorders such as AN, or psychogenic vomiting. Moreover, many of the afflicted individuals were known to be men, rather than adolescent women. Access to food may have also been a key factor to the development of the disease. Historically, food consumed a much larger part of household income, and was possibly more scarce, making binge-eating much more difficult, and/or more likely to occur in men (Keel & Klump, 2003).

Contemporary social trends influencing the development of eating disorders

In the nineteenth century, Charles Lasègue observed the importance of home environment in shaping eating disorder pathology, as well as precipitating emotional stress. Historian Joan Jacob Brumberg points out that during this period in history, middle-class sons and daughters were spending greater amounts of time at home, creating a 'prolonged dependency and intensification of parent–child relationships' (Brumberg, 1989), which she suggests provided fodder for psychological predicaments surrounding individuation. Moreover, as food was becoming more abundant, family meals took centre stage in daily life and perhaps became an accessible (and socially appropriate) venue for daughters to express themselves through their eating patterns. In the twentieth century a new thin ideal for women emerged. Vandereycken notes,

Until the 17th century, the tummy-centered and – by present day standards rather plump – woman was admired. This 'reproductive' type was then replaced by the 'hour-glass' model, with a narrow waist, full bosom, and round bottom. Since the late 19th century, the idealized shape for women has been the lean, almost 'tubular' body type, deprived of any symbolism of fertility and motherhood. (Vandereycken, 2002.)

Fatness became associated with the middle or lower classes in the nineteenth and twentieth centuries. The 'flapper era', where slenderness was stylish, emerged in the 1930s – a time when old established sex roles were being questioned (Boskind-White & White, 1986). Ready-made, mass-produced fashions emerging in the twentieth century favoured lean, more androgynous shapes. The 1960s and 1970s saw the emergence of models such as Twiggy, who personified youthfulness, and asexuality, during a period when pre-adolescents made up a large part of the American population. The emphasis on a thin, possibly pre-adolescent body physique for women, and devaluation of fatness and old age, has generally been embraced by culture since then.

Current conceptualizations

Models for understanding eating disorders based on diagnostic criteria

History illustrates that eating disorders are heterogeneous in presentation as well as in background; such heterogeneity makes it difficult to apply a diagnosis. In clinical practice, our diagnostic efforts are generally guided by

DSM–IV (Diagnostic and Statistical Manual of Mental Disorders, 4th edition; APA, 2000) or ICD–10 (International Classification of Diseases, 10th edition) criteria. The clinician must place the patient and their behaviour into distinct categories, in order to separate normal from pathological behaviour. Currently the DSM–IV includes the following under eating disorders: AN, BN and eating disorder not otherwise specified (EDNOS). Anorexia nervosa is characterized by the refusal to maintain a minimally normal weight. Bulimia nervosa is characterized by repeated episodes of binge eating, followed by inappropriate compensatory behaviour (including vomiting, fasting, excessive exercise, laxatives, diuretics). In addition, the DSM–IV includes fear of becoming fat, and amenorrhoea in postmenarchal women as necessary criteria for AN. Disturbance in perception of one's body weight and size is included as a necessary criterion for both disorders. Two additional diagnoses are included in the DSM–IV: EDNOS and binge-eating disorder (BED), which is included as a provisional category. Eating disorder NOS is essentially any eating disorder which does not fulfil criteria for AN or BN. Obesity, while arguably a result of maladaptive eating patterns, does not appear in the DSM–IV because it has not consistently been associated with a specific psychological or behavioural syndrome.

In addition to guiding our diagnosis of eating disorders, the DSM–IV criteria naturally influence the way we conceptualize disorders. In that respect, it may fall short – it is not designed to focus on pathogenic processes, and therefore does not inform the clinician about aetiologies of disease. Its categorical approach has also been criticized for being both overinclusive and underinclusive. For example, the DSM–IV criterion of weight phobia for AN may not apply across cultures. Weight phobia is more often seen in westernized countries than in other cultures, and has therefore been speculated to be a culture-bound feature of eating disorders. Additionally, individuals with atypical behaviour (i.e. who purge, but do not binge, or who use insulin to control their weight) would be excluded from DSM–IV criteria for either AN or BN. Amenorrhoea may be an overinclusive criterion in that it may be a consequence of malnutrition (not primarily AN), which may occur as a result of numerous medical disorders.

The categorical approach of the DSM–IV has also been criticized for creating artificial boundaries among various eating disorders, and from 'normal'. The developmental perspective argues that the pathological phenomena, which are the criteria for eating disorders, in fact occur quite commonly in so-called normal populations. Descriptive criteria imply a level of independence and stability of disorder that is not justified in the context of rapid changes, such as in adolescence. Sometimes patients fulfil all diagnostic criteria at one point, only to rapidly exit from the illness as they grow older and operate in a different social and temporal context (peer group, family, middle vs. late adolescence). The developmental perspective also challenges the notion that symptoms are sole expressions of internal deficits. It asserts that symptoms are also the function of external environment, represent adaptations to that environment, and thus are impossible to understand without taking psychosocial context into account.

Models for understanding eating disorders based on aetiology

Eating disorders are best understood as final common pathways that result from a wide range of interactions between psychosocial influences and endogenous vulnerabilities. We review diverse fields from genetics to feminist theory, which have contributed to our understanding of eating disorders.

Biological vulnerabilities and conceptualizations

Eating disorders have long been observed to run in families, and genetic epidemiological studies have uncovered evidence that eating disorders are, to some degree, heritable (Wade *et al.*, 2000). Thus far there has been little evidence of genetic main effects. Gene–environment interactions (G × E) with the effect of environment conditional upon the individual's genotype are a promising research area (see Leor, Krispin & Apter, Chapter 6, this volume). Mercer (Chapter 2, this volume) summarizes biological food intake and weight control systems that are potential targets for future single gene, polygenic and G × E research.

Psychological/individual: influences and models

Personality types have often been linked to eating disorders (Wonderlich, 2002). The personality style of patients with restricting type AN is often described as obsessional, socially inhibited, compliant and emotionally restrained (reminiscent of obsessive-compulsive disorder). The personality style of patients with BN is often described as impulsive, interpersonally sensitive and low in self-esteem (more akin to borderline features).

Cognitive behavioural models hold that anorexic and bulimic symptoms are maintained by a characteristic set of beliefs about weight and shape. Core cognitive disturbances are understood in terms of 'schema' (organized cognitive structures) that unite the views of the self and the culturally derived beliefs about the virtue of thinness for female appearance. Such schema give rise to the belief that the solution to a view of the self as unworthy, imperfect and

overwhelmed is thinness and weight loss, which are therefore pursued relent-
lessly (Shafran & de Silva, 2003). This approach does not account well for the
fact that the majority of women holding similar beliefs do not necessarily lead
to eating disorders or even dieting.

Environmental influences and models
Media and social milieu
The 'cult of thinness', a term coined by Gerald Russell, has been observed in
art, fashion and the media in the latter half of the twentieth century. Models,
actresses and Miss America contestants were observed to become thinner in
the twentieth century (Garner & Garfinkel, 1980). A greater emphasis on
dieting emerged in the media, targeting women more than men (Stice, 2002).
Effects of media are particularly profound upon young women who had body
image dissatisfaction at the outset, suggesting a profound interplay between
the individual and environment. The increased prevalence of eating disorders
during the latter half of the twentieth century, as well as the emergence of BN,
have been connected to the emergence of the thin-ideal and the increased
pressure towards dieting. However, Garner & Garfinkel pointed out that the
thin-ideal represented much more than just that – thinness has come to
represent beauty, attractiveness, health and achievement (Garner & Garfinkel,
1980). In addition, parental pressure to lose weight, family criticism of weight
and maternal investment in daughters' slenderness have been positively correlated with adolescent eating disturbance (Stice, 2002).

Dieting leading to eating disorders
Prospective studies have linked dieting to eating disorders (Fairburn et al.,
1997). Whether dieting leads to eating disorders is controversial. The 'continuity theory' suggests that the risk of developing an eating disorder is proportional to the intensity of dieting, and is based on observations that culturally
acceptable dieting may blur or merge with what is considered pathological
thinness (Nasser & Katzman, 2003). Alternatively, the discontinuity theory
suggests that dieting leads to the development of eating disorders only in the
presence of other risk factors (see Stice & Buston, Chapter 4, this volume for
further discussion).

Eating disorders as reaction to changing roles/a voice for women
By the latter half of the twentieth century, Hilde Bruch commented on the
pressure of conflicting feminine roles creating ambivalence in young women

about their bodies. Nasser & Katzman (2003) argue that the increasing incidence of AN during this period existed against the backdrop of decreasing hysteria, and may each have been 'adaptive processes' in the face of particular environmental factors. Specifically, 'hysteria' was commonly thought to be a product of a sexually repressive environment while the anorexic thinness began to be viewed as responding to new environmental demands that promote the desirability for thinness (Nasser & Katzman, 2003).

Culture-bound syndromes

Rising incidence of eating disorders, tendency to afflict young women in westernized countries and gender bias favouring women has given rise to speculation that eating disorders are culture-bound syndromes. Keel & Klump's (2003) meta-analysis investigating eating disorders cross-culturally and cross-historically found little evidence that AN is a culture-bound syndrome, but did find evidence that *weight phobia criteria* may be culture-bound, again calling into question the usefulness of a descriptive approach offered by the DSM–IV. In contrast to their observation of stable rates of AN across time and culture, Keel & Klump's investigation did demonstrate a statistically significant increase of BN over the latter half of the twentieth century, concluding that BN, as well as the weight concerns associated with AN, may be culturally bound phenomena.

Multidisciplinary conceptualizations: the biopsychosocial approach

Biopsychosocial approaches recognize component contributions of biological vulnerabilities, psychological vulnerabilities and environmental triggers. But even this comprehensive perspective is incomplete, because it does not lead us to a carefully integrated account of the various processes leading to the disorders. Ideally, a diagnostic model would provide such an account and may lead the clinician to treat specific processes which have to be ameliorated for a disorder to improve. Biopsychosocial models may be more helpful in retrospectively conceptualizing the contributory aspects to the disease, in a developed adult. However, eating disorders are largely diseases of adolescence with specific risk ages of onset at 14 and 18 and a usual range of 12 to 25, mostly in females (Fichter & Quadflieg, 1995). Conceptualizing these diseases therefore may be most productive if the approach appreciates the temporal development of the disease, with close attention to the development in childhood and adolescence.

Developmental perspective

The developmental approach is the next logical step in the evolution of the diagnosis of eating disorders, which call for a careful consideration of multiple pathogenetic factors in an effort to deliver effective treatments. The perspective replaces a static view of disorder with a model of dynamic pathogenesis. From this perspective, eating disorders are temporary diagnostic clusters that arise out of the confluence of risk factors under the influence of pathogenic endogenous and exogenous influences. Disorder occurs at distinct developmental nodal points when allostatic (i.e. exceptional) load exceeds the individual's capacity to remain in homeostasis (Steiner et al., 1999, 2003).

From a developmental perspective, comparing symptom to normative behaviours is important in determining the clinical significance of a problem. There is no a priori assumption that the presence of any symptom per se is pathognomonic; this determination is made by an active comparison to age-matched groups, not some absolute standard of normality. The second major feature of the model is that it is explicitly nonreductionist and allows for social, psychological and biological processes in the pathogenesis and recovery of disorders. As the disorder is described, an interplay of processes is described which has to be disrupted to restore functioning. These processes are not reducible to only one type (i.e. biological). In the case of AN, endogenous risks, such as an anxious predisposition, obsessive personality organization, avoidant coping and excessive self-regulation, along with a tendency to rigid rhythmicity and avoidance of food under stressful conditions set the stage for the disorder. When embedded in a psychosocial context placing a premium on appearance, fitness, health and idealized images of beauty, such an individual may be ill-prepared for the demands of early adolescence. In the case of BN, the risks differ, while the external demands are similar. Problems present when exit from the family of origin becomes most salient, i.e. late adolescence and young adulthood. Endogenous risks are different; the literature implicates emotional lability, dysthymic mood, irritability, deficient self-regulation and impulsivity, a tendency to internalizing and externalizing behaviours, low rhythmicity of daily habits and eating, and an increased orientation towards food during times of stress and allostatic load, that is a load that puts homeostasis out of balance. (See Fig. 1.1 for a listing of classes of relevant variables.)

The third feature of the model takes the multifactorial approach one step further in that it recognizes that several risk factors contribute to the development of eating disorders over time (as shown in Fig. 1.1). Specifically, it argues

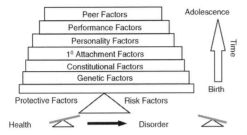

Figure 1.1. The vulnerability/resilience model for the development of eating disorders.

that we must examine the social and temporal context of the individual; without examining it, we will not be able to distinguish between the young woman who will continue to be suffering from major difficulties from the one who will require no treatment at all. For example, excessive preoccupation with appearance in early to mid-adolescence is a normative phenomenon that may not impact the risk of developing an eating disorder. By contrast, the appearance of such concerns in prepubertal girls, especially in the context of attachment problems, may signal the beginning of a potentially pathogenetic pathway (Sharpe *et al.*, 1998). Similarly, the persistence of such excessive concerns in older women, especially those who have had an episode of an eating disorder may be a psychological marker for potential relapse or persistence of disorder.

The developmental view on body image distortion also illustrates its departure from other perspectives. In a descriptive model and biopsychosocial model, body image distortion is seen as a static symptom of a disordered individual. In the developmental model, it is a mutable trait which may be harmless or harmful depending on the circumstance. The majority of children distort to a significant degree the way they conceptualize their bodies, boys equal to girls during the elementary school age (Steiner *et al.*, 1995). Many children also show preoccupation with dieting and appearance in the school age range, especially when they come from a highly privileged social background (Schur *et al.*, 2000). Yet, clearly most children in this age range do not suffer from eating disorders, nor are they at risk to develop such. From a developmental point of view, the significance of these body image problems becomes clearer when we study the outcome of this symptom in adolescence: as boys mature, they tend to underestimate their body size and their dissatisfaction with their appearance is no longer tied to body maturation. As girls mature, they overestimate their bodies and their dissatisfaction with their appearance increases. Dissatisfaction with appearance remains high in women of all ages to a high degree, making this particular diagnostic criterion of eating disorders a weak discriminator between normality and pathology (Steiner *et al.*, 1995).

Attention to the temporal development of eating disorders over time also helps the clinician understand whether the problem can be explained by the phase a patient is in, is a specific risk factor which needs to be tracked and observed or is in fact a disorder which needs to be treated. For example, data from adolescent populations (Killen *et al.*, 1986) suggest that binge–purge behaviour and dieting is quite common in this age range, without any progression to eating disorder. Return to normal functioning occurs by *development proceeding* without clinical intervention.

Attention to temporal development also lends valence to which triggers or vulnerabilities are most important. For example, dieting in an early teen may emerge as comparisons are made to peers in terms of appearance and desirability. Body image problems resurface from childhood. Dieting and weight loss may only become problematic in the wake of a rejection by a peer or in the presence of an extraordinary life stressor, such as a pending parental divorce. While underlying vulnerabilities exist, working through the acute stressor may be most relevant to returning the individual to appropriate levels of functioning.

Finally, the developmental clinician may note disturbances even if symptoms do not add up to a specific disorder, and categorize them along a developmental trajectory in an effort to prevent the onset of full blown disorder. For example, fussiness, colicky digestion, picky eating and a tendency to overeat may be established risk factors for eating problems (Marchi & Cohen, 1990)

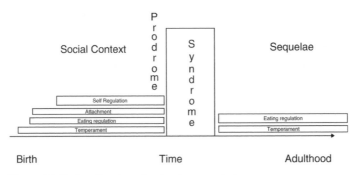

Figure 1.2. Eating disorders: the developmental view.

and may need to be monitored. Prodromal clustering of symptoms, without meeting DSM–IV diagnoses, may alert the clinician to be more sensitive to developmental nodal points which need to be negotiated successfully (see Fig. 1.2).

Conclusions

Eating and food are fundamental aspects of our humanity and of our relationships with our families, peers and self. History demonstrates that eating behaviours are sensitive to stress and environmental demands, particularly in children and adolescents, and particularly in women. The developmental perspective suggests that multiple factors – biological, social, individual, cultural – may coalesce in an individual to, at certain points in life, sway eating patterns into the realm of maladaptation. However, interventions aimed at the most salient of these factors may ultimately redirect the course of an individual's trajectory. Close attention to the individual patient's trajectory rather than simple symptom clusters will assist the clinician in intervening in a timely and relevant manner.

REFERENCES

American Psychiatric Association (2000). Diagnostic and Statistical Manual of Mental Disorders, 4th edition, Text Revision (2000). Washington, DC: American Psychiatric Association.

Boskind-White, M. & White, W. (1986). Bulimarexia: a historical-sociocultural perspective. In *Handbook of Eating Disorders*, ed. Brownell, K. & Foreyt, J. New York: Basic Books, pp. 353–64.

Bruch, H. (1973). *Eating Disorders: Obesity, Anorexia Nervosa, and the Person Within*. New York: Basic Books.

Brumberg, J.J. (1989). *Fasting Girls: The History of Anorexia Nervosa*. New York: Plume.

Fairburn, C.G., Welch, S.L., Doll, H.A. *et al.* (1997). Risk factors for bulimia nervosa: a community based case control study. *Archives of General Psychiatry*, **54**, 509–17.

Fichter, M. & Quadflieg, N. (1995). Psychophysiology of eating disorders. In *Eating Disorders in Adolescence*, ed. Steinhausen, H.C. New York: Walter de Gruyter, pp. 301–37.

Garner, D.M. & Garfinkel, P.E. (1980). Cultural expectation of thinness in women. *Psychological Reports*, **47**, 483–91.

Keel, P. & Klump, K. (2003). Are eating disorders culture-bound syndromes? Implications for conceptualizing their etiology. *Psychological Bulletin*, **129**, 747–69.

Killen, J.D., Taylor, C.B., Telch, M.J. *et al.* (1986). Self- induced vomiting and laxative and diuretic use among teenagers: Precursors of the binge-purge syndrome? *Journal of the American Medical Association*, **255**, 1447–9.

Marchi, M. & Cohen, P. (1990). Early childhood eating behaviors and adolescent eating disorders. *Journal of the American Academy of Child and Adolescent Psychiatry,* **29**, 112–17.

Nasser, M. & Katzman, M. (2003). Sociocultural theories of eating disorders: an evolution of thought. In *Handbook of Eating Disorders,* 2nd edn., ed. Treasure, J., Schmidt, U. & van Furth, E. Chichester: John Wiley & Sons, pp. 139–50.

Schur, E., Sanders, M. & Steiner, H. (2000). Socio-cultural influences on body dissatisfaction and dieting in young children. *International Journal of Eating Disorders,* **27**, 74–82.

Shafran, R. & de Silva, P. (2003). Cognitive-behavioral models. In *Handbook of Eating Disorders,* 2nd edn., ed. Treasure, J., Schmidt, U. & van Furth, E. Chichester: John Wiley & Sons, pp. 121–38.

Sharpe, T.M., Killen, J.D., Bryson, S.W. *et al.* (1998). Attachment style and weight concerns in preadolescent and adolescent girls. *International Journal of Eating Disorders,* **23**, 39–44.

Steiner, H., Kwan, W., Shaffer, T. *et al.* (2003). Risk and protective factors for juvenile eating disorders. *European Child and Adolescent Psychiatry,* **12** (Suppl. 1), 38–46.

Steiner, H., Sanders, M. & Ryst, E. (1995). Precursors and risk factors of juvenile eating disorders. In *Eating Disorders in Adolescence: Anorexia And Bulimia Nervosa,* ed. Steinhausen, H.C. New York: Walter De Gruyter, pp. 95–125.

Steiner, H., Lock, J. & Reisel, B. (1999). Developmental approaches to eating disorders. *Le Prisme,* **30**, 52–67.

Stice, R. (2002). Sociocultural influences on body image and eating disturbance. In *Eating Disorders and Obesity,* 2nd edn, ed. Fairburn, C. & Brownell, K. New York: Guilford Press, pp. 103–7.

Strober, M. (1986). Anorexia nervosa: history and psychological concepts. In *Handbook of Eating Disorders,* ed. Brownell, K. & Foreyt, J. New York: Basic Books, pp. 231–46.

Vandereycken, W. (2002). History of anorexia nervosa and bulimia nervosa. In *Eating Disorders and Obesity,* 2nd edn, ed. Fairburn, C. & Brownell, K. New York: Guilford Press, pp. 151–4.

Wade, T.D., Bulik, C.M., Neale, M. & Kendler, K.S. (2000). Anorexia nervosa and major depression: shared genetic and environmental risk factors. *American Journal of Psychiatry,* **157**, 469–71.

Wonderlich, S.A. (2002). Personality and eating disorders. In *Eating Disorders and Obesity,* 2nd edn., ed. Fairburn, C. & Brownell, K. New York: Guilford Press, pp. 204–9.

World Health Organization (1992). *The ICD-10 Classification of Mental and Behavioural Disorders: Clinical Descriptions and Diagnostic Guidelines.* Geneva: World Health Organization.

Part II

Scientific underpinnings

2

Regulation of food intake and body weight

Julian G. Mercer

The Rowett Research Institute, Aberdeen, UK

Introduction

To thrive, all mammals need to satisfy requirements for energy and nutrients. In order to maintain a stable body weight over an extended period, energy intake as solid or liquid food must be matched with energy expended in metabolism and physical activity with a remarkable degree of accuracy. For example, it has been calculated that the typical change in weight and body composition over a decade by an adult human would require energy supply and demand to be matched to a precision of around 0.2% (Weigle, 1994). This level of accuracy is achieved despite longitudinal variability in availability of, and requirement for, energy. For almost all mammals, other than those maintained under strictly controlled laboratory conditions, the composition, quality and quantity of food that is available for consumption will vary considerably between meals and from day to day, requiring the selection of a suitable combination of food types and quantities over longish periods to smooth out any temporary imbalances, such as a discontinuous supply. Similarly, energy demands will vary widely, being heavily influenced by factors such as developmental state (e.g. growing, reproducing), behaviour (e.g. social influences, migration) and environment (e.g. climate, season). Although the source of food may be discontinuous or irregular, a continuous supply of accessible energy is required for survival, necessitating storage of energy and nutrients, to ensure that supply always meets demand. Energy intake is regulated at both short-term (meals) and longer-term levels, and is influenced by the requirement to establish suitably sized energy stores, firstly to see the animal through the intervals between

Eating Disorders in Children and Adolescents, ed. Tony Jaffa and Brett McDermott. Published by Cambridge University Press. © Cambridge University Press 2007.

meals and secondly to tide the animal over periods when insufficient food can be garnered from the environment. The majority of ingested and absorbed energy not required for more immediate use is deposited into adipose tissue stores as fat. A third variable in the balancing act between energy intake and expenditure, then, is the amount of energy that is maintained in long-term storage. Clearly, the achievement of an adequate level of energy intake, and the establishment and maintenance of appropriately sized energy stores could easily mean the difference between life and death. It is unsurprising, therefore, that sophisticated and active peripheral and central signalling systems exist to regulate food intake and body weight (Schwartz *et al.*, 2000), with the central systems being relatively elevated in the hierarchy of brain function. These systems have considerable redundancy built in as a safeguard.

The increasing global prevalence of obesity, and the medically and economically important diseases and illnesses that are associated with obesity, have propelled research on the regulation of food intake and body weight into the public spotlight. Eating disorders such as anorexia and bulimia nervosa also have a major impact on health and well-being, and represent scenarios where the normal processes of regulation of food intake, energy homeostasis and body weight have effectively broken down. As the introduction to this volume focused on child and adolescent eating disorders, consideration will be given in this chapter to control of energy intake at the level of the individual meal and over the longer term, and to the integration of energy intake and expenditure into body weight regulation, encompassing regulatory events and systems in the periphery and the central nervous system. Mammals regulate food intake and body weight through the integration of a wide range of peripheral and brain signals. These signals may be of neural, metabolic, endocrine and neuroendocrine origin, and our knowledge of interactions between organs and molecules is growing rapidly. Peripheral signals relate the consequences of meal processing, gastrointestinal activity and changes in energy stores, and have predominantly short-duration effects. These signals are relayed to the brain where they are integrated through specific neuronal circuits to influence efferent neuronal activity, higher brain centres, physiology and behaviour, thereby completing the feedback loop. There is good evidence that these regulatory systems are well conserved across mammalian species and many of the signals discussed below have been verified as being active in humans through genetic, physiological or metabolic studies.

Meal feeding and peripheral signals

Most mammals consume food as individual meals, and energy intake must therefore be regulated through the frequency with which meals are taken, and the size of the meals consumed. Within meals, biological signals contribute to meal initiation, the maintenance of feeding, or continuation of the meal, and, importantly, in the context of the development and maintenance of obesity, meal termination (Schwartz, 2004). The latter process is controlled by satiety signals. The stimuli that influence these different phases of the meal-feeding process arise from the food itself, such as its taste, smell and visual appeal, and from the consequences of its ingestion and digestion. Examples of the latter mechanical and chemical stimuli include gastric and intestinal distension, and nutrient concentrations in the gastrointestinal tract and post-absorption in the bloodstream. The arrival of food in the gastrointestinal tract also provokes release of a large number of meal-processing hormones and paracrine factors. One such hormone is cholecystokinin (CCK), which is a proven satiety factor in addition to its other established physiological roles (gut motility, gallbladder contraction, gastric emptying, gastric acid secretion, pancreatic enzyme secretion). A number of these post-ingestive consequences of food intake are able to change the firing rate of the vagus nerve. The importance of the sensory vagus nerve in gut-brain signalling is emphasized by the ability of three quite different stimuli, gastric distension, nutrient infusion (e.g. glucose) and CCK, to alter electrical activity in vagal afferents that innervate the nucleus of the solitary tract (NTS) in the brainstem. The role of CCK in physiological satiety has been subjected to intense scrutiny over the last three decades. Cholecystokinin reduces meal size on peripheral injection, and induces a behavioural satiety sequence, indicative of a physiological satiety event. This effect appears to be mediated via the CCK-A receptor. Conversely, CCK-A receptor antagonists not only block the effect of a CCK injection, but also increase food intake when administered in isolation, suggesting that endogenous meal-released CCK provides negative feedback to induce a physiological state of satiety. These effects are dependent on an intact vagus nerve. An explanation for the effects of CCK on vagal afferent firing rates is provided by the presence of CCK-A receptors on these fibres, relaying signals to the brainstem (Mercer & Lawrence, 1992). Studies of transgenic and mutant rodent strains also support a role for CCK in determining meal size, as does administration of exogenous CCK peptide to non-human primates and humans (see references in Strader & Woods, 2005).

At least 10 gastrointestinal hormones are known to affect meal size in mammals (Strader & Woods, 2005), two of which, ghrelin and peptide YY (PYY_{3-36}), have been characterized only recently. Of these hormones, only ghrelin stimulates food intake, the remainder being satiety agents. Exactly how all these signals interact and how they are regulated is unclear. Ghrelin is the endogenous ligand of the growth hormone secretagogue receptor (GHS-R), and was originally isolated from the rat stomach (Zigman & Elmquist, 2003). Ghrelin is secreted by the stomach in high concentrations during food restriction and is a powerful orexigenic agent that can lead to weight gain and obesity (Tschöp et al., 2000). Ghrelin appears to play a physiological role in hunger and meal feeding in humans as supported by a rise in blood concentration before a meal and a decline thereafter (Cummings et al., 2001). By contrast, the gut-derived hormone, PYY_{3-36}, synthesized in the ileum and colon, inhibits feeding and appears to counter the effect of ghrelin; PYY_{3-36} reduces food intake in rodents, non-human primates and humans (Batterham et al., 2002, 2003). Both ghrelin and PYY_{3-36} have their effect on energy balance by interacting with specific receptors expressed on hypothalamic neurones.

One of the most powerful information sources, produced in the periphery and monitored in the brain, is the adipose tissue-derived hormone, leptin. The cloning of the leptin gene in 1994 (Zhang et al., 1994), and the subsequent cloning of the leptin receptor (Tartaglia et al., 1995) was the catalyst for a re-invigoration of the energy balance field. Although leptin has a wide range of physiological functions (Friedman & Halaas, 1998; Zigman & Elmquist, 2003), it is clear that a primary function of this molecule is to regulate a range of central nervous system (CNS) signalling pathways, and exogenously administered leptin reduces food intake and body weight in laboratory rodents when administered either centrally or peripherally. Endogenous leptin is generally present in the circulation in proportion to body adiposity, and consequently obese humans are generally characterized by high circulating levels of leptin. Leptin therapy in obese adult patients produced only limited weight loss compared with placebo (Heymsfield et al., 1999). Leptin relates information to the hypothalamus about fat mass and energy flux into and out of adipose tissue, thereby providing prompt feedback to those brain centres involved in the regulation of energy balance (Ahima & Flier, 2000). Following transport across the blood–brain barrier, leptin binds to specific receptors (members of the class 1 cytokine receptor family; Friedman & Halaas, 1998) located in key hypothalamic structures. Leptin receptors are also present in the dorsal vagal complex and other hindbrain centres, discrete regions of which have a chemosensory function or are involved in the relaying of satiety and other visceral signals from the periphery. A further link to the periphery is provided by evidence suggesting that leptin may enhance the satiety effect of CCK.

Elevated blood leptin concentrations in obese humans have been interpreted as evidence that obesity is effectively a state of 'leptin resistance' similar to the well-characterized 'insulin resistance' that causes type 2 diabetes. The insulin signal, released from the pancreas in response to food ingestion, like that of leptin, indicates whether energy stores are sufficient (insulin administered directly into the brain reduces food intake), and current evidence indicates that insulin and leptin signals may overlap or converge in the brain, utilizing the same intracellular signalling cascades (Schwartz & Niswender, 2004). In addition to the array of hormonal regulators of food intake, the brain also directly senses levels of nutrients such as glucose and fatty acids. Currently available evidence indicates that this sensory capability contributes to homeostatic energy balance mechanisms.

Central nervous system regulation

Hindbrain

A number of brain regions are involved in the regulation of food intake, energy balance and body weight. One of these regions is the hindbrain, which is a target for signalling from the gastrointestinal tract, processing information in anatomically distinct structures such as the NTS. For example, the NTS receives incoming neural signals from the vagus nerve (such as those influenced by CCK, see above), elicits reflexes that influence gut function and sends signals onwards towards other brain areas. The NTS is also a site of synthesis of neuropeptides destined for transport to the forebrain, such as the products of the preproglucagon gene, glucagon-like-peptide-1 (GLP-1), glucagon-like-peptide-2 (GLP-2) and oxyntomodulin. These peptides are involved in a wide variety of physiological functions (e.g. gastric emptying and insulin secretion), including the regulation of food intake (Larsen et al., 2003). The effect of GLP-1 on gastrointestinal transit and gastric emptying may explain the inhibitory action of this peptide on food intake in humans (Strader & Woods, 2005). Experimental studies have shown that the hindbrain is capable of acting with some autonomy in a reflex manner on information coming from the periphery; CCK can induce satiety in the absence of neural connections to other brain regions (Grill & Smith, 1988). Nevertheless, a substantial body of evidence points to a critical role for the hypothalamus, a complex structure at the base of the forebrain, in the regulation of energy balance.

Hypothalamus

Historically, evidence that the hypothalamus was a major centre in the control of food intake and body weight came from classical lesioning and electrical stimulation studies conducted in the 1950s (Stellar, 1954), and from studies of patients with hypothalamic damage caused by trauma or tumour. From such pioneering studies, 'hunger' and 'satiety' centres were proposed to exist in the lateral hypothalamic area (LHA) and the ventromedial hypothalamic nucleus (VMN), respectively. However, the outcomes of many of these early experimental manipulations have now been subject to some reinterpretation, and these broad regional designations have evolved as we have gained more detailed knowledge of the neuronal populations involved in the regulation of energy balance, the orexigenic (anabolic) and anorexigenic (catabolic) molecular substrates involved, and their regulation and integration (Friedman & Halaas, 1998; Kalra *et al.*, 1999; Schwartz *et al.*, 2000). It is now well established that a network of anatomically distinct hypothalamic structures, and signalling systems contained therein, receive neural, metabolic and hormonal feedback from the periphery and are involved in the maintenance of an appropriate body weight and composition. In addition to the involvement of the LHA and VMN, and another hypothalamic nucleus, the dorsomedial hypothalamic nucleus (DMN; Bernardis & Bellinger, 1998), a key axis within the hypothalamus is now recognized to be that between the arcuate nucleus (ARC) and the paraventricular nucleus of the hypothalamus (PVN). Since the cloning of the leptin gene, several new candidate hypothalamic neuropeptide and receptor systems have been described which appear to be involved in the regulation of energy balance. Some of these signalling systems were previously unknown, whereas, in other cases, peptides with well-established activity in other physiological systems have been demonstrated also to affect energy homeostasis. Furthermore, the activities of many of these recently described neuropeptide systems are regulated by leptin. The ARC appears to be the primary brain target of the circulating leptin signal, although the DMN, VMN, LHA and PVN also express the leptin receptor (Mercer *et al.*, 1996). Leptin-sensitive neuropeptide systems within the hypothalamus play a key role in regulating energy balance (Fig. 2.1).

The energy balance neuropeptides produced in the hypothalamus can be divided into two categories, those that increase food intake, reduce energy expenditure and give rise to positive energy balance and weight gain, and

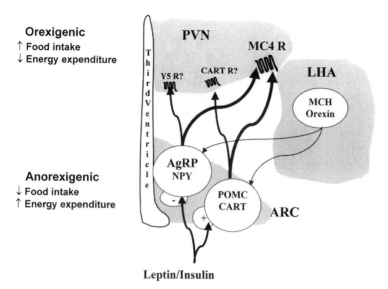

Figure 2.1. Simplified depiction of hypothalamic neuropeptide energy balance systems and their neuroanatomical relationship. Abbreviations: ARC, hypothalamic arcuate nucleus; CART, cocaine and amphetamine-regulated transcript; POMC, proopiomelanocortin; AgRP, agouti-related peptide; NPY, neuropeptide Y; MCH, melanin concentrating hormone; Y5 R, neuropeptide Y Y5 receptor; CART R, CART receptor (uncloned); LHA, lateral hypothalamic area; PVN, paraventricular nucleus of the hypothalamus; MC4 R, melanocortin-4 receptor.

those that have the opposite effect on each side of the energy balance equation, leading to negative energy balance. The ARC contains at least two distinct types of neurones, one of which expresses and synthesizes the complementary orexigenic peptides, neuropeptide Y (NPY) and agouti-related peptide (AgRP; Ollmann *et al.*, 1997), while the other expresses the anorexigenic peptide precursors, proopiomelanocortin (POMC) and cocaine and amphetamine-regulated transcript (CART; Kristensen *et al.*, 1998). Leptin inhibits the activity of these orexigenic systems and stimulates their anorexigenic counterparts. These ARC neurones target the PVN, where receptor fields are located (Fig. 2.1). There is strong evidence supporting the physiological involvement in energy balance regulation of many of these peptides (Friedman & Halaas, 1998; Kalra *et al.*, 1999; Schwartz *et al.*, 2000). For example, for NPY, the exogenous peptide stimulates food intake and reduces energy expenditure on injection into the brain, even in satiated rats, and leads to obesity when administered repeatedly. The orexigenic effect of NPY is concentrated on the PVN. Further evidence of a physiological role for NPY comes from the behaviour of the endogenous peptide system following

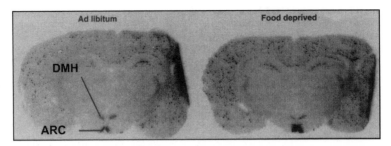

Figure 2.2. Autoradiographs showing up-regulation of neuropeptide Y (NPY) in the ARC, but not in the DMH, of the food-deprived rat. Abbreviations: ARC, hypothalamic arcuate nucleus; DMH, dorsomedial hypothalamic nucleus.

imposed energetic manipulation. Food deprivation or food restriction result in an increase in NPY gene expression in the ARC (Fig. 2.2), driven at least in part by the reduction in blood leptin concentration, and an increase in localized concentrations of NPY peptide in the ARC and PVN. These changes in the activity of the endogenous system are likely to lead to energy conservation while food shortages persist, and prime the animal to over-eat (hyperphagia) in compensation once food availability is restored. Excess energy intake is then stored as fat, leptin levels rise and hypothalamic activity is restored to normal. Although the potential role of the LHA in energy balance regulation has been reassessed in the last 20 years, focus on this hypothalamic structure was reinvigorated following the description of two novel orexigenic systems (see Schwartz et al., 2000; Williams et al., 2004). The LHA synthesizes melanin concentrating hormone (MCH) and the products of the orexin gene, and has connections to and from the ARC (Fig. 2.1).

The above discussion covers only a limited number of the hypothalamic systems involved in energy balance and readers are referred to recent comprehensive reviews for a more detailed description of the full complexity of the regulatory circuitry (Leibowitz & Wortley, 2004; Williams et al., 2004). Nevertheless, the emerging picture is of neuronal circuits in the hypothalamus regulating both appetite and body composition via specific signalling and receptor systems discretely expressed in regional subpopulations of neurones. A critical component of these systems is the melanocortin-4 receptor, downstream from leptin. Activation of this receptor by melanocyte-stimulating hormone (a product of the POMC gene) or synthetic analogues suppresses food intake in rodents, while an additional level of complexity is provided by the demonstration that the orexigenic activity of AgRP is due to its endogenous antagonism of the melanocortin-4 receptor. This receptor is currently the best link between established genetic mutation and severe obesity in man (Hebebrand *et al.*, 2003; see below), and is an active target in drug development. It is important to note that most of our knowledge of the functioning of hypothalamic peptide systems comes from study of in vivo responses following injection of peptides directly into the brain, and from examination of the effect of energy deficit on endogenous gene expression and peptide concentrations through relatively acute imposed manipulations such as complete food deprivation. The effect of spontaneously occurring mutations leading to obesity on the activity of other signalling pathways and the effects of transgenic knockouts have also been examined in some detail. Much less well understood are the sensitivity of energy balance systems to more subtle dietary manipulation and more gradual changes in body weight over longer periods. In short, how do the energy balance systems interact in the longer-term regulation of body weight in the normal animal?

Forebrain regions involved in reward pathways

A substantial and growing body of evidence supports the existence of hypothalamic homeostatic mechanisms for regulating the consumption of food. However, it is equally apparent that taste and reward systems contribute to a hedonic response to food in both humans and laboratory mammals (Saper *et al.*, 2002). The 'pleasure' derived from the consumption of high-energy and sweet foods is likely to have been beneficial during evolution to ensure consumption of such foodstuffs when available. However, in our present environment in which high-calorie foods are available in virtually limitless quantities, it is likely to be contributing to the obesity epidemic. The circuits and molecules underlying the hedonic regulation of feeding are much less well studied than those that underlie the homeostatic mechanisms. Interactions between the homeostatic and hedonic systems are not well understood, but are likely to be important in the overall regulation of food intake and body weight, with competition occurring between the reward value of food and the satiety signals it generates. Several brain areas are involved in reward processing. These include the orbital frontal cortex, central nucleus of the amygdala, hypothalamus, ventral tegmental area, nucleus accumbens (NAc) and NTS. The picture that is emerging is of multiple interconnecting regions involved in the response to natural rewards. The NAc is an important output site, with direct and indirect, two-way communication to relevant regions of the hypothalamus including the PVN and LHA. Manipulation of the NAc may elicit food intake via coordinated stimulation and suppression of orexigenic and anorexigenic peptides in the hypothalamus.

It is likely that the reward attributes of food may override adiposity signals by activating motivational circuitry, with consumption of food being driven by the immediate pleasure it produces rather than by energy deficit. An understanding of how motivational circuitry and its endocrine, neuroendocrine and metabolic regulation contributes to normal energy balance regulation could identify future targets for therapeutic manipulation. There are a number of candidate molecular components of the reward system. The role of endogenous opioid peptides in feeding behaviour and in particular in the modulation of food reward and palatability is relatively well established, with disorders characterized by hyperphagia being associated with aberrant opioid activity. Opioids preferentially enhance intake of palatable foods over less palatable, and increase perceived palatability. Ingestion of food, and especially sweet food, can induce the release of endogenous opiates and regulate opioid gene expression in the NAc. Drugs of abuse also interact with the opioid systems of the brain, suggesting that there may be common neural substrates between food and drug reward. Cannabinoid receptors and their natural ligands, the endocannabinoids, also appear to be involved in CNS reward processes, with a likely role in enhancing food palatability, possibly through interactions with endogenous opioid peptides. Cannabinoid receptor antagonists not only target motivational mechanisms but may also induce advantageous metabolic changes even in animals maintained on a high fat diet. The cannabinoid receptor-1 antagonist, rimonabant, is now licensed in the UK as a human obesity drug.

Conservation of energy balance systems in mammalian species

Research into the mechanisms and metabolic changes underlying obesity is heavily dependent upon the study of experimental animal models. It is therefore critical to establish whether the same mechanisms are present and, more importantly, functional in humans. Much recent insight into the regulation of mammalian energy balance has come from studies of spontaneous single gene mutation and transgenic rodent models. Mutation or targeted deletion of specific genes can cause an obese phenotype in mice and rats, and similar loss of function mutations cause obesity in humans. However, such mutations are very rare in the human population. The melanocortin-4 receptor, for example, is the most common, identified, single gene cause of human obesity, with functionally relevant mutations in the melanocortin-4 receptor accounting for 2–4% of early onset extreme obesity in the human population (Hebebrand et al., 2003). In a relatively small number of additional individuals, the cause of obesity has been pin-pointed to mutations in key energy balance genes that are essential for normal body weight regulation, such as leptin (Montague *et al.*, 1997), the leptin receptor (Clement *et al.*, 1998) and POMC (Krude *et al.*, 1998). Although the existence of these loss of function mutations is probably not directly relevant to the majority of obesity in the human population, they establish the principle that genes that are essential for normal body weight regulation in laboratory rodents are also essential for normal body weight regulation in humans. The successful treatment of the severe childhood obesity resulting from human congenital leptin deficiency with recombinant leptin is proof of principle in this regard (Farooqi *et al.*, 1999). However, the majority of common human obesity is likely to reflect the interaction between a genetic predisposition to weight gain and the prevailing environment, and to be polygenic in nature, with a number of genes involved, each contributing a small effect. The genetic changes summating to susceptibility to obesity are likely to generate numerous small changes in the activity of specific enzymes or pathways within the complex systems that regulate energy homeostasis, rather than a complete loss of function of any one component. This susceptibility then leads to obesity in an obesogenic environment, for example when particular types of diet are available and an increasingly sedentary lifestyle is adopted.

Our developing understanding of the fine detail of energy balance mechanisms in laboratory rodents, and verification of equivalent activity in humans, is likely to bring forward additional new components of the regulatory process, and to reveal hitherto uncharacterized interactions. The potential to manipulate energy balance systems to therapeutic advantage in obesity, metabolic syndrome and eating disorders is fuelling the current frenetic activity within the pharmaceutical industry. However, other opportunities also exist, for example, exploring the interactions between such systems and diet, and in the development of biomarkers of susceptibility. A key question is why the energy balance systems described here, and in particular the homeostatic hypothalamic systems, are unable to prevent the development of inappropriate body composition. The answer to this question may enable us to better harness the endogenous regulatory capacity of the food intake and body weight regulatory systems to widespread benefit.

REFERENCES

Ahima, R.S. & Flier, J.S. (2000). Leptin. *Annual Review of Physiology*, **25**, 413–27.
Batterham, R.L., Cowley, M.A., Small, C.J. *et al.* (2002). Gut hormone PYY3-36 physiologically inhibits food intake. *Nature*, **418**, 650–4.

Batterham, R.L., Cohen, M.A., Ellis, S.M. *et al.* (2003). Inhibition of food intake in obese subjects by peptide YY3-36. *New England Journal of Medicine*, **349**, 941–8.

Bernardis, L.L. & Bellinger, L.L. (1998). The dorsomedial hypothalamic nucleus revisited: 1998 update. *Proceedings of the Society for Experimental Biology and Medicine*, **218**, 284–306.

Clement, K., Vaisse, C., Lahlou, N. *et al.* (1998). A mutation in the human leptin receptor gene causes obesity and pituitary dysfunction. *Nature*, **392**, 398–401.

Cummings, D.E., Purnell, J.Q., Frayo, R.S., Schmidova, K., Wisse, B.E. & Weigle, D.S. (2001). A preprandial rise in plasma ghrelin levels suggests a role in meal initiation in humans. *Diabetes*, **50**, 1714–19.

Farooqi, I.S., Jebb, S.A., Langmack, G. *et al.* (1999). Effects of recombinant leptin therapy in a child with congenital leptin deficiency. *New England Journal of Medicine*, **341**, 879–84.

Friedman, J.M. & Halaas, J.L. (1998). Leptin and the regulation of body weight in mammals. *Nature*, **395**, 763–70.

Grill, H.J. & Smith, G.P. (1988). Cholecystokinin decreases sucrose intake in chronic decerebrate rats. *American Journal of Physiology*, **254**, R853–6.

Hebebrand, J., Friedel, S., Schauble, N., Geller, F. & Hinney, A. (2003). Perspectives: molecular genetic research in human obesity. *Obesity Reviews*, **4**, 139–46.

Heymsfield, S.B., Greenberg, A.S., Fujioka, K. *et al.* (1999). Recombinant leptin for weight loss in obese and lean adults – a randomized, controlled, dose-escalation trial. *Journal of the American Medical Association*, **282**, 1568–75.

Kalra, S.P., Dube, M.G., Pu, S., Xu, B., Horvath, T.L. & Kalra, P.S. (1999). Interacting appetite-regulating pathways in the hypothalamic regulation of body weight. *Endocrine Reviews*, **20**, 68–100.

Kristensen, P., Judge, M.E., Thim, L. *et al.* (1998). Hypothalamic CART is a new anorectic peptide regulated by leptin. *Nature*, **393**, 72–6.

Krude, H., Biebermann, H., Luck, W., Horn, R., Brabant, G. & Gruters, A. (1998). Severe early-onset obesity, adrenal insufficiency and red hair pigmentation caused by POMC mutations in humans. *Nature Genetics*, **19**, 155–7.

Larsen, P.J., Vrang, N. & Tang-Christensen, M. (2003). Central pre-proglucagon derived peptides: opportunities for treatment of obesity. *Current Pharmaceutical Design*, **9**, 1373–82.

Leibowitz, S.F. & Wortley, K.E. (2004). Hypothalamic control of energy balance: different peptides, different functions. *Peptides*, **25**, 473–504.

Mercer, J.G. & Lawrence, C.B. (1992). Selectivity of cholecystokinin (CCK) receptor antagonists, MK-329 and L-365,260, for axonally-transported CCK binding sites on the rat vagus nerve. *Neuroscience Letters*, **137**, 229–31.

Mercer, J.G., Hoggard, N., Williams, L.M., Lawrence, C.B., Hannah, L.T. & Trayhurn, P. (1996). Localization of leptin receptor mRNA and the long form splice variant (Ob-Rb) in mouse hypothalamus and adjacent brain regions by *in situ* hybridization. *FEBS Letters*, **387**, 113–16.

Montague, C.T., Farooqi, I.S., Whitehead, J.P. *et al.* (1997). Congenital leptin deficiency is associated with severe early-onset obesity in humans. *Nature*, **387**, 903–8.

Ollmann, M.M., Wilson, B.D., Yang, Y.K. *et al.* (1997). Antagonism of central melanocortin receptors *in vitro* and *in vivo* by agouti-related protein. *Science*, **278**, 135–8.

Saper, C.B., Chou, T.C. & Elmquist, J.K. (2002). The need to feed: homeostatic and hedonic control of eating. *Neuron*, **36**, 199–211.

Schwartz, G.J. (2004). Biology of eating behavior in obesity. *Obesity Research*, **12**, 102S–6S.

Schwartz, M.W. & Niswender, K.D. (2004). Adiposity signalling and biological defense against weight gain: absence of protection or central hormone resistance? *Journal of Clinical Endocrinology and Metabolism*, **89**, 5889–97.

Schwartz, M.W., Woods, S.C., Porte, D. Jr, Seeley, R.J. & Baskin, D.G. (2000). Central nervous system control of food intake. *Nature*, **404**, 661–71.

Stellar, E. (1954). The physiology of motivation. *Psychological Reviews*, **61**, 5–22.

Strader, A.D. & Woods, S.C. (2005). Gastrointestinal hormones and food intake. *Gastroenterology*, **128**, 175–91.

Tartaglia, L.A., Dembski, M., Weng, X. *et al.* (1995). Identification and expression cloning of a leptin receptor, *OB-R. Cell*, **83**, 1263–71.

Tschöp, M., Smiley, D.L. & Heiman, M.L. (2000). Ghrelin induces adiposity in rodents. *Nature*, **407**, 908–13.

Weigle, D.S. (1994). Appetite and the regulation of body composition. *FASEB Journal*, **8**, 302–10.

Williams, G., Cai, X.J., Elliott, J.C. & Harrold, J.A. (2004). Anabolic neuropeptides. *Physiology and Behavior*, **81**, 211–22.

Zhang, Y., Proenca, R., Maffei, M., Barone, M., Leopold, L. & Friedman, J.M. (1994). Positional cloning of the mouse *obese* gene and its human homologue. *Nature*, **372**, 425–32.

Zigman, J.M. & Elmquist, J.K. (2003). Minireview: from anorexia to obesity – the yin and yang of body weight control. *Endocrinology*, **144**, 3749–56.

3

The development of children's shape and weight concerns

Andrew J. Hill

Leeds University School of Medicine, Leeds, UK

Introduction

Body shape, weight and eating concerns are at the heart of the psychopathology of eating disorders. Journal and magazine surveys report these concerns as commonplace but at their threatening peak during girls' adolescence. The convergence of pubertal growth with social and identity demands underpins body dissatisfaction and fuels behaviours intended to achieve physical change or gain control. Concepts such as thin-ideal internalization help make sense of this process, describing the way an individual cognitively buys into socially defined ideals of attractiveness (Thompson & Stice, 2001). For many, the result is body dissatisfaction since the ideal is some distance from self-appraised reality. And the culprits are easy to identify – fashion models and celebrities, given saturating media coverage and respect by peers and family. However, often overlooked is the way that obesity's negative representation serves to further idealize a thin body.

It is more difficult to say when this process starts, whether these concerns arrive in a rush or have a long gestation. But it seems likely, given the importance of appearance in adult society, that children both ingest and enact these tensions. The purpose of this chapter is to consider what we currently know about the development of children's shape and weight concerns and associated body dissatisfaction. When do they develop and what are their drivers?

Body dissatisfaction

Evaluation

One of the most commonly used methods for describing body dissatisfaction in children is a scale of outline body shapes. These drawings of males and

Eating Disorders in Children and Adolescents, ed. Tony Jaffa and Brett McDermott. Published by Cambridge University Press. © Cambridge University Press 2007.

females range from very thin to extremely fat and were developed for studies of body weight heritability, allowing respondents to describe the body size of parents when alive. Their research profile was accelerated by their use in assessing men and women's choices of ideal and desirable body shapes. Not only were these scales easy to understand, their output was revealing.

Among the first to adapt the drawings and use them with pre-teenagers was Collins. She used scales of seven male or female figures to examine the current and ideal figure choices of over 1000 children, mean age 8 (Collins, 1991). Boys' ideal shape was very close to their choice of current shape. In contrast, the girls' ideal was thinner than either their current perception or the boys' ideal. Even before puberty, girls appeared to be expressing the same body shape preferences found in teenagers and young women.

We have used the original body shape scales to investigate the preferences of 9-year-olds (Hill et al., 1994). Overall, current and ideal body shape choices matched in only 41% of girls and 31% of boys. This congruence of current and ideal shapes is inferred as body satisfaction. Body dissatisfaction is a difference in these two choices and its direction is sex dependent. Of the girls studied, 41% preferred a thinner body shape than their perceived current shape. In contrast, 41% of the boys chose a shape that was broader or heavier than their current shape, only 28% choosing a thinner ideal. Similar patterns of children's body dissatisfaction have been reported by researchers in the UK, North America and Australia.

A development in this methodology is the Children's Body Image Scale in which seven photographs replace the outline drawings (Truby & Paxton, 2002). Evaluated in children aged 7–12 (mean age 9), the authors found that 48% of girls and 36% of boys desired a thinner body than their current perception, with only 10% of girls and 20% of boys desiring a larger figure. One advantage of the photograph scale is that the Body Mass Index (BMI) of each stimulus figure is known. It was of concern that 55% of girls and 45% of boys chose an ideal figure that had a BMI below the 10th BMI percentile. Indeed, this unrealistic idealization of a thin body shape was a major contributor to their apparent dissatisfaction.

Three issues are worthy of comment at this point. First, dissatisfaction is greater in heavier children, with overweight and obese children reasonably accurate in their choice of current shape but having similar ideal shapes to their leaner peers. Second, pubertal growth is a complicating factor. Boys' preference for a broader shape is consistent with their impending growth. For girls, the preference for thinness is in conflict with their gain in body fat and weight, physical changes that happen earlier in girls than boys. Third, ethnicity is an under-researched issue in early body dissatisfaction. We found that more British Asian 9-year-olds expressed a desire to be thinner than their Caucasian peers, despite being significantly lighter (Hill & Bhatti, 1995). Evidence from the US is equivocal, especially when differences in BMI are controlled for.

Younger still

Few studies have looked at very young children's body shape perceptions. Pine (2001) showed the original body figure scales to 5-, 7-, 9- and 11-year-olds. Asked to identify 'The nicest shape for a lady (man) to be', all age groups of girls chose a thinner ideal female figure than did boys. In contrast, girls and boys did not differ at any age in their perception of the ideal male shape. For all ideal choices 5-year-olds selected a thinner figure than any other age group, larger ideals being chosen with increasing age. Importantly, no difference between children's current and ideal body shape was observed in US 5-year-olds (Musher-Eizenman et al., 2003) or 3–6-year-olds (Hendy et al., 2001).

Finally, Davison et al. (2003) have followed the body dissatisfaction of a group of nearly 200 girls from age 5 to 9. At the outset only 9% of the 5-year-olds were dissatisfied with their body shape. But 21% were concerned about weight, primarily assessed as a fear of getting fat. Over the next 4 years, group body dissatisfaction and weight concerns *decreased* significantly and systematically. However, those girls who scored highest on these measures between 5 and 7 were more likely to report dieting at age 9. In addition, heavier girls were more likely to have greater body dissatisfaction and higher weight concern.

Methodological issues

Reviewing the research literature on pre-adolescent body image concerns in 2001, Ricciardelli & McCabe noted that the proportion of girls desiring a thinner body range was between 28 and 55%. In boys, it ranged between 17 and 30%. Generally, these proportions are in line with those observed in adolescents and young adults. However, the degree of variation may also reflect difficulties in understanding the requirements of the assessments used, especially by younger children. For some, the larger body shapes are seen as fat. For others, these shapes suggest a more muscled body, or even a more grown-up person. Careful instructions during the use of these scales can reduce this misunderstanding.

More critical is how cognitive development impacts on these judgements. Smolak (2004) points out that to express body dissatisfaction, a child must be able to assess their own body image and compare it with an internalized ideal. While the research cited earlier may be detecting the early development of a thinness schema, its elaboration is dependent on children's stage of cognitive development. So are pre-operational children able to make the judgements asked in using the body figure scales? Evidence suggests that they have problems. For example, some 5-year-olds are unable to select a figure representing their current shape, apparently distracted by features other than body shape, e.g. 'I don't have hair like that'. Current shape selection may have no relationship to objective body weight, suggesting that some 5-year-olds either don't understand the task or they are not accurate reporters of their current size (Musher-Eizenman et al., 2003). Critically, there are few validity data for the use of figure rating scales in children younger than 8 (Smolak, 2004).

Several other features are missing from this literature. One is the quantitative definition of body dissatisfaction. Observing that 41% of 9-year-old girls place their preferred or ideal body shape at a point thinner than their current perception does not equate to mass dissatisfaction. It is the majority choice of thinness that is impressive rather than the margin of difference and suggests that many children are expressing mild preference not frank dissatisfaction. What these assessments fail to capture is how important it is to the child to have a thinner or larger body. Perceived importance will determine the level of body discontentment and the degree to which body image concerns will influence other aspects of their life (Ricciardelli & McCabe, 2001). Similarly, body dissatisfaction in the absence of measured emotional or behavioural consequences has uncertain meaning. The general conclusion therefore is that we should acknowledge the broad picture of early body shape choices and preferences and accept that these are directed by sex, age and, at least partly, by the child's weight. However, we should reserve the diagnosis of true dissatisfaction for a relative minority of this age group.

Body shape attributions

Views of fatness

Associated with the above literature is a raft of research looking at children's perceptions of and attitudes to overweight and obesity. As already described, thin-ideal internalization does not simply reflect the allure of a thin body shape. Its value is reinforced by the widespread and whole-heartedly negative views of fatness.

The research has its origins in studying perceptions of disability and the personality attributes associated with particular body shapes. In one of the earliest studies, 10–11-year-olds were presented with six line drawings showing a child as physically normal, in leg brace or crutches, in a wheelchair, with facial disfigurement, without a hand, or overweight (Richardson *et al.*, 1961). Asked to choose the picture they liked best, the selection was put to one side and the question repeated to give a rank order of preference. Most preferred was the child with no obvious disability. The overweight child was ranked bottom. In a review of research up to the mid 1980s, DeJong & Kleck (1986) noted the consistency of this rank ordering, with American children almost always placing the overweight child last or next to last. In addition, they observed that the least accepting attitudes to overweight peers were found in industrialized, Western cultures, and that girls appeared less accepting than boys of the overweight child.

In a revealing follow-up, Latner & Stunkard (2003) conducted a replication some 40 years on. Again, the obese child was liked least, placed bottom by even more children than in 1961, especially by girls. In addition, the healthy non-disabled child was more consistently chosen first, again more so than in 1961. It is notable that this polarization of views has occurred against a backdrop of increasing child and adult obesity, suggesting that stigmatization has increased despite obesity's greater visibility and normalization.

Drawings of thin and fat body figures have also been used to assess personality attributes. Staffieri (1967), for example, asked 6–10-year-old boys to assign each of 39 adjectives to the silhouette they best described. The fat body shape was more frequently labelled lazy, stupid, sloppy, dirty, naughty, mean, ugly, and gets teased, and least frequently, best friend and has lots of friends. Research that followed adapted the stimulus materials using photographs with written descriptions or rating as alternatives to the rather artificial forced allocation of attributes. For some traits, fat and thin figures both received fewer positive endorsements than a medium or average shape figure (when included). The message here is clear: some children reject any deviation from normal body shape. Amid this, the greater rejection of fatness is also clear, the labels most commonly attached to fat figures being low intelligence, laziness and social isolation.

A number of more recent studies add to this depiction. In one, fat children's figures were not simply unattractive and friendless, they were rated as extremely unhealthy, unfit and unlikely to eat healthily (Hill & Silver, 1995). Surprisingly, 9-year-olds' ratings were unaffected by their own weight status. Nor does personal body dissatisfaction influence these attributions (Tiggemann & Wilson-Barrett, 1998). However, there is evidence that social class has an impact, with children attending private (fee-paying) schools assigning even fewer positive characteristics to fat figures than state school peers (Wardle *et al.*, 1995). Pre-adolescents appear to have absorbed messages about the unacceptability of overweight, something shaped by their social environment, but the stereotyping process appeared uninfluenced by their own personal attributes.

Early emergence

As regards when these stereotypic views appear, the evidence suggests from the age of 5 and possibly earlier. Musher-Eizenman *et al.* (2004) asked 4–6-year-old children to rate three of the Collins body figure scale drawings. Overall, the fat body shape was the most negatively rated. In addition, the fat body shape was chosen as a friend only 16% of the time (vs. 39% and 45%, thin and average figures respectively) and as best friend only 7% of the time (vs. 55% and 38%).

Using a storyline procedure in which one child was mean, the other nice, Cramer & Steinwert (1998) found that 3–5-year-old children were significantly more likely to choose a drawing of a fat figure as the mean child than a thin or average shape figure. These authors found body size stigmatizing increased with age but was clearly present in 3-year-olds. In addition, girls showed more stigmatization than boys, and while low and average weight children's preferred playmate was average shaped, overweight children were more likely to choose the thin figure. While some very young children have absorbed the prevalent fat-is-bad viewpoint, the degree to which this is internalized, comprehended and acted upon is still unclear.

Acquiring shape and weight concerns

Some of the studies already referred to have sought evidence of the driving forces behind children's idealization of thinness or stigmatizing of fatness. Davison & Birch (2004), for example, hypothesized that anti-fat stereotyping may show intrafamilial resemblance, implying that parents are important vehicles for these attitudes. The outcome was not so simple. There was no association between the stereotyping by 9-year-old girls and their parents. Rather, girls who had negative attitudes to obesity were more likely to rate their parents and peers as talking about body shape issues and weight loss. This suggests a cultivation of attitudes rather than simple mimicry. It also identifies two of the three main socialization agents for children. Outlined below is some of the more recent evidence on their contribution to children's shape and weight cognitions.

Parents

An obvious question to ask in this context is whether children of mothers with a recent eating disorder are more likely to show problems with eating and growth. Stein *et al.* (1999), for example, have shown that infants of mothers with eating disorders have reduced growth compared with controls and that this was related to the amount of mealtime conflict. Continuing to the age of 5, this research group looked at the children's self-representation by video-taping them acting out a family meal in pretend play (Park *et al.*, 2003). Children of mothers with a recent eating disorder represented their mothers more positively in relation to feeding or body shape themes, suggesting that food and eating was a more salient experience for them. On the negative side, the presence of marital disharmony was associated with negative maternal representations, suggesting that children either internalized partner criticisms or their mother's perception of being criticized.

This study is a useful reminder that while research shows such children are at increased risk of psychological disturbance, syndrome development depends on a variety of factors and so is far from inevitable. Nor is the mechanism of intergenerational transmission as straightforward as it may seem. Modelling of maternal shape and weight concerns and behaviours has been a frequently cited reason for family dieting resemblances (Hill & Franklin, 1998). However, direct parental comments to their child about the child's weight or direct encouragement to lose weight appear more powerful than parental modelling (Wertheim *et al.*, 2002).

Some cautions are necessary. First, much of this research deals with normative weight and eating concerns rather than those frankly abnormal and is based on less than complete parental participation. Care is required in generalizing to eating disorders. Second, the effects of modelling may be clearer when behaviours (e.g. dieting) rather than attitudes are the measured variable. Third, some parental comments may be in response to their child's comments. Fourth, studies differ in terms of the informant. Some rely on child reports, others on parental reports, and a few collect both. Different stances on an issue even if recognized, combined with a reluctance to admit problems, can hugely affect outcome. Fifth, the broader family context requires consideration. The contribution of fathers and siblings to a child's weight concerns and behaviours is poorly understood. Likewise, tensions between family food habits and those of the dominant culture, as observed in our study of British-born Asian girls (Hill & Bhatti, 1995), need further investigation. Finally, discordant family relationships and problems in developing secure attachments have both been associated with early weight concerns and body dissatisfaction. It is important to recognize the reciprocal relationship between family functioning and individual dissatisfactions.

Media

The role of the media in the development and prevention of eating disorders has been the subject of several reviews (e.g. British Medical Association, 2000). They distinguish between the media's idealization of thin body shapes in setting a context for the development of eating disorders, the use of the media by individuals with an eating disorder and the potential of the media in eating disorder prevention. But just how great an impact do the media have on children's shape and weight concerns?

A meta-analysis of experimental studies manipulating thin media images concluded that the greatest changes in body satisfaction were seen in participants younger than 19 and in those vulnerable to the activation of thinness schema (Groesz et al., 2002). Media exposure was seen as activating rather than cultivating a thinness schema in females already motivated and cognitively prepared to value themselves in terms of shape, weight and beauty. This triggering role is a valuable perspective. But the priority given to thin body shapes, near absence of fat bodies in fashion media and its potential in cultivating attitudes in younger age groups should not be dismissed. The problem is the relative lack of research. In only one of the 25 studies reviewed were participants pre-teenagers.

Harrison (2000) looked at the relationship between amount of TV viewing, attraction to favourite TV characters, ChEAT (Children's Eating Attitudes Test) scores, body shape standards and stereotyping in around 300 children with a mean age of 7.5. Television viewing was weakly related to ChEAT scores and to boys' negative stereotyping of a fat girl character but was unrelated to either girls' or boys' preference for thinness. Evidence for media-associated thin ideal internalization was apparent in a study of 8–11-year-olds (Cusumano & Thompson, 2001). Using a media influence measure that distinguished internalization, awareness and media pressure, girls scored higher than boys and for girls all three subscales were significantly correlated with a measure of body dissatisfaction. In a yet older sample, Vaughan & Fouts (2003) assessed magazine and TV exposure together with ChEAT scores in a large group of 9–14-year-old girls, and again 16 months later. Girls whose ChEAT scores increased over this period had significantly increased their exposure to fashion magazines but reduced their TV viewing. Girls whose ChEAT scores decreased reduced both magazine and TV exposure.

This very limited set of studies confirms that age is an important factor in understanding media influence. By distinguishing the impact of fashion magazines and TV viewing it confirms an observation made of undergraduates, and is a reminder of the different facets of media influence. However, little can be deduced regarding directional effects. Media exposure could invoke or enhance body dissatisfaction, those already dissatisfied may be drawn to thin idealizing media, or a third variable such as low self-esteem may explain the apparent relationship.

Peers

One of the most striking recent accounts of increasing body dissatisfaction and eating pathology comes from Anne Becker's studies of Fijian adolescent girls (Becker *et al.*, 2002). The impact of Western media exposure via newly introduced TV was apparent in the girls' psychological test scores and their personal comments describing their desire to reshape their bodies to become more like the main programme characters. However, the authors were careful to point out that the response was not a dose effect of TV exposure. Rather, the study showed what effect prolonged exposure to TV had on a peer environment by changing aesthetic ideals and stimulating consumerism.

Peers are hugely influential in the context of children's self-perception, taking over from parents at an increasingly early age. There are several ways that talking about weight and dieting ('fat talk') could be functional in adolescent peer group interactions. One is the giving and receiving of weight control information and advice. Another is the promotion of in-group affiliation, talking about the importance of thinness, sharing dislike of particular body areas, and making these normative. Accordingly, social network analysis that identified patterns of 15-year-old girls' friendship clusters showed higher within-group similarity for body image concern and dieting than occurred between groups (Paxton *et al.*, 1999). In addition, groupings of girls scoring high in body dissatisfaction and dieting showed high levels of peer engagement in weight and shape-related issues.

Research with younger age groups has not asked similarly sophisticated questions. Instead, information about numbers of friends dieting, and talking about weight and weight loss have been combined into single 'peer message' factors for predictive analyses. In one study of 10–14 year old girls this peer message factor was correlated with both dieting and ChEAT scores (Levine *et al.*, 1994). Similarly, the frequency of peer appearance conversations, albeit mediated by thin ideal internalization, predicted body image dissatisfaction in girls and boys aged 12–14 (Jones *et al.*, 2004).

Peer teasing is another potent influence on children. Broadly assessed measures of weight-based teasing have shown peer teasing to be reported by more than a quarter of adolescent girls and boys (Eisenberg *et al.*, 2003).

Teased adolescents were more likely to have low body satisfaction, low self-esteem and more depressive symptoms. Looking specifically at teasing about overweight, we found this to be reported by 21% of pre-adolescent girls and 16% of boys (Hill & Waterston, 2002). Again, these victimized children scored significantly lower on measures of self-competence and self-worth, even after controlling for differences in BMI.

Determination of peer influence needs also to acknowledge that of older and opposite-sex peers. For example, using Junior, Middle and High school systems in the UK to look at exposure to older peers, Wardle & Watters (2004) found girls with regular older peer contact had a thinner ideal figure size, more friends who dieted and a higher ChEAT score. There are also gender differences in the direction of fat talk and fat teasing. Weight-related talk was more frequent between girls but boys were more likely to tease girls about being overweight than girls were to tease boys (Hill & Waterston, 2002). Peer behaviour in relation to children's weight concerns and control deserves far more attention than it has so far received.

Conclusions

This review has considered the early presentation of both shape and weight concerns and their main determinants. The familiar adolescent desire for thinness and associated body dissatisfaction are apparent in girls from 9 and possibly younger. Boys' dissatisfactions, when observed, reflect aspirations for a more muscled body, although overweight boys and girls are united in their dissatisfaction and desire for weight loss. An accurate chronology of body dissatisfaction is unavailable given the lack of recent prospective epidemiological evidence and the need to adequately represent the effects of sex, age and ethnicity (Smolak, 2004). Furthermore, while expressions of dissatisfaction are relatively common their true intensity is uncertain. More obvious is children's distaste for overweight, a reflection of a salient cultural view. In addition, there is research evidence implicating the media, family and peers in the development of these concerns, although causal directions are problematic.

A key question is whether this long gestation of negative feelings about shape, weight and eating actually matter. Does it assist in our understanding of the development of eating disorders? Some patient accounts do identify childhood as a time when some of these feelings, thoughts and associated behaviours started. Many others do not, in terms of shape and weight concern at least. But what the evidence reviewed above suggests is that negative self-evaluation in terms of body weight and appearance is being practised by increasingly younger generations. This includes boys as well as girls, although the direction and associated weight-related behaviours are often different (Cohane & Pope, 2001). A history of meaningful body dissatisfaction may be a largely unrecognized vulnerability, acting later in adolescence when other risks converge, directing the adolescent to express their distress in the form of an eating disorder rather than via a different pathology. As such it does suggest the value of early intervention for the prevention of eating disorders. Exactly what form that should take is still uncertain (see discussion by Noordenbos, Chapter 23, this volume).

REFERENCES

Becker, A. E., Burwell, R. A., Gilman, S. E., Herzog, D. B. & Hamburg, P. (2002). Eating behaviours and attitudes following prolonged exposure to television among ethnic Fijian adolescent girls. *British Journal of Psychiatry,* **180**, 509–14.

British Medical Association (2000). *Eating Disorders, Body Image and the Media.* London: Chameleon Press.

Cohane, G. H. & Pope, H. G. (2001). Body image in boys; a review of the literature. *International Journal of Eating Disorders,* **29**, 373–9.

Collins, M. E. (1991). Body figure perceptions and preferences among preadolescent children. *International Journal of Eating Disorders,* **10**, 199–208.

Cramer, P. & Steinwert, T. (1998). Thin is good, fat is bad: how early does it begin? *Journal of Applied Developmental Psychology,* **19**, 429–51.

Cusumano, D. L. & Thompson, J. K. (2001). Media influence and body image in 8–11 year old boys and girls: a preliminary report on the multidimensional media influence scale. *International Journal of Eating Disorders,* **29**, 37–44.

Davison, K. K. & Birch, L. L. (2004). Predictors of fat stereotypes among 9-year-old girls and their parents. *Obesity Research,* **12**, 86–94.

Davison, K. K., Markey, C. N. & Birch, L. L. (2003). A longitudinal examination of patterns in girls' weight concerns and body dissatisfaction from ages 5 to 9 years. *International Journal of Eating Disorders,* **33**, 320–32.

DeJong, W. & Kleck, R. E. (1986). The social psychological effects of overweight. In *Physical Appearance, Stigma, and Social Behaviour: The Ontario Symposium,* ed. C. P. Herman, M. P. Zanna & E. T. Higgins. Hillsdale, NJ: Lawrence Erlbaum, pp. 65–87.

Eisenberg, M. E., Neumark-Sztainer, D. & Story, M. (2003). Associations of weight-based teasing and emotional well-being among adolescents. *Archives of Pediatric and Adolescent Medicine,* **157**, 733–8.

Groesz, L. M., Levine, M. P. & Murnen, S. K. (2002). The effect of experimental presentation of thin media images on body satisfaction: a meta-analytic review. *International Journal of Eating Disorders,* **31**, 1–16.

Harrison, K. (2000). Television viewing, fat stereotyping, body shape standards, and eating disorder symptomatology in grade school children. *Communication Research*, **27**, 617–40.

Hendy, H. M., Gustitus, C. & Leitzel-Schwalm, J. (2001). Social cognitive predictors of body image in preschool children. *Sex Roles*, **44**, 557–69.

Hill, A. J. & Bhatti, R. (1995). Body shape perception and dieting in pre-adolescent British Asian girls: links with eating disorders. *International Journal of Eating Disorders*, **17**, 175–83.

Hill, A. J., Draper, E. & Stack, J. (1994). A weight on children's minds: body shape dissatisfactions at 9-years old. *International Journal of Obesity*, **18**, 383–9.

Hill, A. J. & Franklin, J. A. (1998). Mothers, pre-adolescent daughters, and dieting: investigating the transmission of weight control. *British Journal of Clinical Psychology*, **37**, 3–13.

Hill, A. J. & Silver, E. (1995). Fat, friendless and unhealthy: 9-year old children's perception of body shape stereotypes. *International Journal of Obesity*, **19**, 423–30.

Hill, A. J. & Waterston, C. L. (2002). Fat-teasing in pre-adolescent children: the bullied and the bullies. *International Journal of Obesity*, **26** (Suppl. 1), 20.

Jones, D. C., Vigfusdottir, T. H. & Lee, Y. (2004). Body image and the appearance culture among adolescent girls and boys. *Journal of Adolescent Research*, **19**, 323–39.

Latner, J. D. & Stunkard, A. J. (2003). Getting worse: the stigmatisation of obese children. *Obesity Research*, **11**, 452–6.

Levine, M. P., Smolak, L. & Hayden, H. (1994). The relation of sociocultural factors to eating attitudes and behaviours among middle school girls. *Journal of Early Adolescence*, **14**, 471–90.

Musher-Eizenman, D. R., Holub, S. C., Edwards-Leaper, L., Persson, A. V. & Goldstein, S. E. (2003). The narrow range of acceptable body types of preschoolers and their mothers. *Applied Developmental Psychology*, **24**, 259–72.

Musher-Eizenman, D. R., Holub, S. C., Miller, A. B., Goldstein, S. E. & Edwards-Leaper, L. (2004). Body size stigmatization in preschool children: the role of control attributions. *Journal of Pediatric Psychology*, **29**, 613–20.

Park, R. J., Lee, A., Woolley, H., Murray, L. & Stein, A. (2003). Children's representation of family mealtime in the context of maternal eating disorders. *Child: Care, Health & Development*, **29**, 111–19.

Paxton, S. J., Schutz, H. K., Wertheim, E. H. & Muir, S. L. (1999). Friendship clique and peer influences on body image concerns, dietary restraint, extreme weight-loss behaviours, and binge eating in adolescent girls. *Journal of Abnormal Psychology*, **108**, 255–66.

Pine, K. J. (2001). Children's perceptions of body shape: a thinness bias in pre-adolescent girls and associations with femininity. *Clinical Child Psychology and Psychiatry*, **6**, 519–36.

Ricciardelli, L. A. & McCabe, M. P. (2001). Children's body image concerns and eating disturbance: a review of the literature. *Clinical Psychology Review*, **21**, 325–44.

Richardson, S. A., Hastorf, A. H., Goodman, N. & Dornbusch, S. M. (1961). Cultural uniformity in reaction to physical disabilities. *American Sociological Review*, **26**, 241–7.

Smolak, L. (2004). Body image in children and adolescents: where do we go from here? *Body Image*, **1**, 15–28.

Staffieri, J. R. (1967). A study of social stereotype of body image in children. *Journal of Personality and Social Psychology*, **7**, 101–4.

Stein, A., Woolley, H. & McPherson, K. (1999). Conflict between mothers with eating disorders and their infants during mealtimes. *British Journal of Psychiatry,* **175**, 455–61.

Thompson, J. K. & Stice, E. (2001). Thin-ideal internalization: mounting evidence for a new risk factor for body-image disturbance. *Current Directions in Psychological Science*, **10**, 181–3.

Tiggemann, M. & Wilson-Barrett, E. (1998). Children's figure ratings: relationship to self-esteem and negative stereotyping. *International Journal of Eating Disorders*, **23**, 83–8.

Truby, H. & Paxton, S. J. (2002). Development of the children's body image scale. *British Journal of Clinical Psychology,* **41**, 185–203.

Vaughan, K. K. & Fouts, G. T. (2003). Changes in television and magazine exposure and eating disorder symptomatology. *Sex Roles*, **49**, 313–20.

Wardle, J., Volz, C. & Golding, C. (1995). Social variation in attitudes to obesity in children. *International Journal of Obesity*, **19**, 562–9.

Wardle, J. & Watters, R. (2004). Sociocultural influences on attitudes to weight and eating; results of a natural experiment. *International Journal of Eating Disorders*, **35**, 589–96.

Wertheim, E. H., Martin, G., Prior, M., Sanson, A. & Smart, D. (2002). Parental influences in the transmission of eating and weight related values and behaviours. *Eating Disorders*, **10**, 321–34.

4

Relation of dieting to eating pathology

Eric Stice[1], Emily Burton[1], Michael Lowe[2] and Meghan Butryn[2]

[1]University of Texas at Austin, Austin, TX, USA
[2]Drexel University, Philadelphia, PA, USA

One of the most widely studied risk factors for eating disorders is dieting. Numerous theorists have posited that dieting increases the risk for onset of binge eating, bulimia nervosa (BN) and anorexia nervosa (AN) (Polivy & Herman, 1985; Fairburn et al., 1986; Huon, 1996; Wilson, 2002).

Dieting is defined as intentional and sustained restriction of caloric intake for the purposes of weight loss or weight maintenance (Herman & Polivy, 1975; Laessle et al., 1989; Wadden et al., 2002; Wilson, 2002). For weight loss to occur, dieting must result in a negative energy balance, whereas weight maintenance necessitates a balance between caloric intake and caloric expenditure (Rosenbaum et al., 1997). For a detailed discussion of the physiology of weight maintenance see Mercer (Chapter 2, this volume). Although this definition is straightforward, dieting is heterogeneous because different people engage in different behaviours to achieve weight loss or weight maintenance. Research suggests that 60–75% of adolescent dieters combine reduced caloric intake with increased physical activity, but a minority reports questionable weight control behaviours, such as meal skipping, and a smaller minority reports unhealthy behaviours such as fasting, vomiting or laxative abuse for weight control purposes (Emmons, 1992; Serdula et al., 1993; French et al., 1995). For example, one study of a large community recruited sample of adolescent females found that 4% reported vomiting, 5% reported diet pill use, 3% reported appetite suppressant use, 2% reported laxative use and 1% reported diuretic use (French et al., 1995). Research suggests that there is also considerable variation in the duration of dieting efforts, ranging from less than a week to 6 months, with a mode of about 1 month (Emmons, 1992; Williamson et al., 1992; French et al., 1999).

Eating Disorders in Children and Adolescents, ed. Tony Jaffa and Brett McDermott. Published by Cambridge University Press. © Cambridge University Press 2007.

Theorists have proposed several mechanisms by which dieting might increase the risk for eating disorder symptoms. According to Polivy & Herman (1985), 'Successful dieting produces weight loss, which in turn might create a state of chronic hunger, especially if such weight loss leaves the dieter at a weight below the set-point weight that is defended physiologically' (p. 196). The chronic hunger experienced by dieters putatively increases the likelihood that they may binge eat. Polivy & Herman (1985) also argue that a reliance on cognitive controls over eating, rather than physiological cues, leaves dieters vulnerable to uncontrolled eating when these cognitive processes are disrupted, for example, during an emotional crisis. Violation of strict dietary rules may also result in the temporary abandonment of dietary restriction because of the abstinence violation effect, a phenomenon in which a minor lapse in behavioural control (e.g. consuming a 'forbidden' food) results in a perceived inability to abstain from a chronic behavioral pattern (e.g. binge eating) (Marlatt & Gordon, 1985). Furthermore, dieting may result in depletion of tryptophan, a precursor of serotonin, which increases the likelihood of binge eating high-carbohydrate food to restore tryptophan levels (Kaye et al., 1998). Binge eating putatively precipitates redoubled dietary efforts and use of radical weight control techniques, such as vomiting and laxative use, which develop into the self-maintaining binge–purge cycle that is the hallmark of BN (Fairburn et al., 1986). Lowe (1993) distinguished between three different facets of dieting – weight suppression (i.e. long-term maintenance of a weight loss), current weight-loss dieting and a history of frequent dieting and overeating – and has argued that weight suppression may be the variable that increases risk for onset of bulimic pathology, rather than current dieting or a history of dieting and overeating (Butryn et al., 2006). Finally, for a subset of vulnerable individuals, successful weight loss induced by dieting may be reinforced by social factors from family and friends and ultimately spiral into AN. Dieting and weight loss can also be reinforcing for some adolescents because of the feeling of control it provides, particularly if an adolescent feels that he or she has little control over other aspects of life (Fairburn et al., 1999).

Dieting has become an increasingly common practice among adolescent and preadolescent females. One study reported that 44% of adolescent females were dieting to lose weight and another 26% of adolescent females were dieting to maintain their weight (Serdula et al., 1993). Another study reported that 56% of females reported at least one intentional weight loss episode by middle adolescence, with an average of 2.5 weight loss episodes (French et al., 1995). Remarkably, these findings have been replicated in even younger samples. Preadolescent girls also report body dissatisfaction and a desire to be thinner (Brodie *et al.*, 1994; Wood *et al.*, 1996; Schur *et al.*, 2000; see Hill, Chapter 3, this volume). For example, 59% of 5–8-year-olds reported that they desired a thinner figure (Lowes & Tiggemann, 2003). This desire appears to be commonly established by age 7 or 8 (Lowes & Tiggemann, 2003) and may be a result of parental modelling. Preadolescent daughters' level of body dissatisfaction and associated weight loss behaviours have been shown to directly correlate with those of their mothers, while preadolescent sons do not show this effect (Ruther & Richman, 1993; Smolak *et al.*, 1999). The mean level of dietary restraint, as evidenced by self-report measures, is also fairly high among preadolescents, and has been shown to be similar in magnitude to dietary restraint levels among younger adolescents (Hill *et al*, 1992). Perhaps most significantly, self-reported dieting behaviours are widespread among preadolescents. One study found that 40% of fourth grade children reported dieting 'at least sometimes' to 'very often', and 80% indicated that they have altered food choices to try to prevent weight gain (Gustafson-Larson & Terry, 1992). Due to the prevalence of dieting behaviours among preadolescents and adolescents, it is important to determine whether dieting practices increase the risk for future eating disorders.

Dozens of studies have found that individuals who score high on dietary restraint scales tend to consume more calories in the laboratory than individuals with low scores on these measures under a variety of conditions, such as after stress inductions and after consumption of high-calorie foods (Polivy & Herman, 1985; Lowe, 1993). However, because these studies have not manipulated dieting or provided evidence of temporal precedence between dieting and future eating behaviours, these findings cannot be unambiguously interpreted. Accordingly, we focus on prospective and experimental studies that have manipulated dieting. Although several of these studies involved adult rather than adolescent participants, such research can nonetheless help answer important questions about dieting in youth.

Consistent with the dieting theory of eating disorders, adolescent girls, regardless of specific age, with elevated scores on various dietary restraint scales or who self-identify as dieters have been found to be at increased risk for future onset of eating disorder symptoms (Stice *et al.*, 1998, 2002; Field *et al.*, 1999) and onset of threshold and subthreshold AN and BN (Patton *et al.*, 1990; Killen *et al.*, 1994, 1996; Santonastaso *et al.*, 1999). Indeed, dieting is the most consistently observed risk factor for eating disorders and the one with the largest effect size (Stice, 2002).

Experiments examining the effects of caloric deprivation on lab-based eating have provided less consistent support for the restraint model. Caloric deprivation produced significant increases in investigator-coded binge eating, but not self-labelled binge eating, in women with binge eating disorder (BED) (Agras & Telch, 1998) and marginally significant increases in ad lib caloric intake for overweight, but not normal weight, participants (Lowe, 1992). However, other studies have found no effect of acute and longer-term dietary restriction on caloric intake (Lowe, 1994; Telch & Agras, 1996; Lowe et al., 2001). Thus, laboratory experiments have provided mixed support for the restraint model and none have assessed all of the DSM–IV symptoms of bulimia nervosa.

Randomized trials that have examined the effects of long-term low-calorie diets on changes in binge eating and DSM–IV bulimic symptoms have generated findings that seem completely at odds with the dieting theory of eating pathology. Randomized trials have found that assignment to low-calorie weight loss diets (e.g. 1200 calories a day) resulted in significantly greater decreases in binge eating for obese (Goodrick et al., 1998; Reeves et al., 2001) and overweight individuals (Klem et al., 1997) relative to wait-list control conditions. Experimental trials have also found that assignment to a weight loss diet (Presnell & Stice, 2003; Groesz & Stice, in press) or a weight maintenance diet (Stice et al., 2005) resulted in significantly greater reductions in bulimic symptoms for normal weight young women relative to wait-list control conditions. Participants in the various dieting conditions of these trials lost significant weight relative to controls, which confirms that dietary restriction was successfully manipulated.

These experimental findings appear to be incompatible with the suggestion that dietary restriction promotes binge eating and bulimic symptoms. They are particularly troublesome for the dieting theory because experiments are more effective than prospective studies in ruling out the possibility that some third-variable explains the dieting–bulimic symptom relation. Within this context, it should also be noted that there are also cross-sectional findings that are similarly incompatible with dieting theory of bulimia nervosa, such as the evidence that dieting intensity is inversely related to binge eating severity in individuals with bulimia nervosa (Lowe et al., 1998). Indeed, a number of investigators over the years have identified empirical findings that do not accord with the dieting theory of eating pathology (e.g. Ruderman, 1986; Tuschl, 1990; Lowe, 1993; Lowe & Timko, 2004).

There are at least three possible explanations for the contradictory findings between the prospective studies reporting that elevated dietary restraint scores predict future onset of bulimic symptoms and the experimental finding that assignment to a diet results in decreased bulimic symptoms. One possible explanation is suggested by the inferential limitations of certain designs. Because randomized experiments rule out third variable explanations and prospective studies do not, the positive relation of self-reported dieting to increases in bulimic pathology may have emerged because some third variable increases the risk for both variables. It has been suggested that a tendency towards caloric overconsumption, a metabolic predisposition to store ingested energy as body fat, or both factors may produce a vulnerability to weight gain (Stice *et al.*, 1999; Lowe & Kral, 2006). In cultures where obesity is stigmatized and thinness is revered, such obesity-prone individuals would be more likely to go on diets and, because diets generally do not produce lasting weight loss, to do so repeatedly. If this were the case, self-reported dieting would be a proxy risk factor for bulimic symptoms solely because it is a marker for weight gain mediated by a tendency to be in positive energy balance (Stice *et al.*, 1999; Lowe & Kral, 2006). In line with this hypothesis, self-reported dieting has consistently been shown to prospectively predict weight *gain* over time (Klesges *et al.*, 1992; French *et al.*, 1994; Stice *et al.*, 1999). More broadly, the fact that it is impossible to rule out third-variable alternative explanations for prospective findings from longitudinal studies serves as a cogent reminder of the importance of using randomized experiments to confirm causal relations suggested by prospective studies.

A second possible explanation for the conflicting findings is that the experimental interventions promote healthy dietary behaviours, but that it is unhealthy dietary behaviours, such as meal skipping, which lead to onset of bulimic pathology. The evidence that many adolescent dieters report skipping meals (Emmons, 1992; Serdula *et al.*, 1993) suggests that such unhealthy dieting behaviours are prevalent. One way to address this possibility would be to manipulate 'dieting as usual' in a randomized experiment with adolescent participants to provide an ecologically valid test of whether dieting, in whatever form it usually takes in the real world in this population, results in increased or decreased bulimic symptoms. It would also be useful to experimentally manipulate dieting behaviours that are thought to be unhealthy, such as meal skipping. However, it is noteworthy that two studies that manipulated meal skipping by assigning participants to a diet involving daily meal skipping or a diet requiring regular meals did not find any experimental effects on change in binge eating frequency or bulimic symptoms (Schlundt *et al.*, 1992; Groesz & Stice, 2005). Within this context it is important to note that many of the dieting behaviours that have been labelled as unhealthy have not actually been investigated in rigorous experimental studies – this is an important direction for future research.

A third possible explanation for the conflicting findings is that prospective studies that have found dieting to be positively related to future risk for eating pathology have used invalid measures of dieting. Numerous studies have found that dieting scales do not show the expected inverse correlations with unobtrusive measures of acute and long-term caloric intake (Klesges *et al.*, 1992; Jansen, 1996; Stice *et al.*, 1999, 2004; Bathalon *et al.*, 2000; van Strien *et al.*, 2000). These results imply that these scales do not assess dietary restriction as suggested by validation studies that relied on self-reported caloric intake (van Strien *et al.*, 1986; Laessle *et al.*, 1989) and the content of the items. For instance, one study found that four widely used measures of dietary restraint did not show the expected inverse correlations with unobtrusive measures of actual caloric intake in a series of four studies (Stice *et al.*, 2004). The importance of this state of affairs cannot be overstated because it implies that the entire literature condemning dieting has been built using apparently invalid measures, which means all findings from studies using these scales must be interpreted in this light.

It should be noted that it is not simply that the field lacks valid measures of dieting, but rather that people generally provide distorted reports of their weight, their caloric intake and their physical activity levels because of strong social desirability pressures in Western culture that favour thinness. For instance, one study found an average under-reporting rate of 20% in a normative sample (Livingstone *et al.*, 1990). Lichtman *et al.* (1992) found that 'diet-resistant' patients, who claimed they could not lose weight on very low calorie diets, underestimated their energy intake by almost 50%.

One possible interpretation of the evidence that dieting scales are invalid measures of dietary restriction is that these scales may be detecting what might be referred to as 'relative dietary restriction'. Perhaps people with an overeating tendency reduce their degree of overeating, but remain in a positive energy balance state and gain weight over time, yet perceive this as dietary restraint. Timmerman & Gregg (2003) and Lowe & Levine (2005) have recently referred to this state as 'perceived deprivation', that is, eating less than one would like to eat but not reducing intake sufficiently to produce weight loss or even avoid weight gain. That is, individuals identified by dieting scales may still be overeating but may think of themselves as dieting because they could eat even more if they 'let themselves go' (i.e. if they reduced what they perceive to be their dietary restraint). This interpretation is suggested by the evidence that individuals with elevated dietary restraint scores consume significantly more calories than those with low dietary restraint scores, but did not feel that they had overeaten (Jansen, 1996). Another possible interpretation of the invalidity findings is that dieting scales may fail to identify those individuals who more regularly practise healthy weight management behaviours. People who are able to consistently maintain a healthy weight through regular consumption of a low-calorie diet and through daily moderate physical activity may not endorse items on dietary restraint scales because they do not conceive of themselves as 'dieting for weight loss or weight maintenance purposes' but rather as living a healthy lifestyle. That is, dieting scales may be missing the people who use weight control behaviours the most consistently. Instead, these scales may identify people who are engaging in transient attempts to control an overeating problem. This interpretation leads to the hypothesis that self-labelled non-dieters may engage in healthy weight control behaviours, such as daily intake of fruit, vegetables and whole-grain foods, and daily physical activity, at a higher frequency than self-labelled dieters.

Before discussing the implications of the foregoing evidence, it is important to point out that the type of dieting that is widely believed to contribute to the development of AN and BN is quite different from the type of dieting studied in most of the research reviewed here. According to retrospective reports AN, and the majority of cases of BN, begin with a period of radical weight loss dieting during which individuals with incipient AN or BN lose a great deal of body weight, especially when considered as a percentage of their starting weights (Russell, 1979; Hsu, 1990). The per cent weight loss from self-reported highest to lowest weight experienced by these individuals during the development of their disorder is often greater than the 25% average weight losses that preceded the development of binge eating in many of Keys' (1950) starving conscientious objectors. Thus the questions raised in this chapter about the causal role of dieting in the development of AN and BN may not apply to the extensive weight losses and ongoing weight suppression experienced by AN and the majority of BN patients.

This review of the extant prospective and experimental findings regarding the relation of dieting to pathology suggests several general conclusions. First, the literature does consistently indicate that adolescents with elevated scores on dieting scales are at elevated risk for future onset of eating pathology. Elevated scores on dieting scales have emerged as the most consistent and robust risk factor for subsequent development of eating disorders. These results suggest that self-labelled adolescent dieters represent an ideal population to target with eating disorder prevention trials. Second, by no means has it been established that dieting causes eating disorders. All of the experimental trials that have directly manipulated dieting have found that initiation of a low-calorie diet results in decreased eating disorder symptoms. Third, rather ironically, low-calorie diet interventions seem to represent a very effective vehicle for reducing eating disorder symptoms. Fourth, advances in our understanding of the relation of dieting to eating pathology has been limited by an over-reliance on cross-sectional and non-experimental findings and an under-reliance on rigorous experimental studies that manipulate dieting and specific dietary behaviours. Indeed, what is perhaps most remarkable about this literature is the confidence that has been placed in the assertion that dieting causes eating pathology in the absence of experimental studies on the matter (e.g. Polivy & Herman, 1985; Fairburn *et al.*, 1986). Finally, much greater attention needs to be devoted to developing valid measures of dieting. It would be highly desirable to develop objective and unobtrusive measures of dieting for use in prospective risk factor studies. Without a valid measure of dieting it will be virtually impossible to make accurate inferences regarding the causes and consequences of dieting.

REFERENCES

Agras, W.S. & Telch, C.F. (1998). The effects of caloric deprivation and negative affect on binge eating in obese binge-eating disordered women. *Behavior Therapy*, **29**, 491–503.

Bathalon, G.P., Tucker, K.L., Hays, N.P. *et al.* (2000). Psychological measures of eating behavior and the accuracy of 3 common dietary assessment methods in healthy postmenopausal women. *American Journal of Clinical Nutrition*, **71**, 739–45.

Brodie, D.A., Bagley, K. & Slade P.D. (1994). Body-image perception in pre- and postadolescent females. *Perceptual and Motor Skills*, **79**, 147–54.

Butryn, M.L., Lowe, M.R., Safer, D. & Agras, W.S. (2006). Weight suppression is a robust predictor of outcome in the cognitive-behavioral treatment of bulimia nervosa. *Journal of Abnormal Psychology*, **115**, 62–7.

Emmons, L. (1992). Dieting and purging behavior in black and white high school students. *Journal of the American Dietetic Association*, **92**, 306–12.

Fairburn, C.G., Cooper, Z. & Cooper, P.J. (1986). The clinical features and maintenance of bulimia nervosa. In *Handbook of Eating Disorders: Physiology, psychology and treatment of obesity, anorexia and bulimia*, ed. Brownell, K.D. & Foreyt, J.P. New York: Basic Books, pp. 389–404.

Fairburn, C.G., Shafran, R. & Cooper, Z. (1999). A cognitive-behavioral theory of anorexia nervosa. *Behaviour Research and Therapy*, **37**, 1–13.

Field, A.E., Camargo, C.A., Taylor, C.B., Berkey, C.S. & Colditz, G.A. (1999). Relation of peer and media influences to the development of purging behaviors among preadolescent and adolescent girls. *Archives of Pediatric Adolescent Medicine*, **153**, 1184–9.

French, S.A., Jeffery, R.W., Forster, J.L., McGovern, P.G., Kelder, S.H. & Baxter, J.E. (1994). Predictors of weight change over two years among a population of working adults: The Healthy Worker Project. *International Journal of Obesity*, **18**, 145–54.

French, S., Jeffery, R.W. & Murray, D. (1999). Is dieting good for you? Prevalence, duration, and associated weight and behavior changes for specific weight loss strategies over four years in US adults. *International Journal of Obesity*, **23**, 320–7.

French, S.A., Perry, C.L., Leon, G.R. & Fulkerson, J.A. (1995). Dieting behaviors and weight change history in female adolescents. *Health Psychology*, **14**, 548–55.

Goodrick, G.K., Poston, W.S., Kimball, K.T., Reeves, R.S. & Foreyt, J.P. (1998). Nondieting versus dieting treatments for overweight binge-eating women. *Journal of Consulting and Clinical Psychology*, **66**, 363–68.

Groesz, L.M. & Stice, E. (in press). An experimental test of the effects of dieting on bulimic symptoms: The impact of meal skipping. *Behavior Research and Therapy*.

Gustafson-Larson, A.M. & Terry, R.D. (1992). Weight-related behaviors and concerns of fourth-grade children. *Journal of the American Dietetic Associaiton*, **92**, 818–22.

Herman, C.P. & Polivy, J. (1975). Anxiety, restraint, and eating behavior. *Journal of Abnormal Psychology*, **84**, 666–72.

Hill, A.J., Oliver, S. & Rogers, P.J. (1992). Eating in the adult world: the rise of dieting in childhood and adolescence. *British Journal of Clinical Psychology*, **31**, 95–105.

Hsu, L.K.G. (1990). *Eating Disorders*. New York: Guilford Press.

Huon, G.F. (1996). Health promotion and the prevention of dieting-induced disorders. *Eating Disorders: The Journal of Treatment and Prevention*, **4**, 257–68.

Jansen, A. (1996). How restrained eaters perceive the amount they eat. *British Journal of Clinical Psychology*, **35**, 381–92.

Kaye, W., Gendall, K. & Strober, M. (1998). Serotonin neuronal function and selective serotonin reuptake inhibitor treatment in anorexia and bulimia nervosa. *Biological Psychiatry*, **44**, 825–38.

Keys, A. (1950). The residues of malnutrition and starvation. *Science*, **112**, 371–3.

Killen, J.D., Hayward, C., Wilson, D.M. *et al.* (1994). Factors associated with eating disorder symptoms in a community sample of 6th and 7th grade girls. *International Journal of Eating Disorders*, **15**, 357–67.

Killen, J.D., Taylor, C.B., Hayward, C. *et al.* (1996). Weight concerns influence the development of eating disorders: A 4-year prospective study. *Journal of Consulting and Clinical Psychology*, **64**, 936–40.

Klem, M.L., Wing, R.R., Simkin-Silverman, L. & Kuller, L.H. (1997). The psychological consequences of weight gain prevention in healthy, premenopausal women. *International Journal of Eating Disorders*, **21**, 167–74.

Klesges, R.C., Isbell, T.R. & Klesges, L.M. (1992). Relationship between dietary restraint, energy intake, physical activity, and body weight: A prospective analysis. *Journal of Abnormal Psychology*, **101**, 668–74.

Laessle, R.G., Tuschl, R.J., Kotthaus, B.C. & Pirke, K.M. (1989). A comparison of the validity of three scales for the assessment of dietary restraint. *Journal of Abnormal Psychology*, **98**, 504–7.

Lichtman, S.W., Pisarska, K., Berman, E.R. *et al.* (1992). Discrepancy between self-reported and actual caloric intake and exercise in obese subjects. *New England Journal of Medicine*, **327**, 1893–8.

Livingstone, M.B., Prentice, A.M. & Strain, J.J. (1990). Accuracy of weighed dietary records in studies of diet and health. *British Medical Journal*, **300**, 708–12.

Lowe, M.R. (1992). Staying on versus going off a diet: effects on eating in normal weight and overweight individuals. *International Journal of Eating Disorders*, **12**, 417–24.

Lowe, M.R. (1993). The effects of dieting on eating behavior: a three-factor model. *Psychological Bulletin*, **114**, 100–21.

Lowe, M.R. (1994). Putting restrained and unrestrained nondieters on short-term diets: effects on eating. *Addictive Behaviors*, **19**, 349–56.

Lowe, M.R., Foster, G.D., Kerzhnerman, I., Swain, R.M. & Wadden, T.A. (2001). Restrictive dieting vs. 'undieting': Effects on eating regulation in obese clinic attenders. *Addictive Behaviors*, **26**, 253–66.

Lowe, M.R., Gleaves, D.H. & Murphy-Eberenz, K.P. (1998). On the relation of dieting and bingeing in bulimia nervosa. *Journal of Abnormal Psychology*, **107**, 263–71.

Lowe, M.R., & Kral, T.V.E. (2006). Stress-induced eating in restrained eaters may not be caused by stress or restraint. *Appetite*, **46**, 16–21.

Lowe, M.R., & Levine, A.S. (2005). Eating motives and the controversy over dieting: eating less than needed versus less than wanted. *Obesity Research*, **13**, 797–805.

Lowe, M.R. & Timko, C.A. (2004). What a difference a diet makes: towards an understanding of differences between restrained dieters and restrained nondieters. *Eating Behaviors*, **5**, 199–208.

Lowes, J. & Tiggemann, M. (2003). Body dissatisfaction, dieting awareness and the impact of parental influence in young children. *British Journal of Health Psychology*, **8**, 135–47.

Marlatt, G.A. & Gordon, J.R. (1985). *Relapse Prevention: Maintenance Strategies in the Treatment of Addictive Behaviors*. New York: Guilford Press.

Patton, G.C., Johnson-Sabine, E., Wood, K., Mann, A.H. & Wakeling, A. (1990). Abnormal eating attitudes in London schoolgirls – a prospective epidemiological study: outcome at 12 month follow-up. *Psychological Medicine*, **20**, 383–94.

Polivy, J. & Herman, C.P. (1985). Dieting and binging: a causal analysis. *American Psychologist*, **40**, 193–204.

Presnell, K. & Stice, E. (2003). An experimental test of the effect of weight-loss dieting on bulimic pathology: tipping the scales in a different direction. *Journal of Abnormal Psychology*, **112**, 166–70.

Reeves, R.S., McPherson, R.S., Nichaman, M.Z., Harrist, R.B., Foreyt, J.P. & Goodrick, G.K. (2001). Nutrient intake of obese female binge eaters. *Journal of the American Dietetic Association*, **101**, 209–15.

Rosenbaum, M., Leibel, R.L. & Hirsch, J. (1997). Medical progress: obesity. *New England Journal of Medicine*, **337**, 396–407.

Ruderman, A.J. (1986). Dietary restraint: a theoretical and empirical review. *Psychological Bulletin*, **99**, 247–62.

Russell, G.F.M. (1979). Bulimia nervosa: an ominous variant of anorexia nervosa. *Psychological Medicine*, **9**, 429–48.

Ruther, N.M. & Richman, C.L. (1993). The relationship between mothers' eating restraint and their children's attitudes and behaviors. *Bulletin of the Psychonomic Society*, **31**, 217–20.

Santonastaso, P., Friederici, S. & Favaro, A. (1999). Full and partial syndromes in eating disorders: a 1-year prospective study of risk factors among female students. *Psychopathology*, **32**, 50–6.

Schlundt, D.G., Hill, J.O., Sbrocco, T., Pope-Cordle, J. & Sharp, T. (1992). The role of breakfast in the treatment of obesity: a randomized clinical trial. *American Journal of Clinical Nutrition*, **55**, 645–51.

Schur, E.A., Sanders, M. & Steiner, H. (2000). Body dissatisfaction and dieting in young children. *International Journal of Eating Disorders*, **27**, 74–82.

Serdula, M.K., Collins, E., Williamson, D.F., Anda, R.F., Pamuk, E. & Byers, T.E. (1993). Weight control practices of US adolescents and adults. *Annals of Internal Medicine*, **119**, 667–71.

Smolak, L., Levine, M.P. & Schermer, E. (1999). Parental input and weight concerns among elementary school children. *International Journal of Eating Disorders*, **25**, 263–71.

Stice, E. (2002). Risk and maintenance factors for eating pathology: a meta-analytic review. *Psychological Bulletin*, **128**, 825–48.

Stice, E., Cameron, R., Killen, J.D., Hayward, C. & Taylor, C.B. (1999). Naturalistic weight reduction efforts prospectively predict growth in relative weight and onset of obesity among female adolescents. *Journal of Consulting and Clinical Psychology*, **67**, 967–74.

Stice, E., Fisher, M. & Lowe, M.R. (2004). Are dietary restraint scales valid measures of acute dietary restriction? Unobtrusive, observational data suggest not. *Psychological Assessment*, **16**, 51–9.

Stice, E., Killen, J.D., Hayward, C. & Taylor, C.B. (1998). Age of onset for binge eating and purging during adolescence: a four-year survival analysis. *Journal of Abnormal Psychology*, **107**, 671–5.

Stice, E., Presnell, K. & Spangler, D. (2002). Risk factors for binge eating onset: a prospective investigation. *Health Psychology*, **21**, 131–8.

Stice, E., Presnell, K., Groesz, L. & Shaw, H. (2005). Effects of a weight maintenance diet on bulimic pathology: An experimental test of the dietary restraint theory. *Health Psychology*, **24**, 402–12.

Telch, C.F. & Agras, W.S. (1996). The effects of short-term food deprivation on caloric intake in eating disordered subjects. *Appetite*, **26**, 221–34.

Timmerman, G.M. and Gregg, E.K. (2003). Dieting, perceived deprivation, and preoccupation with food. *Western Journal of Nursing Research*, **25**, 405–18.

Tuschl, R.J. (1990). From dietary restraint to binge eating: some theoretical considerations. *Appetite*, **14**, 105–9.

van Strien, T., Cleven, A. & Schippers, G. (2000). Restraint, tendency toward overeating, and ice cream consumption. *International Journal of Eating Disorders*, **28**, 333–8.

van Strien, T., Frijters, J.E., van Staveren, W.A., Defares, P.B. & Deurenberg, P. (1986). The predictive validity of the Dutch Restrained Eating Scale. *International Journal of Eating Disorders*, **5**, 747–55.

Wadden, T.A., Brownell, K.D. & Foster, G.D. (2002). Obesity: responding to the global epidemic. *Journal of Consulting and Clinical Psychology,* **70**, 510–25.

Williamson, D.F., Serdula, M.K., Anda, R.F., Levy, A. & Byers, T. (1992). Weight loss attempts in adults: goals, duration, and rate of weight loss. *American Journal of Public Health*, **82**, 1251–7.

Wilson, G.T. (2002). The controversy over dieting. In *Eating Disorders and Obesity: A Comprehensive Handbook*, 2nd edition, ed. Fairburn, C.G. & Brownell, K.D. New York: Guilford Press.

Wood, K.C., Becker, J.A. & Thompson, J.K. (1996). Body image dissatisfaction in preadolescent children. *Journal of Applied Developmental Psychology,* **17**, 85–100.

5

Physical and cognitive changes associated with puberty

Victor M. Fornari and Ida F. Dancyger

North Shore University Hospital, Manhasset, NY, USA

Puberty is perhaps the most important of life transitions. The changes that occur as a result of puberty are both dramatic and universal. It is a process of rapid and simultaneous transformation in biological, social and psychological dimensions of development. Although it may appear that puberty is a discreet event that punctuates the shift from childhood to adulthood, in reality it is a part in a series of events that begins at the time of conception. Our goal in this chapter is to discuss the physical and cognitive changes characteristic of pubertal maturation. New evidence suggests that there are sex differences regarding the biology of puberty that were not previously understood, and this too will be reviewed (Fechner, 2003).

Fetal life

Physical maturation and reproductive functioning are controlled by the endocrine system that operates first through the hypothalamic–pituitary–adrenal axis (HPA system) and then through the hypothalamic–pituitary–gonadal (HPG) axis (Grumbach & Styne, 1998). During the prenatal period, it is the exposure to androgens that organizes the reproductive system (Reiter & Grumbach, 1982). The hypothalamic–gonadotropin releasing hormone (GnRH) pulse generator is initially active during fetal life and early infancy, but is then suppressed during childhood (see Fig. 5.1).

Differences in male and female patterns of gonadotropin secretion have been described during fetal life (Beck-Peccoz et al., 1991). Luteinizing hormone (LH) and follicle-stimulating hormone (FSH) are produced by the gonadotropic cells of the pituitary gland and stimulate the ovaries and testes to secrete oestrogen and testosterone, respectively. The male fetus has a rise in both LH

Eating Disorders in Children and Adolescents, ed. Tony Jaffa and Brett McDermott. Published by Cambridge University Press. © Cambridge University Press 2007.

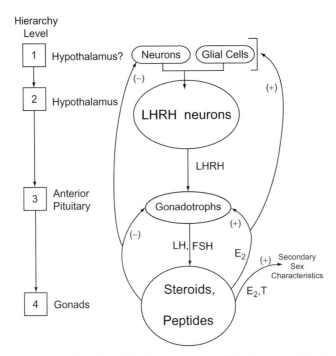

Figure 5.1. The hierarchical arrangement within the hypothalamic-pituitary-gonadal axis at the time of puberty. Puberty is initiated by events that take place within the central nervous system [1]. These events result in an increased pulsatility of LHRH [2], which leads to an increased secretion of pituitary gonadotropins (LH and FSH) [3]. Gonadotropins, in turn, stimulate gonadal development and production of gonadal steroids [4], which are responsible for the development of secondary sex characteristics, and control gonadotropin secretion via negative-feedback loops acting on both the neurons controlling LHRH secretion and pituitary gonadotropins. Oestrogen triggers the first preovulatory surge of gonadotropins (+) by acting on both the neuronal and glial networks controlling LHRH secretion and directly on pituitary gonadotropins.

and FSH by 16 weeks and peaks at 20 weeks, followed by a gradual decline. By contrast, the female fetus has a slightly earlier rise in LH and a more gradual decline. Between 17 and 24 weeks of gestation, LH and FSH levels are higher in female than in male fetuses. Both male and female fetuses are exposed to high levels of oestrogen secondary to maternal feto-placental production. The decrease in LH and FSH seen in both sexes during the third trimester is a result of the maturation of the negative feedback system of the gonadostat (Beck-Peccoz et al., 1991). The brain 'gonadostat' is a model used to describe the regulation of the hypothalamic GnRH pulse generator.

Infancy

At the time of birth, there are elevated gonadotropin levels and sex steroid hormone levels reaching the adult range. This is the result of inhibitory oestrogen levels, produced by the feto-placental unit falling abruptly at the time of birth. Males are born with elevated testosterone levels that decrease quickly in the first day of life and then rise back after one week. In the male infant, LH and FSH return to prepubertal levels by 3 months of age. Females do not have this elevation of testosterone levels. LH is increased for only several months, but FSH remains elevated for the first few years of life. The rise in LH and FSH seen in the first few months of life may be the result of the lack of complete maturity of the gonadostat, thus making it insensitive to the presence of gonadal sex steroids (Beck-Peccoz et al., 1991).

Childhood

During childhood there is quiescence. The gonadostat is very sensitive to low levels of sex steroids and there is inhibition of the GnRH pulse generator. Gonadotropin levels are low in both males and females, as are sex steroids.

Most children begin pubertal development during the middle childhood years. The first increase in adrenal androgens begins at about age 8 for boys and age 6 for girls. Approximately 2 years later, gonadal hormones begin to increase, with a rise in hormones for boys by age 10 and for girls by age 8. The initial rise in hormones is often referred to as adrenarche. It is this event that precedes other hormonal changes as well as the onset of external signs of physical development (Cutler & Loriaux, 1980). Subsequently, it is the maturation of the reproductive system that results in the production of gonadotropin-releasing hormone (GnRH), LH and FSH. Thus, gonadarche follows adrenarche by approximately 2 years, with variable bursts of LH and FSH (Reiter & Grumbach, 1982). Follicle-stimulating hormone and LH are secreted at low levels by the pituitary during childhood, and pulsatile releases of these hormones, particularly during the night-time hours, are characteristic of early puberty.

A factor that has recently been postulated to have an effect on the onset of puberty is leptin (Fechner, 2003). A large body of research regarding leptin has been accumulated in mice. Leptin is produced by adipose cells. It is possible that weight may then play a role in the timing of the onset of puberty.

Puberty

Just prior to puberty, the sensitivity of the gonadostat to the negative feedback of gonadal sex steroids decreases, releasing the hypothalamic-pituitary axis (HPA) from inhibition. It is the consequent GnRH pulses together with the increased sensitivity of the pituitary gonadotropic (LH and FSH producing) cells to GnRH that leads to increased LH and FSH secretion. At the onset of puberty, the pulse generator, controlled by the brain 'gonadostat' is reactivated. It is the LH and FSH pulses that are secreted in response to the GnRH pulses that occur first at night and then during the day as well. The gonads, in response to LH and FSH, enlarge, mature and secrete gonadal sex steroids (Fechner, 2003).

Early in puberty, females have an increase in FSH over LH production secondary to FSH's longer half-life and because of its decreased regulation by GnRH. The increased LH and FSH initiate gonadotropin-dependent follicular development in the ovaries, which stimulates them to produce the sex steroid oestrogen. Oestrogen-sensitive tissues, such as the breasts and uterus, then respond. Breasts have an increase in the glandular, fatty and connective tissues. Males have gonadal and adrenal development approximately 6 months to 1 year later than females. As the testes begin to secrete testosterone under stimulation of LH, they increase in size (Beck-Peccoz et al., 1991).

Increases in LH and FSH are some of the earliest measurable hormonal indications of pubertal development. Follicle-stimulating hormone and LH rise progressively during puberty (Reiter & Grumbach, 1982; Ojeda & Bilger, 2000). Early puberty is characterized by episodic nocturnal bursts of low levels of LH for both boys and girls (Grumbach & Styne, 1998). During the latter stages of pubertal development, LH is released throughout the day in adult-like patterns (Grumbach & Styne, 1998). Follicle-stimulating hormone and LH are important for producing sex hormones, androgens and oestrogens, in order to stimulate the development of reproductive capacities.

In girls, FSH stimulates the production of ovaries to ripen eggs, and LH stimulates the production of the hormones, progesterone and oestrogen, when levels are low (Katchadourian, 1977). Follicle-stimulating hormone has a parallel rise to LH at puberty in boys; FSH rises slightly earlier than LH, and is a sensitive indicator of early pubertal changes in boys. As puberty progresses, FSH is correlated with the maturation of the sertoli cell function, leading to sperm production in boys. The adult-like pattern of tonic release is characteristic of hormonal regulation of reproduction in both girls and boys. It is the hypothalamus that monitors levels of circulating sex steroids, oestrogen and testosterone. The hypothalamus then responds via alterations in release of the gonadotropins. For boys, spermatogenesis occurs when adult levels of androgens and adult-like levels of gonadotropins are attained.

Physical changes occurring at puberty

The changes that occur at puberty have been described by Marshall & Tanner (1974) and classified into five general areas: (1) acceleration followed by deceleration of skeletal growth, or 'growth spurt'; (2) increases in and/or redistribution of body fat and muscle tone; (3) development of the circulatory and respiratory systems, and thus increased strength and endurance; (4) maturation of secondary sexual characteristics and reproductive organs; and (5) changes in hormonal/endocrine systems. It is changes in these core areas which regulate and coordinate the other pubertal events. The pubertal processes are influenced by an interaction of genetic, nutritional and hormonal factors (Brooks-Gunn & Reiter, 1990).

Puberty is heralded by the myriad of physical changes that occur in the body with the advent of the hormonally mediated effects and the cognitive shift associated with them. Puberty encompasses a continuum of development that involves both hormonal and physical maturation that when things go smoothly result in, among other things, both reproductive capacity and adult physical appearance (Tanner, 1962; Grumbach & Styne, 1998).

Growth patterns in developing brains

Growth patterns in developing brains have been detected by interval high-resolution three-dimensional magnetic resonance imaging (MRI) scans (Thompson et al., 2000). Maps of local growth rates revealed the complexity and regional heterogeneity of tissue growth, pruning and maturation of late brain development. Giedd and his colleagues (Giedd et al., 1999; Sowell et al., 1999) demonstrated with longitudinal paediatric neuroimaging using MRI that the volume of white matter increased linearly with age, increasing less in females than in males. By contrast, changes in the volume of grey matter were nonlinear and regionally specific. This MRI study demonstrated a pre-adolescent increase in grey matter. What this represents remains unclear. Whether this grey matter increase is related to changes in neuropil, neuronal size or dendritic or axonal arborization will be best addressed in the future with other scientific methods. There may be a period of brain development when the activities of the teenager may guide selective synapse elimination during adolescence. Animal studies using rats support the role the environment plays in shaping late synaptogenesis (Bourgeois *et al.*, 1989; Kleim *et al.*, 1996).

Factors influencing somatic growth

Growth in stature is continuous and not a linear process over time (Rogol *et al.*, 2002). Evidence suggests that growth proceeds along a pattern characterized by spurts followed by stasis. Over time, this pattern appears as a continuous linear process. Following the rapid growth of the fetus, growth can be divided into three phases: infantile, childhood and pubertal. Each of these three periods has its own distinctive timing and tempo. The infantile phase is characterized by decelerating growth rate during the first 18–24 months. During childhood the growth rate is relatively constant and averages 5–6 cm per year. There is a wide range of variability of normal. Puberty represents the dynamic growth phase marked by rapid changes in body size, shape and composition, some of which are sexually dimorphic while others are not. There is variability based on genetic, nutritional and environmental factors. This period is characterized by the greatest sexual differentiation since fetal life and the most rapid linear growth since infancy. We will now turn away from the biological and toward some psychological aspects of these physical changes.

Timing of maturation

The timing of puberty is highly individual and predicting the onset of puberty is like defining summer: we have a date on the calendar but summer does not really suddenly start on that date, as it is not a single event. Rather, the changing of seasons between spring and autumn is a complex, subtle and variable process. We can see that process more clearly when it has been completed than when it was inaugurated. Also, puberty does not happen in isolation; it occurs within an individual who lives in a social and physical environment.

Assessment of pubertal maturation may refer to objective criteria (such as menarche or age at peak height) according to national reference norms or to subjective criteria based on self-perception in comparison to one's reference group. Does the individual feel 'with the crowd', 'ahead of the crowd' or 'behind the crowd' in terms of his or her bodily changes? The physical changes of puberty (Sarigiani & Petersen, 2000) for any individual may occur at about the same time as those of most adolescent peers or be significantly earlier or later.

For girls and boys, the nature of the physical maturation of puberty, and especially the timing of it, has been the subject of considerable recent research (Brooks-Gunn & Paikoff, 1997; Graber, 1997; Archibald et al., 2003; Hayward, 2003). Puberty in girls is most commonly marked by menarche; however, in boys there is not an equivalent objective physical event (Brooks-Gunn & Warren, 1985; Hayward, 2003). Behavioural changes, psychological development and sexual maturation have been identified as areas of importance for psychosocial adjustment in adolescence.

There are clearly gender differences between boys and girls in these areas. The impact of early maturation on boys can produce both positive and negative consequences. On the one hand, more physically developed males have been found to be more popular, with better self-esteem and higher intellectual abilities (Petersen, 1985). On the other hand, there appears to be increased risk for delinquent or antisocial behaviours, such as drug and alcohol use, truancy and precocious sexual activity (Williams & Dunlop, 1999). It is thought that this increase in problematic behaviours is linked to friendships with older peers (Silbereisen et al., 1989). For females, early maturation probably has fewer benefits and more disadvantages. Early timing of puberty for girls has been associated with more problems with self-image, emotional difficulties and mental health issues, including depression, anxiety and disordered eating behaviours. For some, however, there can be benefits such as increased popularity (together with risky behaviours of drug and alcohol use and early sexual activity) (Ge et al., 2001; King, 2002). In summary, it may be said that early maturation is more advantageous in several respects for boys than for girls. Recent research has indicated that ethnicity may have some influence on puberty development. African-American girls appear to mature earlier by 1 year than Caucasian girls (Herman-Giddens et al., 1997, 1999), who seem to mature earlier than Asian girls (Hammer et al., 1991). At this time, it remains unclear whether sociocultural factors or biological factors best explain these differences (Hayward, 2003).

Physical and environmental factors also impact the timing and course of pubertal maturation. Early pubertal maturation is associated with some health conditions (for example, hypothyroidism, blindness and retardation). Furthermore, some psychosocial stressors, such as depressed mood and family conflict, have been shown to be associated with accelerated pubertal timing (Brooks-Gunn & Warren, 1985; Graber et al., 1995). On the other hand, late menarche is closely linked to physical factors such as decreased nutritional intake, below average weight and increased exercise seen in both normal athletes (for example, gymnasts, figure skaters, dancers and runners) as well as in clinical populations with eating disorders. Other physical and health conditions associated with late pubertal maturation are cystic fibrosis, juvenile onset diabetes, Crohn's disease and sickle-cell anaemia (Sarigiani & Petersen, 2000).

At the extremes of pubertal timing are those individuals who show precocious (very early) or delayed (very late) puberty. Precocious puberty and delayed puberty have been defined by the appearance of any indicator of secondary sexual maturation at more than two standard deviations below or above the mean age of onset, respectively (Grumbach & Styne, 1992). For boys, precocious puberty is less common than for girls, and refers to evidence of increased testicular growth or growth on any other pubertal characteristic prior to 9 years of age. For girls, precocious puberty refers to breast budding before age 8 or pubertal growth spurt before age 7. The absence of pubertal changes by 13 years in girls and 14 years in boys is considered to be delayed puberty (Brooks-Gunn & Reiter, 1990).

In this text on eating disorders, the relationship between puberty and the dramatic physical transformations for girls and boys and the impact of those changes on self-perceptions, body image and body distortion need to be mentioned. In a review paper, Graber and colleagues (1996) found that for girls, body image was influenced not during pubertal changes but rather after the peak pubertal changes had already occurred. There was more negative self-assessment of body image for early maturing girls compared with late and on-time maturating girls from grades six to twelve, according to data from the Adolescent Mental Health Study. Also, it is important to note that these negative perceptions of body image persisted into young adulthood for girls. The tableau is considerably different for boys, who exhibited positive body image with early maturational timing, but this did not persist over time into mid-adolescence. In addition, body dissatisfaction is related to short stature for adolescent boys and overweight for girls. Both of these culturally mediated ideals may be linked to eating disturbances later on in adolescence.

Timing does matter. How do we understand the secular trend to younger ages of physical maturity? Is earlier menses in girls related to higher body weights at younger ages? Has the availability of fast food increased childhood obesity? Are the sedentary activities of today's youth (computers, video games, cell phones) leading to overweight children? Although it appears that these issues may be contributing to an earlier onset of puberty, further research is needed to clarify these and other questions about the changes in timing of physical maturation. How do we cope with younger children having the physical capacity for sexual experimentation, but not yet the maturity or emotional capacity? How does this influence the development of psychological identity and sexuality? These concerns highlight an evolving shift in normative adolescent sexual behaviours that will require future attention from the social science and medical communities. Also, with the recent trend for greater obesity and overweight in children and adolescents, will there be an even younger age for onset of pubertal maturation (associated with higher weights at younger ages) and will this lead to even more difficulties for girls and boys in terms of body image and social expectations? The cultural emphasis on a thin ideal, on sexualizing adolescents, on using younger models in advertising and the general promotion of sex at an earlier and earlier age has consequences.

Cognitive changes associated with puberty

In addition to the momentous changes in physical development in puberty, there are dramatic increases in cognitive abilities. Cognitive development in adolescence is best described in three phases of early (10–13 years), middle (14–16 years) and late (17 years and older). There is a major transformation of cognition in early adolescence in the development of formal operations or abstract reasoning. However, this continues through the middle and late phases and into adulthood as well, where there continue to be significant individual differences in the capacity for formal reasoning. As we now know, the adolescent brain is a brain in transition and continues to develop into and throughout adulthood (Keating & Clark, 1980; Spear, 2000).

Cognitive theory

Piaget described the developmental stages of cognition through childhood and adolescence and characterized the widening scope of intellectual activity and the increased awareness and capacity for insight as the stage of 'formal operations' (Inhelder & Piaget, 1958; Piaget, 1969). As described by Gemelli (1996), this phase sees the emergence of hypothetical thinking, which includes a variety of cognitive abilities necessary for reasoning, planning and processing information and relationships. In Kuhn's review (2000) of recent research, the simple stage model of cognitive development is challenged and expanded to include the processes and dimensions of cognition.

Prominent since the 1970s is the awareness of the contribution of cognitive conceptualizations and their relationship to behaviour. This has led to the emergence of a range of psychotherapeutic approaches that identify the pathological automatic thoughts that interfere with functioning. Behavioural plans are designed to effect a change that requires challenges to the interfering automatic thoughts (Beck, 1976; Meichenbaum, 1977).

Psychological tasks of adolescence

With both the psychological and biological maturity of adolescence come issues of separation and individuation, consolidation of a sense of self, development of a sexual identity and progress toward academic and vocational plans for adult life. Erickson (1950) best described identity formation during adolescence, and Blos has written cogently on separation and individuation from parents, and the importance of friendships with peers and the opposite sex (Blos, 1962).

The most useful framework for this discussion is the biopsychosocial model, which has also been used successfully in so many other domains. Not only is it not theory dependent, but it also has enough elasticity to allow inclusion of a wide range of factors, competing ideas and concepts. The stages of adolescent development include concerns associated with puberty, worries about peer relationships and struggles regarding independence from the family and establishing significant relationships outside the family. For an older adolescent, focus is on increased personal autonomy and separation from parental control.

Recent developments

Changes in technology have impacted on our understanding of the developing brain and cognitive functioning during adolescence. We now know that the brain continues to develop into adulthood. Recent research has begun to document the cognitive correlates of differences in structural brain volumes in adolescents. Magnetic resonance imaging (MRI) has suggested that measurable differences in the medial temporal lobe of adolescents are associated with long-term cognitive abilities, specifically academic skills and the acquisition of intellectual knowledge. However, these relationships may differ as a function of the sex of the adolescent and requires further research with pre-adolescent subjects to help clarify hormonal and developmental factors (Yurgelun-Todd et al., 2003).

So where are we? Like summertime, the myriad of flowers bloom, some early in the season, some late, but together this cacophony of growth, in all its complexity, when it works, is a triumph of sophisticated coordination and timing. In context, normal processes intersect with the realities of life: war, trauma, famine, medical illness, loss of a parent, romantic disappointments and social pressures to be thin, to name only a few. It is a wonder that puberty proceeds as smoothly as it usually does. Throughout adolescence, the work of development that was made possible by the physical, cognitive and psychological changes induced by puberty continues unabated.

REFERENCES

Archibald, A.B., Graber, J.A. & Brooks-Gunn, J. (2003). Pubertal processes and physiological growth in adolescence. In *Blackwell Handbook of Adolescence*, ed. Adams, G.R. & Berzonsky M. D. Malden, MA: Blackwell Publishers, pp. 24–47.

Beck, A. (1976). *Cognitive Therapy and Emotional Disorders*. New York: International Universities Press.

Beck-Peccoz, P., Padmanabhan, V., Baggiani, A.M. *et al.* (1991). Maturation of hypothalamic-pituitary gonadal function in normal human fetuses: circulating levels of gonadotropins, their common alpha subunit and free testosterone, and discrepancy between immunological and biological activities of circulating follicle-stimulating hormone. *Journal of Clinical Endocrinology and Metabolism*, **73**, 525–32.

Blos, P. (1962). *On Adolescence*. New York: The Free Press.

Bourgeois, J.P., Jatreboff, P.J. & Rakic, P. (1989). *Proceedings of the National Academy of Science*, **86**, 4297–301.

Brooks-Gunn, J. & Paikoff, R. (1997). Sexuality and developmental transitions during adolescence. In *Health Risks and Developmental Transitions during Adolescence*, ed. Schulenberg, J., Maggs, J.L. & Hurrelmann, K. Cambridge: Cambridge University Press, pp. 190–219.

Brooks-Gunn, J. & Reiter, E.O. (1990). The role of pubertal processes in the early adolescent transition. In *At the Threshold: The Developing Adolescent*, ed. Feldman, S. & Elliott, G. Cambridge, MA: Harvard University Press, pp. 16–53.

Brooks-Gunn, J. & Warren, M.P. (1985). Measuring physical status and timing in early adolescence: a developmental perspective. *Journal of Youth and Adolescence*, **14**, 163–89.

Cutler, G. & Loriaux, D.L. (1980). Adrenarche and its relationship to the onset of puberty. *Federation Proceedings*, **39**, 2384–90.

Erikson, E.H. (1950). *Childhood and Society*. New York: Norton.

Fechner, P.Y. (2003). The biology of puberty: new developments in sex differences. In *Gender Differences at Puberty*, ed. Hayward, C. Cambridge: Cambridge University Press, pp. 17–28.

Ge, X., Conger, R.D. & Elder, G.H. (2001). The relation between puberty and psychological distress in adolescent boys. *Journal of Research on Adolescence*, **11**, 49–70.

Gemelli, R. (1996). Adolescent phase of mental development: age 12 years to age 19 years. In *Normal Child and Adolescent Development*, ed. Gemelli, R. Washington, DC: American Psychiatric Press, pp. 445–552.

Giedd, J.N., Blumenthal, J., Jeffries, N.O. *et al.* (1999). Brain development during childhood and adolescence: a longitudinal MRI study. *Neuroscience*, **2**, 861–3.

Graber, J.A. (1997). Is psychopathology associated with the timing of pubertal development? *Journal of the American Academy of Child and Adolescent Psychiatry*, **36**, 1768–76.

Graber, J.A., Brooks-Gunn, J. & Warren, M.P. (1995). The antecedents of menarcheal age: heredity, family environment, and stressful life events. *Child Development*, **66**, 346–59.

Graber, J.A., Petersen, A.C. & Brooks-Gunn, J. (1996). Pubertal processes: methods, measures, and models. In *Transitions through Adolescence: Interpersonal Domains and Context*, ed. Graber, J.A., Brooks-Gunn, J. & Petersen, A.C. Mahwah, NJ: Lawrence Erlbaum Associates, pp. 23–53.

Grumbach, M.M. & Styne, D. (1992). Puberty: ontogeny, neuroendocrinology, physiology, and disorders. In *Williams Textbook of Endocrinology*, 8th edition, ed. Wilson, J.D. & Foster, D.W. Philadelphia: W. B. Saunders, pp. 1139–221.

Grumbach, M.M. & Styne, D.M. (1998). Puberty: ontogeny, neuroendocrinology, physiology, and disorders. In *Williams Textbook of Endocrinology*, ed. Wilson, J.D., Foster, D.W. & Kronenberg, H.M. Philadelphia: W. B. Saunders, pp. 1509–625.

Hammer, L., Wilson, D., Litt, I.F. *et al.* (1991). Impact of pubertal development on body fat distribution among White, Hispanic and Asian female adolescents. *Journal of Pediatrics*, **118**, 975–80.

Hayward, C. (2003). *Gender Differences at Puberty*. Cambridge: Cambridge University Press.

Herman-Giddens, M.E., Slora, E.J., Wasserman, R.C. *et al.* (1997). Secondary sexual characteristics and menses in young girls seen in office practice: a study from the Pediatric Research Office Settings Network. *Pediatrics*, **99**, 505–12.

Herman-Giddens, M.E., Slora, E.J., Wasserman, R.C. *et al.* (1999). Reexamination of the age limit for defining when puberty is precocious in girls in the United States: implications for evaluation and treatment. *Pediatrics*, **104**, 936–41.

Inhelder, B. & Piaget, J. (1958). *The Growth of Logical Thinking*. New York: Basic Books.

Katchadourian, H. (1977). *The Biology of Adolescence*. San Francisco: W.H. Freeman.

Keating, D.P. & Clark, L.V. (1980). Development of physical and social reasoning in adolescence. *Developmental Psychology*, **16**, 23–30.

King, R.K. (2002). Adolescence. In *Child and Adolescent Psychiatry*, 3rd edition, ed. Lewis, M. New York: Lippincott Williams & Williams, pp. 332–42.

Kleim, J.A., Lussnig, E., Schwarz, E.R., Comery, T.A. & Greenough, W.T. (1996). Synaptogenesis and fos expression in the motor cortex of the adult rat after complex motor skill acquisition. *Journal of Neuroscience*, **16**, 4529–35.

Kuhn, D. (2000). Adolescent thought processes. In *Encyclopedia of Psychology*, ed. Kazdin, A.E. Washington, DC: American Psychological Association, Oxford University Press, pp. 52–9.

Marshall, W.A. & Tanner, J.M. (1974). Puberty. In *Scientific Foundations of Pediatrics*, ed. Douvis, J.D. & Drobeing, J. London: Heinemann, pp. 124–51.

Meichenbaum, D. (1977). *Cognitive-behavior Modification*. New York: Plenum Press.

Ojeda, S.R. & Bilger, M. (2000). Neuroendocrine regulation of puberty. In *Neuroendocrinology in Physiology and Medicine*, ed. Conn, P.M. & Freeman, M.E. New Jersey: Humana Press, p. 212.

Petersen, A.C. (1985). Pubertal development as a cause of disturbance: myths, realities, and unanswered questions. *Genetic, Social and General Psychology Monographs*, **111**, 205–32.

Piaget, J. (1969). The intellectual development of the adolescent. In *Adolescence: Psychosocial Perspectives*, ed. Caplan, G. & Lebovici, S. New York: Basic Books, pp. 22–26.

Reiter, E.O. & Grumbach, M.M. (1982). Neuroendocrine control mechanisms and the onset of puberty. *Annual Review of Physiology*, **44**, 595–613.

Rogol, A.D., Roemmich, J.N. & Clark, P.A. (2002). Growth at puberty. *Journal of Adolescent Health*, **31**, 192–200.

Sarigiani, P.A. & Petersen, A.C. (2000). Puberty and biological maturation. In *Encyclopedia of Psychology*, ed. Kazdin, A.E. Washington, DC: American Psychological Association, Oxford University Press, pp. 39–46.

Silbereisen, R.K., Petersen, A.C., Albrecht, H.T. & Kracke, B. (1989). Maturational timing and the development of problem behavior: longitudinal studies in adolescence. *Journal of Early Adolescence*, **9**, 247–68.

Sowell, E.R., Thompson, P.M., Holmes, C.J., Jernigan, T.L. & Toga, A.W. (1999). In vivo evidence for post-adolescent brain maturation in frontal and striatal regions. *Neuroscience*, **2**, 859–61.

Spear, L.P. (2000). The adolescent brain and age-related behavioral manifestations. *Neuroscience and Biobehavioral Reviews*, **24**, 417–63.

Styne, D.M. & Grumbach, M.M. (1991). Disorders of puberty in the male and female. In *Reproductive Endocrinology: Pathophysiology and Clinical Management*, ed. Yen, S.S.C. & Jaffe, R. B. Philadelphia: W. B. Saunders, pp. 511–54.

Tanner, J.M. (1962). *Growth at Adolescence*. New York: Lippincott.

Thompson, P.M., Giedd, J.N., Woods, R.P., MacDonald, D., Evans, A.C. & Toga, A.W. (2000). Growth patterns in the developing brain detected by using continuum mechanical tensor maps. *Nature*, **404**, 190–3.

Williams, J.M. & Dunlop, L.C. (1999). Pubertal timing and self-reported delinquency among male adolescents. *Journal of Adolescence*, **22**, 157–71.

Yurgelen-Todd, D., Killlgore, W.D.S. & Cintron, C.B. (2003). Cognitive correlates of medial temporal lobe development across adolescence: a magnetic resonance imaging study. *Perceptual and Motor Skills*, **96**, 3–17.

6

Genetic influences in the development of eating disorders

Shani Leor, Orit Krispin and Alan Apter

Schneider Children's Medical Center, Petach Tikva, Israel

Introduction

Eating disorders (EDs) presenting in childhood are complex conditions. Current aetiological models thus emphasize multifactorial determinants. This chapter focuses on the genetic factors influencing the development of EDs. Further details can be found in this volume on family factors (see Lock & Couturier, Chapter 19), individual factors (see Bryant-Waugh, Chapter 9; Hay & McDermott, Chapter 18) and environmental issues including emotional trauma (see Brewerton, Chapter 13).

Evidence of genetic influences

Family and twin studies

Family studies have shown that anorexia nervosa (AN) is more common among relatives of probands than among relatives of normal controls or among relatives of non-anorexic psychiatric patients (reviewed in Gorwood et al., 2003). Similarly, studies on probands with bulimia nervosa (BN) have shown higher rates of BN among first-degree relatives (Strober et al., 2000).

Twin studies have been used to distinguish between the genetic and the environmental contributions to the familial liability observed in EDs. About 38–55% of the identical (monozygotic, MZ) twins described in the literature were concordant for AN (Kipman et al., 1999). This rate is greater than would be expected from prevalence data, and is also much higher than the fraternal (dizygotic, DZ) twins concordance rate (0–11%). Systematic controlled twin studies have also reported a higher concordance rate among MZ twin sisters than among DZ (55–56% vs. 5–7%) (Holland et al., 1984, 1988). In contrast,

Eating Disorders in Children and Adolescents, ed. Tony Jaffa and Brett McDermott. Published by Cambridge University Press. © Cambridge University Press 2007.

Walters & Kendler (1995) could not detect a genetic component to AN. In their analysis of a large population-based female twin sample (n = 2163) DZ concordance rates were higher than MZ rates. Still, co-twins of twins with AN were at significantly higher risk for lifetime AN, BN, major depression and current low body mass index. For BN, again, reported concordance rates for MZ twins (23–100%) are greater than for DZ twins (0–33%) (Kendler et al., 1991). Overall, twin studies report heritability estimates for AN and BN of between 54% and 83%.

Eating disorder symptoms also appear to be heritable. In studies among twin population-based samples, pathologic attitudes including drive for thinness, eating and weight concerns, body dissatisfaction, and weight preoccupation showed heritabilites of approximately 32% to 72% (Klump et al., 2000b). Twin studies of binge eating, self-induced vomiting and dietary restraint have found heritabilities for these behaviours of between 46 and 82% with nonshared environmental factors explaining the rest of the variance (Reichborn-Kjennerud et al., 2004). Also, there seem to be age-developmental differences in the genetic effects on eating attitudes and behaviours (Klump et al., 2000c).

Shared genetic diathesis with other disorders or traits

One strategy for identifying the genetic influence on EDs has been to determine whether particular psychiatric disorders or traits are expressions of a shared genetic diathesis.

Other forms of psychopathology

In a population-based female twin sample, Wade et al. (2000) found a modest overlap (34%) in the genetic liability that predisposes an individual to both AN and major depression. They proposed that there are both shared and unique genetic effects in the aetiology of the two disorders. Despite excess of alcohol and drug use disorders in the families of both forms of EDs, particularly BN (Bulik, 1987; Lilenfeld et al., 1997), more recent evidence (Kendler et al., 1995; Lilenfeld et al., 1998) suggests that BN and substance use disorders are transmitted independently in families. Rates of obsessive-compulsive personality disorder (OCPD) among relatives of AN probands with and without OCPD were virtually identical and significantly greater than among relatives of controls suggesting shared familial transmission of AN and OCPD (Lilenfeld et al., 1998). Shared diathesis between obsessive-compulsive disorder (OCD) and BN (Kaye et al., 1998) as well as AN (Cavallini et al., 2000) has been suggested.

Personality traits

Psychometric studies have consistently linked both AN and BN to a cluster of moderately heritable traits suggesting that these phenotypes are based on shared genetic factors. Individuals with AN and BN exhibit characteristic personality traits such as high levels of harm avoidance, perfectionism, obsessionality, stress reactivity and negative emotionality (Klump et al., 2000a). While these traits may be exaggerated by starvation, their persistence after recovery from the disorder independently of body weight has prompted the speculation that they may be premorbid traits acting as vulnerability factors contributing to the pathogenesis of EDs. Studies examining familial relationships between personality traits and EDs have suggested familial transmission. Lilenfeld et al. (2000) reported increased rates of perfectionism and stress reactivity in first degree relatives of bulimic probands. Woodside et al. (2002) found that mothers of EDs probands showed elevated levels of perfectionism and more concerns about weight and shape compared with controls.

Body weight

The high heritability of body weight leads to questions of shared genetic transmission between body weight and eating abnormalities. Klump et al. (2000c) examined this possibility by investigating shared genetic transmission of body mass index (BMI) and disordered eating. Their findings suggested some shared genetic transmission, though most genetic influence on the disordered eating variables was independent. Genetic implications also arise when conceptualizing AN as an extreme variant on the weight scale (with obesity at the other end of the scale) as suggested by Hebebrand & Remschmidt (1995).

Shared transmission of AN and BN

There seems to be cross-transmission between AN and BN suggesting at least some shared underlying psychopathology (Strober et al., 2000). Several studies (Lilenfeld et al., 1998; Strober et al., 1990, 2000) have reported greater frequency of BN in relatives of anorexic probands than in the relatives of comparison subjects. Likewise, in family studies of BN, AN was more frequent in the families of bulimic probands (Stein et al., 1999; Strober et al., 2000). An epidemiological sample of twins obtained via the Virginia Twin Registry (Kendler et al., 1991; Walters & Kendler, 1995) adds to the evidence of a strong association between AN and BN. It was found that the co-twin of a twin with AN was 2.6 times more likely to have a lifetime diagnosis of BN than were co-twins of unaffected twins. Nonetheless, BN is more common in families of

BN probands, and the opposite is true for AN. Moreover, the frequency of BN among relatives of anorexic patients was found to increase only when the anorexic probands were of the binge-purge type (Rivinus *et al.*, 1984).

Molecular genetic studies

Two genetic strategies have predominantly been used to identify susceptibility loci for eating disorders on the human genome: linkage-type analyses and association studies. Briefly, linkage studies test the hypothesis of co-segregation between a marker locus and a trait within families. For EDs the preferable type of analysis is nonparametric methods which are based on the number of alleles shared at the marker locus between pairs of relatives. In contrast to linkage-type studies, association studies test whether an allele and a phenotypic trait show correlated occurrence within a population. This is accomplished by comparing the frequency of the alleles of the gene in individuals with and without the disorder (case-control) or by examining the frequency of transmission of alleles from parents to children with EDs.

Association studies

One way to map out the nature of the genetic susceptibility to EDs is to examine the relative influence of a specific gene or genetic marker ('candidate gene'). The task is complex. Whilst disturbances of neurotransmitters, neuropeptides and neuroendocrine systems have been reported in ill and recovered persons with AN and BN, the aetiological significance of many findings remains unclear. Furthermore, it is difficult to disentangle primary abnormalities, which may reflect genetic variability in vulnerability from secondary consequences of drastic weight loss and chaotic eating. The unknown phenotypic boundaries of AN and BN pose yet another problem in depicting the genes potentially involved. Still, candidate gene studies, based on the current understanding of the pathophysiology of AN and BN, are being undertaken to identify the underlying loci and genes. These studies have focused on genes linked to central monoamine functioning and on genes related to weight control, feeding and energy expenditure.

Serotonin-linked genes

The serotonin (5-hydroxytryptamine; 5-HT) system may play an important role in the pathophysiology of eating disorders (Brewerton, 1995). For example, underweight patients with AN have reduced cerebrospinal fluid (CSF) levels of the 5-HT metabolite 5-hydroxyindoleacetic acid (5-HIAA) (Kaye *et al.*, 1988).

Cerebrospinal fluid 5-HIAA values tend to normalize with weight restoration (Kaye *et al.*, 1988) and have been found to be higher than normal in women who have recovered from AN (Kaye *et al.*, 1991). These elevated levels of CSF 5-HIAA have been suggested to reflect a premorbid trait of hyperserotonergic function among individuals with AN (Kaye, 1997). In view of the female predominance in EDs, the hypothesis of 5-HT involvement in EDs has further support from the fact that 5-HT circuits and 5-HT related behaviours show sexual dimorphism (Goodwin *et al.*, 1987). Thus, association studies have focused on polymorphisms in 5-HT related genes. One of the most popular associations investigated has been between the *-1438G/A* polymorphism in the 5-HT$_{2A}$ receptor gene promoter and AN or BN. Several studies have found a higher frequency of the 'A' allele and the 'AA' genotype in individuals with AN (primarily the restricting subtype – AN-R) than in controls. However, other studies could not confirm this association (reviewed in Hinney *et al.*, 2004). The heterogeneous, inconsistent results represent the story of association studies of complex traits. Sample size, genetic and clinical heterogeneity, ethnic admixture, and very low prior probability of any particular candidate gene to be associated with a complex disorder are among the factors that contribute to this pattern of sporadic reports of significance followed by nonreplication.

A range of other 5-HT polymorphisms have been investigated but no associations with eating disorders have yet been clearly replicated, or confirmed in a family study or by meta-analysis (reviewed in Hinney *et al.*, 2004). In a multicentre family-based study, our group found no direct associations between any of the 5-HT genes and AN in the Israeli population (Leor *et al.*, unpubl. data).

Dopamine-linked genes
The dopaminergic (DA) system has been implicated in regulation of feeding behaviour and motor activity. It has also been recognized to play a role in more specific characteristics of EDs such as amenorrhea, distortion of body image, hyperactivity, ritualized behaviours, novelty seeking, reward and reinforcement processes as well as addictive tendency (reviewed in Gorwood *et al.*, 1998). As such, the DA system has been hypothesized to play a role in the development of EDs, especially AN (Kaye *et al.*, 1999). Studies of D$_3$ (Bruins-Slot *et al.*, 1998) and D$_4$ (Hinney *et al.*, 1999; Karwatz *et al.*, 2001) receptor genes have failed to find any evidence for involvement of DA polymorphisms in AN. However, a study by our group (Frisch *et al.*, 2001) suggests that the COMT gene, which produces an enzyme involved in dopamine catabolism, is associated with genetic susceptibility to AN. Individuals homozygous for

the high activity allele have two-fold increased risk for the development of the disorder. This finding has not been replicated in European populations (Karwautz *et al.*, 2001; Gabrovsek *et al.*, 2004). A Japanese research group has recently reported an association between the short allele of the dopamine transporter 3′UTR-VNTR polymorphism and EDs with binge-eating behaviour (AN binge-eating/purging type and BN) (Shinohara *et al.*, 2004).

Other candidate genes

Sex hormones have been implicated in weight problems and affective states. Furthermore, the female predominance of AN and BN and the frequent onset around puberty point to a possible involvement of female sex hormones in the development of these EDs, particularly AN (Young, 1990). Two studies (Rosen-kranz *et al.*, 1998; Eastwood *et al.*, 2002) explored the association between EDs and oestrogen receptor polymorphisms, yielding conflicting results. Genes involved in energy balance and body weight regulation such as UCP-2 and UCP-3 protein products, melanocortic system (POMC and MC-4R), leptin, agouti-related protein (AGRP) and neuropeptide Y, have been studied for associations with EDs. No significant associations have yet been found, except in one study on AGRP gene (Vink *et al.*, 2001) and in one study on the UCP-2/UCP-3 gene cluster (Campbell *et al.*, 1999). Following the Vink *et al.* (2001) study, the GG genotype of the *199G/A (Ala-67-Thr) AGRP* polymorphism was described as significantly associated with fatness and abdominal adiposity in a group of individuals with a mean age of 53 years, but not in a group of younger individuals (mean age 25 years) (Argyropoulos *et al.*, 2002). This polymorphism could, therefore, play a role in body weight regulation, feeding or the development of EDs in an age-dependent fashion. There is evidence suggesting that the BDNF (brain-derived neurotrophic factor) gene may play a role in the susceptibility to EDs. Ribases *et al.* (2003) reported a strong association of the *Met* allele of the *Val66Met* BDNF polymorphism with restrictive AN and low minimum BMI. In a larger sample, this polymorphism was found to be associated with all ED subtypes (Ribases *et al.*, 2004). A Japanese group reported an association between a different BDNF polymorphism (*196G/A*) and EDs, specifically AN-R and BN-purging type (as opposed to non-purging type) (Koizumi *et al.*, 2004). Using both case-control and family-based designs, our group found a significant association between the calcium-activated potassium channel gene (hSKCa3) and AN (Koronyo-Hamaoui *et al.*, 2002, 2004).

A relatively new and promising research direction in psychiatric genetics is not solely to examine associations between genes and broadly defined, categorical diagnostic criteria but to include also clinical endophenotypes based on quantifiable, continuous traits or dimensions. For example, studies have reported both positive (Hu *et al.*, 2003) and negative (Karwautz *et al.*, 2001) results regarding an association between 5-HT$_{2c}$R and AN. Westberg *et al.* (2002) reported an association between the 5-HT$_{2c}$R's *cys23ser* polymorphism and weight loss in teenage girls regardless of diagnosis of AN, consequently suggesting that the polymorphism is not specifically associated with AN, but with a general proneness in young women to experience rapid weight loss due to reduced food intake. Support for this supposition comes from a subsequent study, also examining the *cys23ser* polymorphism, where in addition to association with AN, significant correlation between genotype and minimum BMI was found (Hu *et al.*, 2003). Similarly, it has been proposed that the discrepancy in findings regarding the 5-HT$_{2A}$R *-1438G/A* polymorphism can be resolved when considering the 'A' allele as a modifying rather than a vulnerability allele (Kipman *et al.*, 2002). In their study, Kipman *et al.* confirmed the absence of the 'A' allele's association with AN but found that patients with the 'A' allele had a significantly later age of onset of the disorder. Compatible with this line of reasoning, Ricca *et al.* (2004) have recently reported that AN and BN patients with the 'AA' genotype showed higher scores on the EDE Weight and Shape Concern scales, as well as greater overall severity of the eating disorder psychopathology (EDE total score). Nishiguchi *et al.* (2001) have proposed that the *-1438G/A* distribution differs by eating behaviour and AN clinical subtype. They found a significantly higher 'G' allele frequency in a group of patients with AN-BP and BN, compared to controls.

Another plausible research direction, especially when investigating polygenic conditions such as EDs, is to search for associations while considering together different genes, which might be involved. For example, Urwin *et al.* (2003) found no association between the MAO-A gene and AN-R. But when stratifying the MAO-A data according to the NETpPR polymorphism within the promoter region of the norepinephrine transporter gene significant gene-gene interaction in AN-R was found, suggesting important involvement of the noradrenergic system in the biological underpinnings of AN-R.

Linkage studies

No unequivocal susceptibility genes have been identified for either eating disorder, yielding systematic model-free genome-wide screens warranted. In the first genome-wide linkage analysis to be performed, only weak evidence for linkage in AN was noted, the highest nonparametric linkage score being for a marker on chromosome 4 (Grice *et al.*, 2002). In families of probands with restricting subtype of AN (i.e. those with no bingeing or purging) there was modest evidence of linkage to chromosome 1p33–36. A further analysis, which covaried for related behavioural traits (drive-for-thinness, obsessionality), came up with a different locus on chromosome 1, as well as loci on chromosomes 2 and 13 (Devlin et al., 2002). When additional single nucleotide polymorphisms identified at two positional candidate genes located on chromosome 1p33–36 (the 5-HT$_{1D}$ receptor and the opioid delta receptor genes) were incorporated in the restricting AN linkage analysis the evidence for linkage was further increased (Bergen et al., 2003a, 2003b). All these findings must be judged preliminary and should be investigated in additional samples. Recently, this same research group – the Price Foundation Collaborative Group – conducted a second genome-wide linkage scan, this time of 308 multiplex families with a BN proband (Bulik et al., 2003). Significant linkage was detected on chromosome 10p. Suggestive linkage occurred on chromosome 14. A second scan, conducted in a subset of families in which at least two affected relatives reported self-induced vomiting, revealed a stronger linkage signal on chromosome 10p and again suggestive linkage on chromosome 14. It is interesting to note that evidence for linkage to chromosome 10p has also been observed in obesity (Price et al., 2001). The coincident linkages may reflect shared underlying biological mechanisms such as a tendency toward weight gain which could be associated both with obesity and the onset of the unhealthy eating and weight-loss behaviours characteristic of BN (Bulik et al., 2003). It is also noteworthy that the two genome scans, one based on ascertainment of probands with AN and the second based on ascertainment of probands with BN, yielded different linkage results (Bulik et al., 2003). This further supports the argument that AN and BN are related but not identical conditions with differences in the genetic susceptibility.

Conclusions

It can be seen that while there is much learned on the genetic causes of AN and BN much remains to be learned. The available data strongly suggest that the genetic influences reside in multiple genes and reflect interaction between multiple genes and the environment. Furthermore, it is most likely that what is inherited is not a disorder per se but risk factors for the development of a disorder, such as perhaps a tendency toward obsessionality, a disturbance of body image, a regulation dysfunction of neurotransmitters or certain personality traits acting as endophenotypes. The identification and analysis of endophenotypes related to EDs can therefore be of great importance for determining the

genetic mechanism underlying EDs. Additionally, genetic–environment interaction studies, such as those of Caspi *et al.* (2005), especially if they can be
done in the context of a longitudinal cohort study, are likely to be the most
profitable type of study in elucidating the genetic vulnerability to EDs.

REFERENCES

Argyropolos, G., Rankinen, T., Neufeld, D.R. *et al.* (2002). A polymorphism in the human
agouti-related protien is associated with late-onset obesity. *Journal of Clinical Endocrinology and
Metabolism*, **87**, 4198-202.

Bergen, A.W., van den Bree, M.B.M., Yeager, M. *et al.* (2003a). Candidate genes for anorexia
nervosa in the 1p33–36 linkage region: serotonin 1D and delta opioid receptor loci exhibit
significant association to anorexia nervosa. *Molecular Psychiatry*, **8**, 397–406.

Bergen, A.W., Yeager, M., Welch, R. *et al.*; The Price Foundation Collaborative Group (www.
anbn.org) (2003b). Candidate gene analysis of the Price Foundation anorexia nervosa affected
relative pair dataset. *Current Drug Targets – CNS and Neurological Disorders*, **2**, 41–51.

Brewerton, T.D. (1995). Towards a unified theory of serotonin dysregulation in eating and
related disorders. *Psychoneuroendocrinology*, **20**, 561–90.

Bruins-Slot, L., Gorwood, P., Bouvard, M. *et al.* (1998). Lack of association between anorexia
nervosa and D3 dopamine receptor gene. *Biological Psychiatry*, **43**, 76–8.

Bulik, C.M. (1987). Drug and alcohol abuse by bulimic women and their families. *American
Journal of Psychiatry*, **144**, 1604–6.

Bulik, C.M., Devlin, B., Bacanu, S.A. *et al.* (2003). Significant linkage on chromosome 10p in
families with bulimia nervosa. *American Journal of Human Genetics*, **72**, 200–7.

Campbell, D.A., Sundaramurthy, D., Gordon, D., Markham, A.F. & Pieri, L.F. (1999). Association between a marker in the UCP-2/UCP-3 gene cluster and genetic susceptibility to
anorexia nervosa. *Molecular Psychiatry*, **4**, 68–70.

Caspi, A., Moffitt, T.E., Cannon, M. *et al.* (2005). Moderation of the effect of adolescent-
onset cannabis use on adult psychosis by a functional polymorphism in the catechol-
O-methyltransferase gene: longitudinal evidence of a gene X environment interaction.
Biological Psychiatry, **57**, 1117–27.

Cavallini, M.C., Bertelli, S., Chiapparino, D., Riboldi, S. & Bellodi, L. (2000). Complex segregation
analysis of obsessive-compulsive disorder in 141 families of eating disorder probands, with and
without obsessive-compulsive disorder. *American Journal of Medical Genetics*, **96**, 384–91.

Devlin, B., Bacanu, S.A., Klump, K.L. *et al.* (2002). Linkage analysis of anorexia nervosa
incorporating behavioral covariates. *Human Molecular Genetics*, **11**, 689–96.

Eastwood, H., Brown, K.M.O., Markovic, D. & Pieri, L.F. (2002). Variation in the *ESR1* and
ESR2 genes and genetic susceptibility to anorexia nervosa. *Molecular Psychiatry*, **7**, 86–9.

Frisch, A., Laufer, N., Danziger, Y. *et al.* (2001). Association of anorexia nervosa with the high activity
allele of the COMT gene: a family-based study in Israeli patients. *Molecular Psychiatry*, **6**, 243–5.

Gabrovsek, M., Brecelj-Anderluh, M., Bellodi, L. *et al.* (2004). Combined family trio and case-control analysis of the COMT Val158Met polymorphism in European patients with anorexia nervosa. *American Journal of Medical Genetics Part B (Neuropsychiatric Genetics)*, **124B**, 68–74.

Goodwin, G. M., Fairburn, C. G. & Cowen, P. J. (1987). Dieting changes serotonergic function in women, not in men: implications for etiology of anorexia nervosa. *Psychological Medicine*, **17**, 839–42.

Gorwood, P., Bouvard, M., Mouren-Siméoni, M. C., Kipman, A. & Ades, J. (1998). Genetics and anorexia nervosa: a review of candidate genes. *Psychiatric Genetics*, **8**, 1–12.

Gorwood, P., Kipman, A. & Foulon, C. (2003). The human genetics of anorexia nervosa. *European Journal of Pharmacology*, **480**, 163–70.

Grice, D. E., Halmi, K. A., Fichter, M. M. *et al.* (2002). Evidence for a susceptibility gene for anorexia nervosa on chromosome 1. *American Journal of Human Genetics*, **70**, 787–92.

Hebebrand, H. J. & Remschmidt, H. (1995). Anorexia nervosa viewed as an extreme weight condition: genetic implications. *Human Genetics*, **95**, 1–11.

Hinney, A., Friedel, S., Remschmidt, H. & Hebebrand, J. (2004). Genetic risk factors in eating disorders. *American Journal of Pharmacogenomics*, **4**, 209–23.

Hinney, A., Schneider, J., Ziegler, A. *et al.* (1999). No evidence for involvement of polymorphisms of the dopamine D4 receptor gene in anorexia nervosa, underweight, and obesity. *American Journal of Medical Genetics*, **88**, 594–7.

Holland, A. J., Hall, A., Murray, R., Russell, G. F. M. & Crisp, A. H. (1984). Anorexia nervosa: a study of 34 twin pairs and one set of triplets. *British Journal of Psychiatry*, **145**, 414–19.

Holland, A. J., Sicote, N. & Treasure, J. (1988). Anorexia nervosa: evidence for a genetic basis. *Journal of Psychosomatic Research*, **32**, 561–71.

Hu, X., Giotakis, O., Li, T., Karwautz, A., Treasure, J. & Collier, D. A. (2003). Association of the 5-HT2c gene with susceptibility and minimum body mass index in anorexia nervosa. *Neuroreport*, **14**, 781–3.

Karwautz, A., Rabe-Hesketh, S., Hu, X. *et al.* (2001). Individual-specific risk factors for anorexia nervosa: a pilot study using a discordant sister-pair design. *Psychological Medicine*, **31**, 317–29.

Kaye, W. H. (1997). Anorexia nervosa, obsessional behavior, and serotonin. *Psychopharmacology Bulletin*, **33**, 335–44.

Kaye, W. H., Frank, G. K. & McConaha, C. (1999). Altered dopamine activity after recovery from restricting-type anorexia nervosa. *Neuropsychopharmacology*, **21**, 503–6.

Kaye, W. H., Gwirtsman, H. E., George, D. T. & Ebert, M. H. (1991). Altered serotonin activity in anorexia nervosa after long-term weight restoration. *Archives of General Psychiatry*, **48**, 556–62.

Kaye, W. H., Gwirtsman, H. E., George, D. T., Jimerson, D. C. & Ebert, M. H. (1988). CSF 5-HIAA concentrations in anorexia nervosa: reduced values in underweight subjects normalize after weight gain. *Biological Psychiatry*, **23**, 102–5.

Kendler, K. S., MacLean, C., Neale, M., Kessler, R., Heath, A. & Eaves, L. (1991). The genetic epidemiology of bulimia nervosa. *American Journal of Psychiatry*, **148**, 1627–37.

Kendler, K. S., Walters, E. E., Neale, M. C., Kessler, R. C., Heath, A. C. & Eaves, L. J. (1995). The structure of the genetic and environment risk factors for six major psychiatric disorders in women. *Archives of General Psychiatry*, **52**, 374–83.

Kipman, A., Bruins-Slot, L., Boni, C. *et al.* (2002). 5-HT(2A) gene promoter polymorphism as a modifying rather than a vulnerability factor in anorexia nervosa. *European Psychiatry*, **7**, 227–9.

Kipman, A., Gorwood, P., Mouren-Siméoni, M.C. & Adès, J. (1999). Genetic factors in anorexia nervosa. *European Psychiatry*, **14**, 189–98.

Klump, K.L., Bulik, C.M., Pollice, C.M.P.H. *et al.* (2000a). Temperament and character in women with anorexia nervosa. *Journal of Nervous and Mental Disorders*, **188**, 559–67.

Klump, K.L., Holly, A., Iacono, W.G., McGue, M. & Wilson, L.E. (2000b). Physical similarity and twin resemblance for eating attitudes and behaviors: a test of the equal environments assumption. *Behavior Genetics*, **30**, 51–8.

Klump, K.L., McGue, M. & Iacono, W.G. (2000c). Age differences in genetic and environmental influences on eating attitudes and behaviors in preadolescent and adolescent twins. *Journal of Abnormal Psychology*, **109**, 239–51.

Koizumi, H., Hashimoto, K., Itoh, K. *et al.* (2004). Association between the brain-derived neurotrophic factor 196G/A polymorphism and eating disorders. *American Journal of Medical Genetics Part B (Neuropsychiatric Genetics)*, **127B**, 125–7.

Koronyo-Hamaoui, M., Danziger, Y., Frisch, A. *et al.* (2002). Association between anorexia nervosa and the hsKCa3 gene: a family-based and case control study. *Molecular Psychiatry*, **7**, 82–5.

Koronyo-Hamaoui, M., Gak, E., Stein, D. *et al.* (2004). CAG repeat polymorphism within the KCNN3 gene is a significant contributor to susceptibility to anorexia nervosa: a case-control study of female patients and several ethnic groups in the Israeli Jewish population. *American Journal of Medical Genetics, Part B (Neuropsychiatric Genetics)*, **131B**, 76–80.

Lilenfeld, L.R., Kay, W.H., Greeno, C.G. *et al.* (1997). Psychiatric disorders in women with bulimia nervosa and their first-degree relatives: effects of comorbid substance dependence. *International Journal of Eating Disorders*, **22**, 253–64.

Lilenfeld, L.R., Kay, W.H., Greeno, C.G. *et al.* (1998). A controlled family study of anorexia nervosa and bulimia nervosa: psychiatric disorders in first-degree relatives and effects of proband comorbidity. *Archives of General Psychiatry*, **55**, 603–10.

Lilenfeld, L.R., Stein, D., Bulik, C.M. *et al.* (2000). Personality traits among currently eating disordered, recovered and never ill first-degree female relatives of bulimic and control women. *Psychological Medicine*, **30**, 1399–410.

Nishiguchi, N., Matsushita, S., Suzuki, K., Murayama, M., Shirakawa, O. & Higuchi, S. (2001). Association between 5HT2A receptor gene promoter region polymorphism and eating disorders in Japanese patients. *Biological Psychiatry*, **50**, 123–8.

Price, R.A., Li, W.D., Bernstein, A. *et al.* (2001). A locus affecting obesity in human chromosome region 10p12. *Diabetologia*, **44**, 363–6.

Reichborn-Kjennerud, T., Bulik, C.M., Tambs, K. & Harris, J.R. (2004). Genetic and environmental influences on binge eating in the absence of compensatory behaviors: a population-based twin study. *International Journal of Eating Disorders*, **36**, 307–14.

Ribases, M., Gratacos, M., Armengol, L. *et al.* (2003). Met66 in the brain-derived neurotrophic factor (BDNF) precursor is associated with anorexia nervosa restrictive type. *Molecular Psychiatry*, **8**, 745–51.

Ribases, M., Gratacos, M., Fernandez-Aranda, F. *et al.* (2004). Association of BDNF with anorexia, bulimia and age of onset of weight loss in six European populations. *Human Molecular Genetics*, **13**, 1205–12.

Ricca, V., Nacmias, B., Boldrini, M. *et al.* (2004). Psychopathological traits and 5-HT2A receptor promoter polymorphism (-1438 G/A) in patients suffering from Anorexia Nervosa and Bulimia Nervosa. *Neuroscientific Letters*, **365**, 92–6.

Rivinus, T.M., Biederman, J., Herzog, D.B. *et al.* (1984). Anorexia nervosa and affective disorders: a controlled family history study. *American Journal of Psychiatry*, **141**, 1414–18.

Rosenkranz, K., Hinney, A., Ziegler, A. *et al.* (1998). Systematic mutation screening of the estrogen receptor beta gene in probands of different weight extremes: identification of several genetic variants. *Journal of Clinical Endocrinology and Metabolism*, **83**, 4524–7.

Shinohara, M., Mizushima, H., Hirano, M. *et al.* (2004). Eating disorders with binge-eating behaviour are associated with the s allele of the 3′-UTR VNTR polymorphism of the dopamine transporter gene. *Journal of Psychiatry and Neurosciences*, **29**, 134–7.

Stein, D., Lilenfeld, L., Plotnicov, K. *et al.* (1999). Familial aggregation of eating disorders: results from a controlled family study of bulimia nervosa. *International Journal of Eating Disorders*, **26**, 211–15.

Strober, M., Freeman, R., Lampert, C., Diamond, J. & Kaye, W. (2000). Controlled family study of anorexia nervosa and bulimia nervosa: evidence of shared liability and transmission of partial syndromes. *American Journal of Psychiatry*, **157**, 393–401.

Strober, M., Lampert, C., Morrell, W., Burroughs, J. & Jacobs, C. (1990). A controlled family study of anorexia nervosa. Evidence of familial aggregation and lack of shared transmission with affective disorders. *International Journal of Eating Disorders*, **9**, 239–53.

Urwin, R.E., Bennetts, B.H., Wilcken, M.B. *et al.* (2003). Gene-gene interaction between the monoamine oxidase A gene and solute carrier family 6 (neurotransmitter transporter, noradrenalin) member 2 gene in anorexia nervosa (restrictive subtype). *European Journal of Human Genetics*, **11**, 945–50.

Vink, T., Hinney, A., van Elburg, A.A. *et al.* (2001). Association between an agouti-related protein gene polymorphism and anorexia nervosa. *Molecular Psychiatry*, **6**, 325–8.

Wade, T.D., Bulik, C.M., Neale, M. & Kendler, K.S. (2000). Anorexia nervosa and major depression: shared genetic and environmental risk factors. *American Journal of Psychiatry*, **157**, 469–71.

Walters, E.E. & Kendler, K.S. (1995). Anorexia nervosa and anorexic-like syndromes in a population-based female twin sample. *American Journal of Psychiatry*, **152**, 64–71.

Walters, E.E., Neale, M.C., Eaves, L.J., Heath, A.C., Kessler, R.C. & Kendler, K.S. (1992). Bulimia nervosa and major depression: a study of common genetic and environmental factors. *Psychological Medicine*, **22**, 617–22.

Westberg, L., Bah, J., Råstam, M. *et al.* (2002). Association between a polymorphism of the 5-HT2C receptor and weight loss in teenage girls. *Neuropsychopharmacology*, **26**, 789–93.

Woodside, D.B., Bulik, C.M., Halmi, K.A. *et al.* (2002). Personality, perfectionism, and attitudes toward eating in parents of individuals with eating disorders. *International Journal of Eating Disorders*, **31**, 290–9.

Young, J.K. (1990). Estrogen and the etiology of anorexia nervosa. *Neuroscience and Biobehavioral Reviews*, **15**, 327–31.

7

Epidemiology of eating disorders

Søren Nielsen

Storstrom County Hospital, Naestved, Denmark

Eating disorders in children and adolescents might be the only psychiatric condition with some positive connotations in the Westernized 'cult of thinness'. Nevertheless, these conditions are not free from stigmatization (Russell, 2004). Furthermore, the victims and their families suffer a lot, much developmental potential is not fulfilled, a huge burden of care is placed on both families and healthcare delivery systems (Nielsen & Bará-Carrill, 2003) and excess mortality in anorexia nervosa (AN) is well documented (Nielsen *et al.*, 1998; Nielsen, 2001). Findings from a few centres of excellence deviate from the general pattern in that excess mortality is not reported for AN (Korndörfer *et al.*, 2003; Crisp *et al.*, 2006).

I will focus on publications reporting findings for children and adolescents, but I cannot avoid touching upon themes of a more general epidemiological nature. As always when you are synthesizing evidence, you are standing on the shoulders of giants. My major inspirations are Szmukler (1985), Hodes (1993), Hoek (1993), van't Hoff (1994), Fombonne (1995), Hsu (1996) to whom I shall refer the interested reader.

As the findings differ dependent on source population, screening instruments and diagnostic system, I shall be clear about the type of population behind the data presented here. Hoek (1993) defined the following sources of data – level 1 'community'; level 2 'total in primary care'; level 3 'conspicuous in primary care'; level 4 'total psychiatric patients'; level 5 'psychiatric inpatients only'.

Register studies – referred and treated cases

In Denmark Nielsen (1990) found peak incidence of AN in the age range 14–19 years, using a nationwide psychiatric admission register. That is, data are from

Eating Disorders in Children and Adolescents, ed. Tony Jaffa and Brett McDermott. Published by Cambridge University Press. © Cambridge University Press 2007.

what Hoek (1993) terms 'level 5' psychiatric inpatients only. For females the Poisson (incidence) rate, based on first admissions, in this age group is 9.87 per 100 000 person-years of observation (exact 95% CI: 8.83–10.98). Rates are homogeneous across the age range 14–19 years (P = 0.97). For each individual year of age the rates are homogeneous across the 15-year observation period, i.e. 1973 to 1987, P-values ranging from 0.25 to 0.91. The population of Denmark in this period was around 5 million. All computations used *StatXact6.1* (Cytel, 2003).

In Switzerland the most recent study (Milos *et al.*, 2004) yielded significantly higher Poisson rates in 12–25-year-old females (17.41 (95% CI: 14.51–20.71)) per 100 000 person-years of observation. An increase in incidence was reported for the first three study periods, i.e. 1956–58, 1963–65 and 1973–75, but for the three latest study periods, i.e. 1973–75, 1983–85 and 1993–95, the Poisson rates were homogeneous (P = 0.65). The population of this region of Switzerland is about 1 million. A long-term population-based study from Rochester, Minnesota (Lucas & Holub, 1995), is pertinent as it reports detailed findings for the 10–14-year-olds and the 15–19-year-olds. For the latter group there is a positive trend in incidence, per quinquennium the incidence increased 9.16 (per 100 000 person-years of observation). This increase is statistically signifi-cant (t = 2.69; df 8; P = 0.027). For the 10–14-year-old females the changes in incidence is best described by two linear trends joined around 1 April 1951 (Jones & Dey, 1995). From 1935 to 1951 the trend is strongly negative, and then it changes into a clearly positive value; the improvement over a straight line is significant (F = 15.47; dfnum 2, dfden 6; P = 0.004). In the period under study the population of Rochester increased from 23 000 in 1935 to 60 000 in 1985. The authors have kindly supplied me with unpublished details of the study (J. Melton Lee III, pers. comm.) including the latest period 1985–1989. The incidence estimates for the period 1935–1989 are based on 22 female and 3 male cases aged 10–14 years and 80 female and 5 male cases aged 15–19 years. Another interesting unpublished observation is an unusual M/F ratio (male-to-female ratio) for the 15–19-year-olds and for the 20–24-year-olds. Across the period 1935 to 1979 there is a consistent pattern with a 'too low' M/F ratio around 0.6–0.75 for the 15–19-year-olds, and $\sim$ 0.5 for the 20–24-year-olds. In the last two 5-year periods the M/F ratio still has the minimum in the 20–24-year age group, but at a slightly higher level, i.e. 0.67 and 0.75 respect-ively. The explanation is a 'large influx of young females due to the health care industry' (J. Melton Lee III, pers. comm.).

In the UK, Currin *et al.* (2005) used the General Practice Research Database (GPRD; http://www.gprd.com) to update and extend earlier work by

Turnbull *et al.* (1996) so that the years 1988 to 2000 were included in the analyses. This database covers some 280 general practitioners and over 3 million patients. The database is broadly representative of the UK population with respect to age and gender, but small practices and inner London are slightly under-represented. This register is on Hoek's (1993) level 3 – 'conspicuous in primary care'. The incidence for AN was remarkably stable in the years studied (1988–2000); for 10–19-year-old females a value of 34.6 per 100 000 person-years (95% CI: 22.0–47.1) was obtained. In males the corresponding value was 2.3 (95% CI: 0–5.4). For bulimia nervosa (BN) a different picture emerges, from 1988 a significant increase, and then there seems to be a break point (Jones & Dey, 1995) around 1995–1996. Since this peak there has been a decrease of nearly 40% in BN incidence for females. For the year 2000 the incidence of AN and BN in 10–19-year-old females is remarkably similar. The figure for AN is given above; the incidence for BN is 35.8 (95% CI: 23.0–48.6). A formal statistical test (Santner & Duffy, 1989) confirms this impression. Common Poisson rate 35.2 (95% exact CI: 26.8–45.4), exact test of homogeneity of the two Poisson rates (AN and BN) $P = 1.00$, OR 1.03 (exact 95% CI: 0.6–1.79). The finding of similar rates in AN and BN was replicated for males in this age group, the Poisson rates are on a much lower level – 2.8 (95% exact CI: 0.9–6.6). Exact $P_{HOMOGENEITY} = 1.000$. The authors would do well to analyse their data in smaller age bands, e.g. 10–14 years, 15–19 years and 20–24 years to facilitate comparisons with other published reports.

Sør-Trøndelag study, Norway

Using a modified version of the Survey for Eating Disorders (SEDs) (Götestam & Agras, 1995), an instrument which was validated by Ghaderi & Scott (2002), Kjelsås *et al.* (2004) tried to reach 1987 adolescents aged 14 and 15 years from 13 different schools in the Sør-Trøndelag County, Norway. This was a population-based one stage self-report survey (Hoek, 1993; level 1 – 'community'). Ten of the schools were in the city of Trondheim. As 11 children did not get parental permission to participate and 16 returned inconsistent forms 1960 correctly completed forms were collected. This gives a response rate of 1026 (99.2%) girls and of 934 (98.0%) boys. This sample represents 64.2% of the 14- and 15-year-olds in Trondheim, and 34.0% of this age group in Sør-Trøndelag County. The total number in this age group in Norway was 105 619 at the time of the study, i.e. the sample is 1.9% of the total number of 14- and 15-year-olds in Norway. Demographic data and self-reported weight and height for all probands were collected. Both DSM–III–R and DSM–IV eating disorder diagnoses were generated by the SEDs. Lifetime prevalences for girls were 18.6% (n = 191) for 'any DSM–III–R ED', 0.7% (n = 7) for AN, 3.6% (n = 37) for BN, 1.5% (n = 15) for BED and 12.9% (n = 132) for EDNOS. For boys the corresponding figures are 6.5% (n = 61) for 'any ED', 0.2% (n = 2) for AN, 0.6% (n = 6) for BN, 0.9% (n = 8) for BED, 4.8% (n = 45) for EDNOS. These numbers change when DSM–IV ED-diagnoses are generated – see Table 2 in the original publication.

Göteborg study, Sweden

This and the following surveys described are population-based two stage epidemiological surveys (Hoek, 1993), level 1 – 'Community'. All 4291 children (2136 girls, 2155 boys) born in 1970 and living in Göteborg (population ∼ 450 000) in 1985 were measured and weighed, and longitudinal growth charts were available in the screening process (Råstam et al., 1989; supplemented by personal communications from Maria Råstam, 2005). The pupils also completed a short questionnaire. On the basis of this screening 43 were selected for a full psychiatric assessment, and 23 females and two males fulfilled the DSM–III–R criteria for AN. The research group interpreted this finding as 'an accumulated population prevalence of AN in those aged 17 years and under (defined as prevalence at age 15 plus incident cases up to age 17) of 1.08% for females and 0.09% for males'.

New Jersey County, USA

In a single New Jersey County all ninth through twelfth grades, i.e. ages 14–17 years (n = 5596), were screened (Whitaker et al., 1990). Population of the county was 84 429. There were 2564 boys and 2544 girls that took part in the study (91%). DSM–III criteria were used. Six cases of AN, 6 cases with AN and BN and 18 cases of normal weight BN were found. Weighted prevalences (sampling weights to ensure that the prevalences reported reflect the prevalence of the source population) was reported as 0.3, 0.2 and 4.0 % respectively, for females (one male only had normal weight BN).

Haute-Marne study, France

In this study 3527 pupils from 153 classes, aged 11 to 20 years were offered a screening questionnaire; 3311 (93.9%) participated, and of these 3287 (93.2%) completed the questionnaire (Flament et al., 1995). Stage II was a clinical interview; 209 of 242 were actually interviewed. Fifty-nine were selected due to eating-related problems, of these 45 were interviewed. Three girls fulfilled diagnostic criteria for AN, which is equivalent to a prevalence of 0.5%. Seven girls (all aged from 16–19 years) fulfilled DSM–III–R criteria for BN, which gives a prevalence of 1.1%. Other forms of disturbed eating were frequent. What the authors termed 'prandial hyperphagia' was found in 21 subjects, and 'excessive snacking' in 90 subjects.

Buskerud study, Norway

In Buskerud county, southern part of Norway (population 226 453), a sample of 1000 15-year-olds were randomly selected (400 boys and 600 girls) from the total of 2762 adolescents in the catchment area (Rosenvinge *et al.*, 1999). Consent was obtained from 913 students (330 boys and 583 girls). The timing of the screening was kept secret until the actual screening. Due to misunderstandings between teachers and research team 235 pupils missed the screening (116 boys and 119 girls). A careful investigation by teachers and school health staff resulted in identifying 16 students with suspected eating disorders symptoms out of a total of 332 dropouts (binomial proportion = 0.0482). The girls in the group screened (n = 464) resulted in identifying 19 similar cases (binomial proportion = 0.0409). Risk difference (RD), also known as the difference of (binomial) proportions, = −0.0072. This RD is not statistically significant (exact P = 0.64), thus the drop-out should not result in significant bias. Stage 1 screening consisted of three subscales from the EDI (Garner *et al.*, 1983), 'drive for thinness', 'bulimia' and 'body dissatisfaction', and the scales 'perfectionism' and 'general dissatisfaction' from the SCANS (Slade & Dewey, 1986; Slade *et al.*, 1990). The pupils were also asked to report weight and height, which was used to estimate BMI. Of the total sample (n = 678) 73 fulfilled the EDI 'drive for thinness' criterion of a score of 10 or above. All of these were successfully interviewed. A gender-, age- and BMI-matched group of 73 was selected, and all of these were successfully interviewed. This screening resulted in two disparate distributions across the eating disorder categories (Rosenvinge *et al.*, 1999; Table 1) (My re-analysis of the author's data gives the following result – Fisher's Exact Test statistic 47.71; P < 0.000 000.) DSM–IV diagnostic criteria were used. The discriminative power of the chosen screening method seems to be sufficient for the categories 'clinical ED' (P = 0.000 06) and 'at risk' (P = 0.000 008), whereas the category 'sub-clinical BN' is distributed fairly evenly (P = 0.44) in the two groups. The P-values are from analyses of 2 × 2 tables using Fisher's Exact Test (Cytel, 2003).

The prevalence estimates in this study are based on 14 'clinical' cases of ED (anorexia nervosa, restrictive subtype (AN-R) none; anorexia nervosa, binge-purging subtype (AN-B) two; BN five; binge eating disorder (BED) 7), and five cases of subclinical BN. Furthermore an 'at risk' group was defined as 'subjects who were dieting, or explicitly considered dieting, as a way to handle personal problems and a slim body as the solution'. Twenty-four from the high scorers and three from the control group of low scorers were identified. None of the cases were in treatment for eating disorder. Prevalences for girls are AN 0.4%; BN 1.1%; subclinical BN 1.1%; BED 1.5%.

Navarra study, Spain

In a region of Spain with a population of about 500 000, Pérez-Gaspar et al. (2000) selected a representative sample of female adolescents aged 12–21 years. Forty-three schools were selected, and of these 39 schools agreed to partici-pate. The potential study population was 3472, but as 610 girls did not complete the screening questionnaire, the study cohort was 2862 girls (82.4%). All high scorers (> 30 on EAT-40) were subjected to a clinical interview and diagnosed according to DSM–IV criteria. In all 119 clinical cases of ED were found: AN 9 cases, BN 22 cases and EDNOS 88 cases. The resulting prevalences were AN 0.3% (95% CI: 0.1–0.6), BN 0.8% (0.5–1.2) and EDNOS 3.1% (2.5–3.8).

Ontario, Canada

Two Canadian studies are pertinent, both from Ontario. One (Jones et al., 2000) reports findings from a nondiabetic sample of 1098 12–19-year-old females. No case of AN was found, but 5 cases of BN, 44 cases of EDNOS and 84 cases of sub-threshold eating disorder were identified in this population. Extensive screening procedures and EDE-interviews led to mutually exclusive DSM–IV diagnostic categories. The other study (Colton et al., 2004) reports findings from a slightly younger population – 303 9–14-year-old females. Only 3 cases of sub-threshold eating disorders were reported, and no cases of AN, BN or EDNOS appeared in this population. The children's version of the EDE (Cooper & Fairburn, 1987) was used in the interviews.

Summary

Findings from the studies outlined above are summarized in Table 7.1.

Table 7.1. Raw data on female eating disorders from two-stage population-based surveys

Source	Flament et al. (1995)	Pérez-Gaspar et al. (2000)	Jones et al. (2000)	Colton et al. (2004)	Rosenvinge et al. (1999)	Santonastaso et al. (1996)	Patton et al. (1990)
Origin	Haute-Marne, France	Navarra, Spain	Ontario, Canada	Toronto, Canada	Buskerud, Norway	Padova, Italy	London, UK
Age range (years)	11–20	12–21	12–19	9–14	15	16	15
Diagnoses	DSM–III–R	DSM–IV	DSM–IV	DSM–IV	DSM–IV	DSM–IV	Russell criteria
AN	3	9	0	0	2	0	0
BN	7	22	5	0	5	0	4
EDNOS	0	88	44	0	0	4	0
BED	0	0	0	0	7	0	0
Sub-thresh	111	0	84	3	5	12	18
NO ED	3166	2743	965	300	445	343	988
Σ	3287	2862	1098	303	464	359	1010

Source	Rathner & Messner (1993)	Wlodarczyk-Bisaga et al. (1996)	Whitaker et al. (1990)	Råstam et al. (1989)	Råstam et al. (1989)
Origin	Bressanone, Austria	Warsaw, Poland	New Jersey, USA	Göteborg, Sweden	Göteborg, Sweden
Age range	11–20	14–16	14–17	15	15
Diagnoses	DSM–III–R	DSM–III–R	DSM–III	DSM–III–R	DSM–III
AN	2	0	6(+6 AN/B)	15	10
BN	0	0	17	3	3
EDNOS	0	0	0	0	0
BED	0	0	0	0	0
Sub-thresh	5	16	0	3[a]	3[a]
NO ED	510	731	2515	2115	2120
Σ	517	747	2544	2136	2136

[a]AN partial syndrome.

Distribution across the diagnostic spectrum is not uniform from site to site, even when the study of Colton *et al.* (2004), which covers a younger age range, is omitted. This difference persists even when the cells for EDNOS and subthreshold ED are collapsed. Asymptotic and Monte Carlo estimate of the exact P-value gave uniform results $P = 0.000\,000$ (99% CI: 0–0.000 46). Flament *et al.* (1995) used DSM–III–R for the clinical diagnoses and had two other categories for subthreshold ED 'prandial hyperphagia' and 'excessive snacking', all others used DSM–IV diagnoses. As the methodology of these studies are of a similar and high quality, the causes of these robust differences ought to be elucidated.

Across reported epidemiological studies of eating disorders in child and adolescent samples the following picture emerges: incidence of AN seems to have levelled off since 1970. Prevalence and incidence are strongly dependent on source population, i.e. the figures are much higher in 'community' samples than in 'treated' samples. Variations in availability of services and in treatment-seeking behaviour have a significant influence on reported figures in register studies. Incidence of BN is not yet stable. Incidence and prevalence of BED in children and adolescents is not well elucidated.

Implications for research

There are two arguments against the widespread habit of reporting a common incidence or prevalence rate for both sexes combined. First, you belong to either one or the other of the two genders, and there is a 10-fold difference in risk for most clinical eating disorders. Second, you cannot safely assume that the M/F ratio is close to unity, at least not without investigating it. Please note the M/F ratios for the different age groups reported from Rochester, Minnesota (see above).

Clinical implications

Some of the population-based studies report treatment-seeking behaviour, and thus contribute important supplementary information to the estimates given by Hoek (1993). Råstam *et al.* (1989) mention that half (9/18) of their defined AN cases were in treatment. Whitaker *et al.* (1990) reported that for AN and AN + BN 5 out of 6 were in treatment. For normal weight bulimia only 5 of 18 were in treatment, even though 13 of 18 had a CGAS-score in the clinical range (< 71). Rosenvinge *et al.* (1999) were concerned as none of their identified cases had sought treatment.

Diagnostic issues

Although the two major diagnostic systems (WHO, 1992; APA, 1994) are approaching each other, quite a few inconsistencies await resolution (Nielsen & Palmer, 2003). The DSM–IV term EDNOS is to this author not as helpful clinically as the ICD-10 terms 'atypical' AN resp. BN, as these terms hint at the type of treatment that might be useful. In children there are specific and deep problems with the prevailing diagnostic systems (Doyle & Bryant-Waugh, 2000), and hence with the relevance of epidemiological estimates.

REFERENCES

American Psychiatric Association. (1994). *Diagnostic and Statistical Manual of Mental Disorders,* 4th edition. Washington, DC: American Psychiatric Association.

Colton, P., Olmsted, M., Daneman, D., Rydall, A. & Rodin, G. (2004). Disturbed eating behavior and eating disorders in preteen and early teenage girls with type 1 diabetes. *Diabetes Care,* **27,** 1654–9.

Cooper, Z. & Fairburn, C. (1987). The eating disorder examination: a semi-structured interview for the assessment of the specific psychopathology of eating disorders. *International Journal of Eating Disorders,* **6,** 1–8.

Crisp, A.H., Gowers, S., Joughin, N. *et al.* (2006). Death, survival and recovery in anorexia nervosa. A thirty five year study. *European Eating Disorders Review,* **14,** 168–75.

Currin, L.A., Schmidt, U., Treasure, J. & Jick, H. (2005). Time trends in eating disorder incidence. *British Journal of Psychiatry,* **186,** 132–5.

Cytel Software Corporation (2003). *StatXact Version 6.1 with Cytel Studio.* Cambridge, MA: Cytel Software Corporation.

Doyle, J. & Bryant-Waugh, R. (2000). Epidemiology. In *Anorexia Nervosa and Related Eating Disorders in Childhood and Adolescence,* ed. Lask, B. & Bryant-Waugh, R. Hove: Psychology Press, pp. 41–61.

Flament, M. F., Ledoux, S., Jeammet, P., Choquet, M. & Simon, Y. (1995). A population study of bulimia nervosa and subclinical eating disorders in adolescence. In *Eating Disorders in Adolescence,* ed. Steinhausen, H.-C. Berlin: Walter de Gruyter, pp. 21–36.

Fombonne, E. (1995). Eating disorders: time trends and possible explanatory mechanisms. In *Psychosocial Disorders in Young People: Time Trends and Their Causes,* ed. Rutter, M. & Smith, D. J. Chichester: John Wiley & Sons, pp. 615–85.

Garner, D.M., Olmstead, M.P. & Polivy, J. (1983). Development and validity of a multidimensional eating disorder inventory for anorexia nervosa and bulimia. *International Journal of Eating Disorders,* **2,** 15–34.

Ghaderi, A. & Scott, B. (2002). The preliminary reliability and validity of the self-report for eating disorders (SEDs): A self-report questionnaire for diagnosing eating disorders. *European Eating Disorders Review*, **10**, 61–76.

Götestam, K. G. & Agras, W. S. (1995). General population-based epidemiological study of eating disorders in Norway. *International Journal of Eating Disorders*, **18**, 119–26.

Hodes, M. (1993). Anorexia nervosa and bulimia nervosa in children. *International Review of Psychiatry*, **5**, 101–8.

Hoek, H. W. (1993). Review of the epidemiological studies of eating disorders. *International Review of Psychiatry*, **5**, 61–74.

Hoek, H. W. & van Hoeken, D. (2003). Review of the prevalence and incidence of eating disorders. *International Journal of Eating Disorders*, **34**, 383–96.

Hsu, L. K. G. (1996). Epidemiology of the eating disorders. *Psychiatric Clinics of North America*, **19**, 681–700.

Johnson, J. G., Cohen, P., Kasen, S. & Brook, J. S. (2002). Eating disorders during adolescence and the risk for physical and mental disorders during early adulthood. *Archives of General Psychiatry*, **59**, 545–52.

Jones, J. M., Lawson, M. L., Daneman, D., Olmsted, M. P. & Rodin, G. (2000). Eating disorders in adolescent females with and without type 1 diabetes: cross sectional study. *British Medical Journal*, **320**, 1563–6.

Jones, R. H. & Dey, I. (1995). Determining one or more change points. *Chemistry and Physics of Lipids*, **76**, 1–6.

Kjelsås, E., Bjørnstrøm, C. & Götestam, K. G. (2004). Prevalence of eating disorders in female and male adolescents (14–15 years). *Eating Behaviors*, **5**, 13–25.

Korndörfer, S. R., Lucas, A. R., Suman, V. J., Crowson, C. S., Kraahn, L. E. & Melton III, L. J. (2003). Long-term survival of patients with anorexia nervosa: a population-based study in Rochester, Minnesota. *Mayo Clinic Proceedings*, **78**, 278–84.

Lucas, A. R. & Holub, M. I. (1995). The incidence of anorexia nervosa in adolescent residents of Rochester, Minnesota, during a 50-year period. In *Eating Disorders in Adolescence*, ed. Steinhausen, H.-C. Berlin: Walter de Gruyter, pp. 3–19.

Milos, G., Spindler, A., Schnyder, U., Martz, J., Hoek, H. W. & Willi, J. (2004). Incidence of severe anorexia nervosa in Switzerland: 40 years of development. *International Journal of Eating Disorders*, **35**, 250–8.

Nielsen, S. (1990). The epidemiology of anorexia nervosa in Denmark from 1973 to 1987: a nationwide register study of psychiatric admission. *Acta Psychiatrica Scandinavica*, **81**, 507–14.

Nielsen, S. (2001). Epidemiology and mortality of eating disorders. *Psychiatric Clinics of North America*, **24**, 201–14.

Nielsen, S. & Bará-Carrill, N. (2003). Family, burden of care and social consequences. In *Handbook of Eating Disorders*, 2nd edition, ed. Treasure, J., Schmidt, U. & van Furth, E. Chichester: John Wiley & Sons, pp. 191–206.

Nielsen, S. & Palmer, B. (2003). Editorial – diagnosing eating disorders – AN, BN and the others. *Acta Psychiatrica Scandinavica*, **108**, 161–2.

Nielsen, S., Møller-Madsen, S., Isager, T., Jørgensen, J., Pagsberg, K. & Theander, S. (1998). Standardized mortality in eating disorders – a quantitative summary of previously published and new evidence. *Journal of Psychosomatic Research*, **44**, 413–34.

Patton, G.C., Selzer, R., Coffey, C., Carlin, J.B. & Wolfe, R. (1999). Onset of adolescent eating disorders: population based cohort study over 3 years. *British Medical Journal*, **318**, 765–8.

Pérez-Gaspar, M., Gual, P., de Irala-Estevez, J., Martinez-Gonzalez, M.A., Lahortiga, F. & Cervera, S. (2000). Prevalence of eating disorders in a representative sample of female adolescents from Navarra (Spain). *Medica Clinica (Barc)*, **114**, 481–6.

Råstam, M., Gillberg, C. & Garton, M. (1989). Anorexia nervosa in a Swedish urban region. A population-based study. *The British Journal of Psychiatry*, **155**, 642–6.

Rathner, G. & Messner, K. (1993). Detection of eating disorders in a small rural town: an epidemiological study. *Psychological Medicine*, **23**, 175–84.

Rosenvinge, J.H., Sundgot-Borgen, J. & Börresen, R. (1999). The prevalence and psychological correlates of anorexia nervosa, bulimia nervosa and binge eating among 15-year-old students: a controlled epidemiological study. *European Eating Disorders Review*, **7**, 382–91.

Russell, G. (2004). The stigmatisation of eating disorders. In *Every Family in the Land*, Revised Edition, ed. Crisp, A.H. London: Royal Society of Medicine Press, pp. 180–7.

Santner, T.J. & Duffy, D.E. (1989). *The Statistical Analysis of Discrete Data*. New York: Springer Verlag.

Santonastaso, P., Zanetti, T., Sala, A. et al. (1996). Prevalence of eating disorders in Italy: a survey on a sample of 16-year-old female students. *Psychotherapy and Psychosomatics*, **65**, 158–62.

Slade, P.D. & Dewey, M.E. (1986). Development and preliminary validation of SCANS: a screening test for identifying individuals at risk of developing anorexia nervosa and bulimia nervosa. *International Journal of Eating Disorders*, **5**, 517–38.

Slade, P.D., Dewey, M.E., Kiemle, G. & Newton, T. (1990). An update on SCANS: a screening test for identifying individuals at risk of developing an eating disorder. *International Journal of Eating Disorders*, **9**, 583–4.

Szmukler, G.I. (1985). The epidemiology of anorexia nervosa and bulimia. *Journal of Psychiatric Research*, **19**, 143–53.

Turnbull, S., Ward, A., Treasure J., Jick, H. & Derby, L. (1996). The demand for eating disorder care. An epidemiological study using the general practice research database. *British Journal of Psychiatry*, **169**, 705–12.

van Hoeken, D., Seidell, J. & Hoek, H.W. (2003). Epidemiology. In *Handbook of Eating Disorders*, 2nd edition, ed. Treasure, J. Schmidt, U. & van Furth, E. Chichester: John Wiley & Sons, pp. 11–34.

van't Hoff, S.E. (1994). *Anorexia Nervosa: The Cultural and Historical Specificity. Fallacious Theories and Tenacious 'Facts'*. Lisse (NL): Swets & Zeitlinger.

Whitaker, A., Johnson, J., Schaffer, D. et al. (1990). Uncommon troubles in young people: Prevalence estimates of selected psychiatric disorders in a nonreferred adolescent population. *Archives of General Psychiatry*, **47**, 487–96.

Wlodarczyk-Bisaga, K. & Dolan, B. (1996). A two-stage epidemiological study of abnormal eating attitudes and their prospective risk factors in Polish schoolgirls. *Psychological Medicine*, **26**, 1021–32.

World Health Organization (1992). *The ICD-10 Classification of Mental and Behavioural Disorders: Clinical Descriptions and Diagnostic Guidelines*. Geneva: WHO.

8

Neuroimaging

Janet Treasure[1] and Hans-Christoph Friederich[2]

[1]Guy's Hospital, London, UK
[2]Heidelberg University, Heidelberg, Germany

Introduction

Neuroimaging studies have provided new insights in neural brain circuits and neuroreceptor functions of eating disorders and as a consequence have contributed to a change of the conceptual framework of the pathophysiology and aetiology of eating disorders. Most research has been collected for the two distinct DSM–IV defined eating disorders: anorexia (AN) and bulimia nervosa (BN). To our knowledge only three studies have specifically investigated teenagers with an eating disorder (Gordon *et al.*, 1997; Chowdhury *et al.*, 2003; Wagner *et al.*, 2003), although in many studies a wide age range of the participants is found, including adolescents. This chapter is substantially based on findings in adulthood. Task and provocation using eating disorder-related stimulus material have been used to unravel the disorder-specific neural circuits. However, eating disorders show a high psychiatric comorbidity including depression, anxiety and obsessive-compulsive disorders. Therefore, overlap with other psychiatric disorders is likely and may impact on the interpretation of the findings.

Neural basis of hunger, satiety and reward value of food

Motivation for food intake and eating behaviour is not only dependent on internal factors sensing recent energy intake and energy homeostasis, but is also determined by the incentive value ('wanting') and hedonic pleasure ('liking') of food (Fig. 8.1). Motivational aspects of food intake involve higher mental processes such as emotional, motivational and cognitive processing, which are poorly understood (see also Mercer, Chapter 2). Neuroimaging

Eating Disorders in Children and Adolescents, ed. Tony Jaffa and Brett McDermott. Published by Cambridge University Press. © Cambridge University Press 2007.

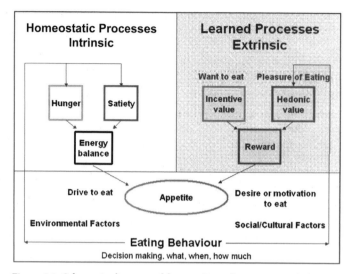

Figure 8.1. Schematic diagram of factors that influence eating behaviour.

techniques have been employed to link subcortical and cortical brain regions to various aspects of food intake as well as to the subjective reward and pleasure value of food in healthy controls.

Neural networks involved in meal initiation (orexigenic network) and meal termination (anorexigenic network) have been investigated in neuroimaging studies by focusing on the comparison between internal states of extreme hunger and satiety. A common finding of most studies is that satiety was associated with increased perfusion of the ventromedial and dorsolateral prefrontal cortex (Liu *et al.*, 2000; Del Parigi *et al.*, 2002). The prefrontal cortex (PFC) is known to be a critical structure for mediating emotional and motivational behaviours and interacts with the limbic system. There are direct projections between the PFC and the limbic system.

In the fasted state, relatively higher perfusion was observed in several subcortical regions such as hypothalamus as well as insular and temporal cortices (Liu *et al.*, 2000; Del Parigi *et al.*, 2002). The importance of the hypothalamus for the short-term and long-term energy regulation is well established (see Mercer, Chapter 2). Changes in activation of the insular and temporal cortex are thought to deal with gustatory information.

Furthermore, hedonic and reward values of taste and olfactory stimuli have been investigated using fMRI and PET studies. These studies consistently have found reward value representation and processing in the amygdala and orbitofrontal cortex (OFC) (for review see Kringelbach, 2004). Moreover, a functional segregation of the neural representation for pleasant and aversive responses to food is postulated. Small and colleagues for example used a paradigm, where chocolate was consecutively eaten beyond satiety. Initially subjects rated the chocolate as very pleasant, corresponding to an activation of the medial OFC, the insula and striatum. In contrast, eating chocolate beyond satiety was associated with aversive ratings, paralleled by an activation of the lateral OFC, prefrontal regions and the parahippocampal gyrus (Small et al., 2001). Moreover, associations between aversive ratings in response to food and odours and the left amygdala have been reported (Zald et al., 2002).

In summary, neuroimaging studies provide a new method to investigate the complex higher order processes of motivational food intake. These studies suggest that eating behaviour is regulated centrally by a complex network, including orexigenic and anorexigenic neural circuits. Based on the present literature the following simplified model of cortical structures involved in motivational food intake can be derived. Sensory information (vision, taste, smell) is conveyed for further multimodal integration in brain structures such as the orbitofrontal cortex and the amygdala, where their reward value is assigned. The information then is passed on to the ventromedial prefrontal and the dorsolateral prefrontal cortex, which play a role in monitoring learning and memory mechanisms as well as in controlling behaviour. The hedonic experience of food cues and motivation of food intake is furthermore modulated by hunger and other internal states conveyed predominantly from the hypothalamus (Fig. 8.2).

Structural changes ('Pseudoatrophy')

Brain lesions studies have revealed that prefrontal, temporal, mesiotemporal regions and the hypothalamus predominantly on the right-hand side are particularly linked with pathological eating behaviours and amount of food intake (for review see Uher & Treasure, 2005).

There are several lines of evidence from structural CT and MRI studies that underweight AN patients show enlarged ventricular volume, dilated sulci and reductions in both white (mainly myelinated axons) and grey matter (cell bodies of neurons and glia cells) (Katzman et al., 1996; Swayze et al., 2003). Bulimia nervosa patients show similar changes with respect to widened cerebral sulci (cortical atrophy) but with less pronounced loss of brain volume. However, the ventricles and midbrain areas in BN are normal in size (Krieg et al., 1987; Hoffman et al., 1989, 1990). Noteworthy in AN is that, despite good reversibility of white matter deficits with weight gain and normalisation of

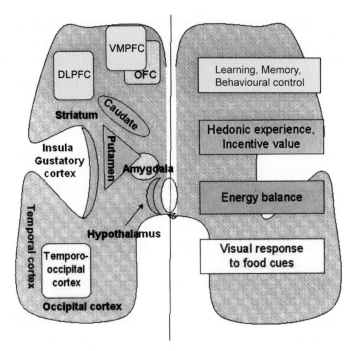

Figure 8.2. Simplified schematic illustration of cortical brain regions involved in motivational food intake.

The schema is based on findings in human PET and fMRI studies on hunger, satiety and reward regulation. Brain regions: OFC (orbitofrontal cortex), VMPFC (ventromedial prefrontal cortex), DLPFC (dorsolateral prefrontal cortex).

eating behaviour, a significant grey matter reduction seems to persist beyond recovery (Golden *et al.*, 1996; Katzman *et al.*, 1996). Further evidence of a grey matter deficit in weight-recovered AN comes from a postmortem study (Neumarker *et al.*, 2000).

The reason for structural changes in normal weight BN and recovered AN is unknown. It is also a matter of debate, whether the mentioned alterations include the whole brain or are regional. There is evidence for example that the pituitary gland as well as the amygdala-hippocampal formation are decreased in volume (Giordano *et al.*, 2001). Hypercortisolaemia in AN may contribute to a reduction in brain mass, especially in the hippocampus-amygdala region. The hippocampus-amygdala formation is a crucial target for glucocorticoid effects during stress (for review of this system in relation to feeding see Peters *et al.*, 2004). Another potential explanation for the brain atrophy might be alterations in brain metabolism in eating disorders. Magnetic resonance spectroscopy studies showed several differences in brain chemicals. However, these changes were either closely related to BMI or reversible with weight recovery, suggesting they are most likely induced by nutritional deficits (Schlemmer et al., 1998; Roser et al., 1999).

Brain function in eating disorders

Resting state

Brain function during resting conditions was mainly assessed using positron emission tomography (PET) and single photon spectroscopy (SPECT). A globally reduced glucose metabolism in BN and AN, with normalization after recovery, was shown in PET studies. The reduction of glucose metabolism was most prominent in parietal brain regions in BN and parietal as well as frontal brain regions in AN. In contrast to AN, overall brain metabolism was not decreased in BN. Thus as expected, overall brain glucose metabolism was dependent on the nutritional state and BMI. A relatively increased glucose metabolism instead was found in the caudate nucleus of AN and BN. Perfusion studies using SPECT found relative hypoperfusions in frontal, temporal and parietal regions in AN. Furthermore, there have been reports of a diminished cerebral blood flow pattern in AN restricting and purging type. The AN restricting subtype showed a decreased blood flow in the frontal and anterior cingulate region and an increased perfusion in the amygdala, hippocampus and thalamus regions. This differential pattern was not found in the AN purging subtype. With respect to recovery after weight gain, inconsistent findings are reported for SPECT studies. Råstam and colleagues report temporoparietal and frontal hypometabolism persisting years after recovery from AN (for review see Uher et al., 2002).

Findings in BN are less consistent. PET studies identified parietal hypometabolism and a loss of the normal right>left asymmetry in brain glucose metabolism. These resting functional abnormalities tend to resolve with recovery. Based on the high prevalence of depressive comorbidity in BN, another study directly compared resting brain activity of patients with major depressive disorders and BN. Differences in basal ganglia and right hemispheric activation were used as arguments against a shared pathophysiology of these two disorders (for review see Uher et al., 2002).

In summary, in AN most frequently alterations of the frontal, temporal and parietal cortex as well as basal ganglia during the ill state have been reported. The mesial temporal and anterior cingulate cortex are important regions within the fear network and it is possible that these changes may reflect an increased anxiety level in AN. The caudate nucleus is involved in obsessive-compulsive behaviour in humans (Rauch, 2000) and alterations of AN and BN in this region might correspond to obsessional behaviours predominantly related to symmetry, exactness and order in eating disorders (Srinivasagam et al., 1995). However, the interpretation of resting brain studies can be difficult. First of all, it is not possible to control for the patient's cognition during the experiment. Second, metabolic changes may depend on the nutritional state and differences in blood flow (low blood pressure and heart rate in AN).

Behavioural challenge

Changes in brain structure and metabolism during resting conditions showed several brain alterations in eating-disordered patients, but their specificity for the genesis, the maintenance and the core symptoms of eating disorders remain unclear. To assess functional changes relevant to ED psychopathology, specific provocation paradigms have been employed including either food, eating or body image paradigms.

Food challenge

The first AN food provocation study was conducted by Nozoe and colleagues (1993) using SPECT and finding an increased frontal lobe perfusion in response to eating a cake. The same paradigm was used to demonstrate a differential activation pattern in AN and BN. In BN there was an increased frontotemporal perfusion observed in the resting state, which decreased upon eating cake. AN patients in contrast showed an increased perfusion of the frontotemporal region during eating.

More recent studies used functional MRI (fMRI) and showed an activation of limbic structures, including the amygdala and insula region in AN, in response to labelled high caloric drinks (Ellison et al., 1998). The authors interpreted their findings as an activation of the fear network, corresponding to the clinical observation of a 'caloric phobia' in AN women. This finding was not replicated in a later PET study, which showed as a single difference between healthy controls and patients an increased activation of the visual associative cortex (Gordon et al., 2001). Using fMRI, our research group recently demonstrated an activation in the ventromedial prefrontal and anterior cingulate cortices in response to food images in people with AN and BN, but not in healthy controls. This abnormal reaction was specific to disease-related stimuli and did not generalize to the disease-unrelated emotional stimuli (Uher et al., 2004). It was also present in women long-term recovered

Table 8.1. Brain activation in response to food stimuli

	No	VM-PFC	ACC	PCC	L-PFC	IPL	Precuneus	Cerebell.
ED	26	↑	↑		↓	↓	↓	↓
BN	10	↑	↑	↑	↓		↓	
AN	16	↑	↑			↓	↓	↓
BPAN	7	↑	↑			↓		↓
RAN	9	↑						
Rec RAN	9	↑	↑			↓		↑

Brain regions significantly differentially activated in eating disorders (ED) and its subgroups (BPAN: binge-purge AN, RAN: restrictive AN, Rec RAN: recovered from restrictive AN) as compared with controls. Brain regions: VM-PFC (ventromedial prefrontal cortex), ACC (anterior cingulate cortex), PCC (posterior cingulate cortex), L-PFC (lateral prefrontal cortex), IPL (inferior parietal lobule), Cerebell. (cerebellum). ↑ significantly more active than in controls; ↓ significantly less active than in controls. The data are based on fMRI studies (Uher et al., 2003, 2004).

from AN (Uher et al., 2003). Interestingly, there is evidence that brain lesions in this area have caused eating disorder-like syndromes (Uher & Treasure, 2005). The ventromedial prefrontal cortex and the anterior cingulate are abundantly interconnected and are a convergence zone for emotional processing and storing of subjectively significant and self-related stimuli (Bechara et al., 2000). Abnormal activation in this area is also found in response to disease-related cues in obsessive-compulsive disorder (Rauch et al., 1994) and in addiction (Volkow & Fowler, 2000).

Bulimia nervosa patients in our study were additionally characterized by lower levels of activation to food cues in the lateral prefrontal cortex (Uher et al., 2004). This aspect of brain reactivity differentiated the patients with BN from both healthy controls and from those with AN. As the lateral prefrontal cortex is involved in cognitive inhibition and suppression of undesirable behaviour (Aron et al., 2003), this decreased lateral prefrontal involvement in food processing in BN is interpreted as corresponding to the lack of control over eating. Table 8.1 and Fig. 8.3 illustrate the mentioned findings of our recent study.

Body image challenge

Body schema and body image are related terms that are very often used synonymously. Body schema is understood as an abstract internal representation of the body in space, which helps to locate the exact position of body parts

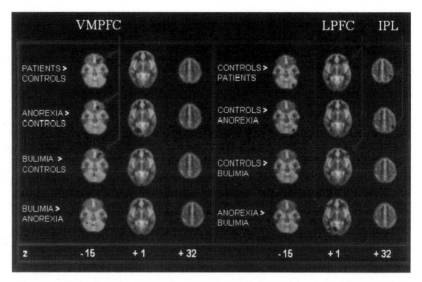

Figure 8.3. Brain activation maps in response to food stimuli.

Differences in brain activation between eating disordered patients and healthy controls are shown on three representative axial slices. The vertical position of the slices is determined by the z coordinate, which is given at the bottom of the picture. It is based on fMRI studies (Uher *et al.*, 2003, 2004). Brain regions: VMPFC (ventromedial prefrontal cortex), LPFC (lateral prefrontal cortex), IPL (inferior parietal lobule).

(Paillard, 1991). Injury and lesion studies showed that the left parietal lobe and its connections to the thalamus are important for body schema representation (McGlynn & Schacter, 1989).

To our knowledge, there is only one fMRI study with a representative patient sample published. In this, cerebral reactions to distorted own or other female bodies were recorded in adolescent patients with AN and age-matched healthy controls (Wagner *et al.*, 2003). Anorexia nervosa patients showed greater activation in response to distorted female bodies in the dorsolateral prefrontal cortex and inferior parietal lobule (IPL). Interestingly, a more detailed analysis showed that the increased activation in the IPL was only found in response to the presentation of their own but not others' distorted body. The authors interpreted their findings as higher activations in regions involved in attentional processing (prefrontal cortex) and visuo-spatial integration (inferior parietal lobule) in AN compared with healthy controls. While further studies are of course necessary, this finding raises hopes that brain imaging might be a suitable tool to shed light on the controversial and complex construct of body image disturbance in eating disorders.

Neurotransmission

Brain imaging studies using neurotransmitter ligands have offered new opportunities to study neurotransmitter functions and pathways, as well as their relation to pathological behaviour. Neuromediators such as dopamine (DA) and serotonin (5-HT) are believed to be involved in eating disorder pathology. Eating or food cues as naturally pleasurable stimuli trigger release of the pleasure and reward messenger DA. Alterations within the reward circuit are considered as a vulnerability factor for restraint or disinhibited eating, similar to addictive behaviours (e.g. drug abuse). Volkow and colleagues (2003) for example showed that restrained eating in healthy subjects was associated with an increased DA responsivity in the striatum. People recovered from AN showed an increased D2/D3 receptor binding in the antero-ventral striatum (Frank *et al.*, 2005). In contrast a reduction in dopamine transporter levels in the striatum has been found in BN (Tauscher *et al.*, 2001). However, DA research in eating disorders is still in its infancy and further studies are required.

Serotonin among other functions is involved in satiety regulation and food intake. In AN and BN, PET and SPECT studies have examined receptor binding in ill and recovered patients. Ill AN patients showed a reduced receptor activity in the left frontal, bilateral parietal and occipital cortex. Recovered restrictive AN patients showed a reduced 5-HT2A binding in mesial temporal and parietal cortical areas as well as in the cingulate cortex. Recovered binge-purge AN showed reduced receptor binding in the left subgenual cingulate, left parietal and right occipital cortex. In recovered BN subjects a reduced 5-HT2A receptor binding was found only in the orbitofrontal cortex. In the ill state, no differences in 5-HT2A binding between BN patients and healthy controls were found. These studies support an alteration of 5-HT2A brain activity in AN as a trait marker, whereas alterations in BN are uncertain, and larger replications will be needed. Experimental studies suggest that the antidepressant effect of SSRIs is mediated via 5-HT1A receptors. To study 5-HT1A in BN is therefore of particular interest. In BN patients an increased 5-HT1A receptor binding was found, localized in frontal, cingulate and temporal regions. Furthermore, in another study a significant reduction of serotonin transporter density in ill BN patients in the thalamic and hypothalamic regions was found (for review see Frank *et al.*, 2004).

In summary, brain imaging studies revealed alterations in serotonergic function most consistently shown in recovered and weight-restored women. These findings argue against the hypothesis that changes in neurotransmission of serotonin are merely a consequence of malnutrition or starvation. However, an unanswered question remains whether alteration in serotonin function is a product of the disease (scar-effect) or a potential cause. Findings from studies using different radioligands suggest that several different components of the serotonin neurotransmitter circuit are affected. Most studies in AN patients report significant changes of serotonin activity in mesial temporal (amygdala) regions and in the subgenual cinguli. The subgenual cinguli as well as the amygdala have been implicated in depression and anxiety disorders and possibly reflect the high comorbidity for mood disorders in AN.

Summary

In this chapter, we have summarised findings of neuroimaging research in eating disorders across a wide range of different methods and tools. No localized macroscopic brain damage has been found, rather there is a more generalized atrophy, probably resulting from inadequate nutrition. Fortunately much of the brain volume loss is reversible although some loss of grey matter may persist.

Functional alterations are most commonly found in the prefrontal area, including the anterior cingulate cortex, in the mesial temporal (amygdala-hippocampal formation) cortex and in the inferior parietal lobule. Some specificity between the ED-subgroups is found; BN patients in comparison with AN and healthy controls show less activation of the dorsolateral pre-frontal cortex. This is of great interest, since this area is implicated in the inhibition and suppression of disliked behaviour and is also activated in satiation.

Persistent changes in a distributed network involving the prefrontal cortex and limbic systems remain despite recovery in task activation studies and receptor imaging studies. This would support a neurodevelopmental causal model of eating disorders. The alternative explanation is that these findings are a 'scar' from the illness. A promising challenge in the future will be to consider how genetic, developmental and environmental influences shape brain circuit structure and function.

Acknowledgements

Dr Hans-Christoph Friederich was supported by the Christina Barz Fellowship 2004 and the Nina Jackson Eating Disorders Research Fund, in conjunction with the Psychiatry Research Trust (registered charity no. 284286).

REFERENCES

Aron, A.R., Fletcher, P.C., Bullmore, E.T., Sahakian, B.J. & Robbins, T.W. (2003). Stop-signal inhibition disrupted by damage to right inferior frontal gyrus in humans. *Nature Neuroscience*, **6**, 115–16.

Bechara, A., Damasio, H. & Damasio, A.R. (2000). Emotion, decision making and the orbito-frontal cortex. *Cerebral Cortex*, **10**, 295–307.

Chowdhury, U., Gordon, I., Lask, B., Watkins, B., Watt, H. & Christie, D. (2003). Early-onset anorexia nervosa: is there evidence of limbic system imbalance? *International Jownal of Eating Disorders*, **33**, 388–96.

Del Parigi, A., Gautier, J.F., Chen, K. *et al.* (2002). Neuroimaging and obesity: mapping the brain responses to hunger and satiation in humans using positron emission tomography. *Annals of the New York Academies of Science*, **967**, 389–97.

Ellison, Z., Foong, J., Howard, R., Bullmore, E., Williams, S. & Treasure, J. (1998). Functional anatomy of calorie fear in anorexia nervosa. *Lancet*, **352**, 1192.

Frank, G.K., Bailer, U.F., Henry, S., Wagner, A. & Kaye, W.H. (2004). Neuroimaging studies in eating disorders. *CNS Spectra*, **9**, 539–48.

Frank, G.K., Bailer, U.F., Shannan, E.H. *et al.* (2005). Increased dopamine D2/D3 receptor binding after recovery from anorexia nervosa measured by positron emission tomography and [11C]Raclopride. *Biological Psychiatry*, **58**, 908–12.

Giordano, G.D., Renzetti, P., Parodi, R.C. *et al.* (2001). Volume measurement with magnetic resonance imaging of hippocampus-amygdala formation in patients with anorexia nervosa. *Journal of Endocrinology Investigation*, **24**, 510–14.

Golden, N.H., Ashtari, M., Kohn, M.R. *et al.* (1996). Reversibility of cerebral ventricular enlargement in anorexia nervosa, demonstrated by quantitative magnetic resonance imaging. *Journal of Pediatrics*, **128**, 296–301.

Gordon, I., Lask, B., Bryant-Waugh, R., Christie, D. & Timimi, S. (1997). Childhood-onset anorexia nervosa: towards identifying a biological substrate. *International Journal of Eating Disorders*, **22**, 159–65.

Gordon, C.M., Dougherty, D.D., Fischman, A.J. *et al.* (2001). Neural substrates of anorexia nervosa: a behavioral challenge study with positron emission tomography. *Journal of Pediatrics*, **139**, 51–7.

Hoffman, G.W., Ellinwood, E.H., Jr., Rockwell, W.J., Herfkens, R.J., Nishita, J.K. & Guthrie, L.F. (1989). Cerebral atrophy in bulimia. *Biological Psychiatry*, **25**, 894–902.

Hoffman, G.W., Ellinwood, E.H., Jr., Rockwell, W.J., Herfkens, R.J., Nishita, J.K. & Guthrie, L.F. (1990). Brain T1 measured by magnetic resonance imaging in bulimia. *Biological Psychiatry*, **27**, 116–19.

Katzman, D.K., Lambe, E.K., Mikulis, D.J., Ridgley, J.N., Goldbloom, D.S. & Zipursky, R.B. (1996). Cerebral gray matter and white matter volume deficits in adolescent girls with anorexia nervosa. *Journal of Pediatrics*, **129**, 794–803.

Krieg, J.C., Backmund, H. & Pirke, K.M. (1987). Cranial computed tomography findings in bulimia. *Acta Psychiatrica Scandinavica*, **75**, 144–9.

Kringelbach, M.L. (2004). Food for thought: hedonic experience beyond homeostasis in the human brain. *Neuroscience*, **126**, 807–19.

Liu, Y., Gao, J.H., Liu, H.L. & Fox, P.T. (2000). The temporal response of the brain after eating revealed by functional MRI. *Nature*, **405**, 1058–62.

McGlynn, S.M. & Schacter, D.L. (1989). Unawareness of deficits in neuropsychological syndromes. *Journal of Clinical Experimental Neuropsychology*, **11**, 143–205.

Neumarker, K.J., Bzufka, W.M., Dudeck, U., Hein, J. & Neumarker, U. (2000). Are there specific disabilities of number processing in adolescent patients with anorexia nervosa? Evidence from clinical and neuropsychological data when compared to morphometric measures from magnetic resonance imaging. *European Child and Adolescent Psychiatry*, **9** (Suppl. 2), II111–II121.

Nozoe, S., Naruo, T., Nakabeppu, Y., Soejima, Y., Nakajo, M. & Tanaka, H. (1993). Changes in regional cerebral blood flow in patients with anorexia nervosa detected through single photon emission tomography imaging. *Biological Psychiatry*, **34**, 578–80.

Paillard, J. (1991). Motor and representational framing of space. In *Brain and Space*, ed. Paillard, J. Oxford: Oxford University Press, pp. 163–82.

Peters, A., Schweiger, U., Pellerin, L. *et al.* (2004). The selfish brain: competition for energy resources. *Neuroscience and Biobehavioral Reviews*, **28**, 143–80.

Rauch, S.L. (2000). Neuroimaging research and the neurobiology of obsessive-compulsive disorder: where do we go from here? *Biological Psychiatry*, **47**, 168–70.

Rauch, S.L., Jenike, M.A., Alpert, N.M. *et al.* (1994). Regional cerebral blood flow measured during symptom provocation in obsessive-compulsive disorder using oxygen 15-labeled carbon dioxide and positron emission tomography. *Archives in General Psychiatry*, **51**, 62–70.

Roser, W., Bubl, R., Buergin, D., Seelig, J., Radue, E.W. & Rost, B. (1999). Metabolic changes in the brain of patients with anorexia and bulimia nervosa as detected by proton magnetic resonance spectroscopy. *International Journal of Eating Disorders*, **26**, 119–36.

Schlemmer, H.P., Mockel, R., Marcus, A. *et al.* (1998). Proton magnetic resonance spectroscopy in acute, juvenile anorexia nervosa. *Psychiatry Research*, **82**, 171–9.

Small, D.M., Zatorre, R.J., Dagher, A., Evans, A.C. & Jones-Gotman, M. (2001). Changes in brain activity related to eating chocolate: from pleasure to aversion. *Brain*, **124**, 1720–33.

Srinivasagam, N.M., Kaye, W.H., Plotnicov, K.H., Greeno, C., Weltzin, T.E. & Rao, R. (1995). Persistent perfectionism, symmetry, and exactness after long-term recovery from anorexia nervosa. *Americal Journal of Psychiatry*, **152**, 1630–4.

Swayze, V.W., Andersen, A.E., Andreasen, N.C., Arndt, S., Sato, Y. & Ziebell, S. (2003). Brain tissue volume segmentation in patients with anorexia nervosa before and after weight normalization. *International Journal of Eating Disorders*, **33**, 33–44.

Tauscher, J., Pirker, W., Willeit, M. *et al.* (2001). [123I] beta-CIT and single photon emission computed tomography reveal reduced brain serotonin transporter availability in bulimia nervosa. *Biological Psychiatry*, **49**, 326–32.

Uher, R., Brammer, M.J., Murphy, T. *et al.* (2003). Recovery and chronicity in anorexia nervosa: brain activity associated with differential outcomes. *Biological Psychiatry*, **54**, 934–42.

Uher, R., Murphy, T., Brammer, M.J. *et al.* (2004). Medial prefrontal cortex activity associated with symptom provocation in eating disorders. *American Journal of Psychiatry*, **161**, 1238–46.

Uher, R. & Treasure, J. (2005). Brain lesions and eating disorders. *Journal of Neurology, Neurosurgery and Psychiatry*, **76**, 852–7.

Uher, R., Treasure, J. & Campbell, I. (2002). Neuroanatomical bases of eating disorders. In *Biological Psychiatry*, ed. D'Haenen, H.A.H., den BoerBoer, J.A. & Willner, P. Chichester: John Wiley & Sons, pp. 1173–80.

Volkow, N.D. & Fowler, J.S. (2000). Addiction, a disease of compulsion and drive: involvement of the orbitofrontal cortex. *Cerebral Cortex*, **10**, 318–25.

Volkow, N.D., Wang, G.J., Maynard, L. *et al.* (2003). Brain dopamine is associated with eating behaviors in humans. *International Journal of Eating Disorders*, **33**, 136–42.

Wagner, A., Ruf, M., Braus, D.F. & Schmidt, M.H. (2003). Neuronal activity changes and body image distortion in anorexia nervosa. *Neuroreport*, **14**, 2193–7.

Zald, D.H., Hagen, M.C. & Pardo, J.V. (2002). Neural correlates of tasting concentrated quinine and sugar solutions. *Journal of Neurophysiology*, **87**, 1068–75.

Part III

Abnormal states

9

Anorexia nervosa in children and adolescents

Rachel Bryant-Waugh

Great Ormond Street Hospital for Children NHS Trust, London, UK

Introduction

This chapter focuses on diagnostic, classification and presentation issues in relation to children and adolescents with anorexia nervosa (AN). It includes a discussion of current diagnostic criteria, and difficulties applying these to a younger age group; reference to the ongoing debate around nosological and classification issues; a consideration of factors related to early identification; and a description of common presentations from a clinical perspective. Co-morbid non-eating disorders psychopathology is discussed by Brewerton in Chapter 13 of this volume. Treatment of AN is dealt with in Part IV of this volume. In line with the UK eating disorders guideline developed under the auspices of the National Institute for Clinical Excellence (NICE, 2004), this chapter relates to young people from the age of 8 years and over.

Diagnosis and classification

Diagnostic criteria for anorexia nervosa

The two diagnostic systems most commonly used throughout the world are those drawn up by the American Psychiatric Association (DSM-IV; APA, 1994), and the World Health Organization's ICD–10 (WHO, 1993). Both use the term 'anorexia nervosa' to denote full syndrome presentations, and DSM–IV further distinguishes between a restricting subtype and a binge-eating/purge subtype (see Tables 9.1 and 9.2). Restricting AN is commonly seen in younger patients, and is characterized by consistent restriction of food intake, often accompanied by excessive exercising. Binge-eating/purge subtype of AN is characterized by regular binge-eating episodes in the context of dietary

Eating Disorders in Children and Adolescents, ed. Tony Jaffa and Brett McDermott. Published by Cambridge University Press. © Cambridge University Press 2007.

Table 9.1. DSM–IV diagnostic criteria for anorexia nervosa

A: Refusal to maintain body weight at or above a minimally normal weight for age and height (e.g. weight loss leading to maintenance of body weight less than 85% of that expected; or failure to make expected weight gain during period of growth, leading to body weight less than 85% of that expected).

B: Intense fear of gaining weight or becoming fat, even though underweight.

C: Disturbance in the way in which one's body weight or shape is experienced, undue influence of body weight or shape on self-evaluation, or denial of the seriousness of the current low body weight.

D: In postmenarcheal females, amenorrhea, i.e. the absence of at least three consecutive menstrual cycles. (A woman is considered to have amenorrhea if her periods occur only following hormone, e.g. oestrogen, administration.)

From American Psychiatric Association (1994). *Diagnostic and Statistical Manual of Mental Disorders*, 4th edition. Washington, DC: APA.

Table 9.2. ICD–10 Diagnostic criteria for anorexia nervosa

A. There is weight loss or, in children, a lack of weight gain, leading to a body weight at least 15% below the normal or expected weight for age and height.

B. The weight loss is self-induced by avoidance of 'fattening foods'.

C. There is a self-perception of being too fat, with an intrusive dread of fatness, which leads to a self-imposed low weight threshold.

D. A widespread endocrine disorder involving the hypothalamic-pituitary-gonadal axis is manifest in women as amenorrhoea and in men as a loss of sexual interest and potency.

E. The disorder does not meet criteria A and B for bulimia nervosa.

From World Health Organization (1993). *The ICD-10 Classification of Mental and Behavioural Disorders. Diagnostic Criteria for Research*. Geneva: WHO.

restriction OR episodes of vomiting, laxative misuse or other purging behaviours (see further section on presentation below). Thus an individual who restricts her intake and does not binge, but does engage in self-induced vomiting (with or without excessive exercise), would be classified as AN binge-eating purging subtype.

Atypical anorexia nervosa and eating disorder not otherwise specified

Individuals not meeting full diagnostic criteria but presenting with a clinical eating disorder fall in the ICD–10 system under the heading 'atypical anorexia nervosa', whilst in the DSM–IV system such patients would receive a diagnosis of 'eating disorder not otherwise specified', more commonly referred to as

EDNOS. Someone presenting with amenorrhoea and typical eating disorder psychopathology, but not quite meeting the weight criterion, would receive a diagnosis of EDNOS or atypical AN. However, someone presenting with extreme weight loss, amenorrhoea and loss of appetite or minimal food intake due to depression would clearly not receive such a diagnosis.

Dissatisfaction and problems with current diagnostic criteria

The diagnostic criteria for AN are currently the topic of much discussion and debate within the field of eating disorders. A number of observations and research findings have fuelled this debate. It can be argued that any valid axis-I diagnosis (such as AN) should organize individuals into clinically distinct subgroups (Steiger, 2004). However, clinical reality suggests that a high percentage of patients migrate between the eating disorder diagnoses of AN, bulimia nervosa (BN) and their atypical forms (Fairburn & Harrison, 2003). Furthermore, evidence-based proposals have been put forward for more clinically relevant groupings across eating disorder diagnostic categories (e.g. Western & Harnden-Fischer, 2001), leading some to suggest that eating disorder subtypes may be more clearly determined on the basis of factors other than eating behaviours, such as personality traits (Steiger, 2004).

While many clinicians and researchers would agree that diagnostic criteria in general, and those for AN in particular, can be useful, they are very often not literally applied, and, if they are, present considerable problems. Some authors argue that existing criteria do not adequately describe the central features of AN (e.g. Hebebrand *et al.*, 2004). These authors suggest that terms such as 'refusal' (DSM–IV criterion A) and the weight phobia criterion (DSM–IV B) lack empirical support, and put forward a proposal for alternative criteria, which they suggest allows a 'better integration of biologically derived hypotheses addressing the nosology and the symptomatology of anorexia nervosa'. Others have made alternative suggestions, for example, Palmer (2003) proposes that the concept of 'motivated eating restraint' might be a better way to conceptualize the 'weight concern' currently regarded as a marker of core eating disorder psychopathology.

In addition to concerns about the diagnostic criteria for full syndrome AN, the definition of its atypical variants also causes difficulty – EDNOS or atypical AN should only be used as a diagnosis where the patient presents with a clinical eating disorder, thus technically not for 'subclinical' cases. This raises problems in terms of definition of 'clinical eating disorder' and practical issues in terms of precisely where the lines should be drawn in the strict application of criteria. DSM–IV and ICD–10 are non-directive in this respect, recommending that appropriately defined criteria be drawn up for research purposes. There continues to be a lack of clarity concerning the issue of 'clinical severity', with researchers actively exploring the boundary between normality and clinical syndrome (Palmer, 2000). The notion of 'functional impairment' has become important in this respect, with a clinical eating disorder being associated with a degree of functional impairment. In children this might entail impairment of physical development or social functioning.

There is now good evidence that a large number of patients of all ages presenting for treatment fall into the 'not otherwise specified' or 'atypical' categories of either AN or BN (Nicholls *et al.*, 2000; Turner & Bryant-Waugh, 2004), further supporting calls for a revision of the current system. It does seem rather unhelpful that up to a half of patients seen in clinics fall into a residual category. Fairburn & Harrison (2003) describe the existing classification scheme for eating disorders as 'unsatisfactory and anomalous' and identify it as a high priority for review.

Diagnosing anorexia nervosa in children and adolescents

Current diagnostic criteria for AN are often difficult to apply to younger individuals. Some of the main practical difficulties are reviewed here.

Weight criterion (DSM–IV A; ICD–10 A)

DSM–IV is actually less precise than ICD–10 about the weight cut-off for a diagnosis. The well-known 'less than 85% of that expected' is given as an example, but tends to be used in practice as a diagnostic cut-off. In children, this is often taken to mean less than 85% weight for height, but this would imply that 100% is 'expected'. ICD–10 is more explicit with its requirement that weight is 'at least 15% below the normal or expected weight for age and height'. There are, however, real difficulties delineating precisely how to determine whether a young person's weight is less than 85% or at least 15% below expected. Children's expected weights are usually calculated on the basis of their age, height and gender using population norms, plotting values on standard growth and development charts. When a child loses weight, or fails to gain weight because of inadequate dietary intake, growth rates may be impaired. Slowed growth velocity may result in measured height at assessment being less than expected height for that child, compared with premorbid growth trajectory and percentiles. Nevertheless, this measured value is then used to calculate expected weight, to determine whether the 85%/15% criterion is met, but as it may be a compromised height this can result in an underestimation of the true expected body weight.

In adults, this criterion is rarely strictly applied as set out in the diagnostic criteria; instead body mass index (BMI) of 17.5 or below is commonly used as a guideline in the diagnosis of AN, being easier to apply than the 'less than 85% of expected/at least 15% below normal' rule. Body mass index is however not a static measurement, and norms vary according to age, as well as between boys and girls, making absolute BMI values unsuitable for children and adolescents. Increasingly BMI percentiles (Cole *et al.*, 1995) and related charts (Child Growth Foundation, 1997) are used for this younger age group, as these allow the interpretation of BMI values in relation to peer population reference data regarding BMI distribution. Unfortunately, all too often clinicians working with children and adolescents mistakenly apply the 17.5 cut-off (which will overestimate severity of weight loss), or report absolute BMI values which must then be read off an appropriate percentile chart before they can acquire any useful meaning. Hebebrand *et al.* (2004) have proposed that the weight criterion should read 'Weight is below a minimally normal weight for age and height. As a guideline, [this] is defined as a BMI $\leq$ 10th percentile of the reference population.' Others have argued that such a cut-off would be too high, and propose that a BMI below the 2nd percentile would be both closer to the current absolute value of 17.5 in adults, and result in fewer false positive identifications (Royal College of Psychiatrists, 2002). Clearly these issues are extremely complex, and as yet, there remains a lack of agreement and consistency in this respect which inevitably leads to variation in the use of a full diagnosis of AN.

Core cognitive disturbances (DSM–IV B and C; ICD–10 C)

With regard to central psychopathology of AN, it has been demonstrated that childhood-onset AN is very similar to the more typical later adolescent-onset disorder in terms of level of concern and distorted cognitions related to eating, weight and shape (Cooper *et al.*, 2002). However, particularly in the case of children, it can be extremely difficult to reliably elicit the presence of core psychopathology precisely as specified in the diagnostic criteria. With regard to the DSM–IV system, confirming that there is 'undue influence on body weight or shape on self-evaluation' can be extremely complex. The whole concept of having a scheme for self-evaluation is one that many younger children may not have consciously encountered. Often clinicians infer this to be present or absent rather than formally evaluate whether it is present or not. A careful, detailed assessment of the child's thoughts, attitudes and behaviours are crucial to the formal process of diagnosing AN in children and adolescents. Whilst this might appear an obvious statement, the potential difficulty encountered in reliably eliciting the presence of features without resort to inference cannot be overemphasized.

Amenorrhoea criterion (DSM–IV D; ICD–10 D)

This criterion is not applicable to pre-pubertal children, and in those who have entered puberty but who have not yet established a regular menstrual cycle. A significant number of young people who develop AN between the ages of 8 and 14 will fall into these categories. In some, puberty itself may have been delayed through the reduction in energy intake and concomitant weight loss. Hebebrand *et al.* (2004) suggest that this criterion might be more usefully rephrased to include the presence of known physiological adaptations to inadequate energy intake, which could include amenorrhoea of a minimum of three months in postmenarcheal females, but which could also include other adaptations to semi-starvation such as bradycardia, hypothermia and hypotension. This would seem a sensible suggestion, which could be applied to patients across the age range.

Wider issues related to classification

The classification of eating disturbances in childhood more generally remains a subject of much discussion, with two main strands to the debate: first, the increasing level of dissatisfaction around diagnostic and classification issues in eating disorders mentioned above, and second, the issues related to classifying mental illness of any type in children and adolescents (Rosen, 2003). As with other mental illness diagnoses, diagnostic criteria for AN have been derived largely from adult clinical samples, raising the question of whether they are sufficiently flexible and developmentally appropriate to use with younger patients. It seems fairly clear that in the context of child and adolescent eating disturbances more generally, existing diagnostic systems are rather limited in their scope and do not satisfactorily capture the full range of clinical presentations seen. With regard to AN in particular, Lask & Bryant-Waugh proposed on the basis of their extensive clinical experience of younger patients the 'Great Ormond Street (GOS) Checklist' – not intended to replace formal diagnostic criteria, but to represent working definitions that adequately described most of their patients (Bryant-Waugh, 2000). The GOS criteria, which undoubtedly have good face validity, have contributed towards prompting further efforts to derive more developmentally sensitive criteria for AN in children and younger adolescents (see Table 9.3).

Early identification

In 2002 the US National Institutes of Health convened a workshop on overcoming barriers to treatment research in AN. One of its recommendations

Table 9.3. Great Ormond Street Checklist for anorexia nervosa

1. Determined weight loss, achieved through one or more of the following:
   a. Food avoidance/restriction.
   b. Self-induced vomiting.
   c. Excessive exercising.
   d. Abuse of laxatives.
2. Abnormal cognitions around weight and/or shape.
3. Morbid preoccupation with weight and/or shape, food and/or eating.

From Bryant-Waugh, R. (2000). Overview of the eating disorders. In: *Anorexia Nervosa and Related Eating Disorders in Childhood and Adolescence*, 2nd edition, ed. Lask, B. & Bryant-Waugh, R. Hove: Psychology Press, p. 38.

related to the need to improve early recognition of AN in adolescents (Agras *et al.*, 2004). Although sensible as a suggestion in the light of the general finding that the less time between the onset of the disorder and the start of appropriate treatment, the more favourable the outcome, this may be easier said than done. It may be relatively straightforward to identify full syndrome AN, but it is much more difficult to accurately identify young people who are on the way to developing a full syndrome disorder. Clinical observation suggests that some children who present with depressive and/or oppositional features may be struggling with issues of control, which over time become more focused on weight/shape issues. Such presentations may represent a prodrome of AN, but the necessary longitudinal research has not been conducted to clarify this. Furthermore, we know that even when the full disorder is correctly identified, there may often be a delay in the initiation of appropriate treatment, or too relaxed an approach to lack of progress, which can be particularly problematic for younger patients due to the disruption of puberty and developmental processes that accompany it. Surprisingly little is known about the early stages of AN generally, and almost nothing in relation to children and adolescents specifically. In an attempt to try to address this gap in knowledge, one recent study aimed to identify whether there were any specific patterns in the timing or content of visits to the general practitioner (GP) in children who went on to develop AN (Lask *et al.*, 2005). These authors found that children with AN had visited their GPs more frequently than controls, particularly in the year prior to diagnosis, with main reason for consultation being concerns around eating or weight. Thus in late childhood/early adolescence even a single consultation around weight loss, or eating difficulties, for which there is no obvious medical cause, should alert the GP to the possibility of an eating disorder, and prompt a more detailed assessment. The NICE guidelines suggest that one of the key factors in relation to early identification is the GP considering it a possibility (NICE, 2004, p. 74). For further discussion on early identification see Noordenbos' discussion of secondary prevention in this volume.

Presentation

Anorexia nervosa is seen in clinical settings in children from around the age of 8 years upwards, and occurs in both boys and girls. Although the clinical features, and even the physical appearance of such young people when they are in an emaciated state, bear strong similarities, each young person's illness will be related to a unique pattern of traits, circumstances and triggers.

The most obvious presenting feature in AN is low weight. The majority of children will actually lose weight, but the diagnostic criteria do allow for lack of weight gain during a period of growth. Children vary in terms of stated reasons for their low weight. Some will maintain that they have always been small, and that they like being small. Some will be more overt about body image disturbance, and describe themselves as fat and needing to lose weight. Others may have had a period of illness, which has resulted in some weight loss, and somehow maintaining that low weight becomes a goal in itself after the original illness has resolved. Still others will simply argue with you that they are not at a low weight, and tell you they know plenty of other people who weigh less than them.

This core discrepancy between the child's strongly held belief that her (or his) weight is not a cause for concern, and the professionals' knowledge that it is, represents an important aspect of the presentation of AN, and one that has acquired greater prominence in recent years (Tan *et al.*, 2003). The area of consent to treatment and treatment refusal, related to the young person's capacity to make decisions, is a complex one. A young person with AN may not view herself as ill, may not wish to gain weight, and may not want to engage in a treatment process that appears to have as a main aim to make her fat. People of any age who suffer from AN are mostly fearful or ambivalent about engaging in treatment, leading some to view them as 'resistant', 'manipulative' or 'in denial' – terms which really have no place in attempts to work with patients to help them to move on from the grip of their anorexia. It can be extremely difficult at times to maintain a therapeutic alliance with an ambivalent young person, and the ethical dilemmas that arise in the case of health deteriorating further present a considerable challenge to clinicians. The difficulty that young people have in coming to terms with the fact that they have an eating disorder, and the confusion they experience around 'recovery', can significantly hamper engagement and subsequent treatment. The NICE guidelines recommend that in the case of essential treatment being refused, either the use of legislation enabling patients to be detained (in the UK, the Mental Health Act) should be invoked, or the right of those with parental authority to override the child's refusal. However, the guidelines also recommend that it is inadvisable to rely indefinitely on parental consent to treatment in the case of young patients (NICE, 2004). Manley *et al.* (2001) have helpfully set out a proposed framework for ethical decision-making in an attempt to address some of the complex legal and ethical issues that can arise in the treatment of young people with AN.

Weight loss is achieved primarily by dietary restriction. This can start with a bang or can be a slow gradual process for which it is hard in retrospect to identify a start point. Very often children will decide to eat more healthily – sometimes triggered by curriculum-based input at school on a whole range of issues that might touch on diet, weight and exercise, sometimes triggered by health problems in family members, sometimes triggered by teasing, or other difficult or unpleasant events in the child's life. There is a wide range of triggers, none of which should be confused with causes. 'Healthy eating' in practice often means cutting out fat and carbohydrates as much as possible or, perhaps more accurately, these components of a normal balanced diet are avoided under the guise of the more socially acceptable healthy eating. Sometimes children are quite secretive about their dietary restriction, hiding or throwing away food (especially packed lunches), other children may request smaller helpings or claim they are full and do not want pudding, etc. Many parents describe this process as happening without them really noticing at first. The end result is that these children invariably end up with both an energy deficient and an unbalanced intake.

Alongside dietary restriction, children and adolescents may present with a range of other weight management strategies. By far the commonest in the younger age group are excessive exercising and self-induced vomiting. Laxative misuse and misuse of other substances such as appetite suppressants, diuretics and amphetamines are less common than in older adolescents and adults, perhaps because it is much harder for children to obtain such substances.

Excessive exercising can take the form of secretive workouts, but can also include running and overenthusiastic participation in sports and fitness regimes. Amongst children receiving inpatient treatment for AN, it is not uncommon to find ballet dancers, athletes, gymnasts and runners – young people who have sporting achievements at a high level. However, there are also young people who have never been particularly sporty, but who develop a compulsion to run or to exercise as part of their illness. Excessive exercising as a feature of AN can be extraordinarily difficult to manage, and in some cases can be dangerous. Buchowski *et al.* (2004) describe recurrent self-induced syncope in two adolescent patients with AN who engaged in isometric exercises, alongside other forms of overexercising, drawing attention to the importance of assessing all forms of exercise, not just the obvious ones. Nurses and other staff caring for young people receiving inpatient treatment are well aware of the full range of possibilities in this respect including repeated rapid muscle clenching, always standing up, leg jiggling, etc. Holtkamp *et al.* (2004) investigated the relationships between dietary restriction, physical activity and psychopathology in 30 adolescents admitted for treatment of AN. They concluded that anxiety symptoms and dietary restriction may synergistically contribute to increased levels of exercise, and in their discussion of the clinical implications of their findings caution that restriction of physical activity during refeeding may further increase anxiety and stress, which in turn can create problems for full engagement in treatment. Thus one of the best ways to approach excessive exercising as a main presenting feature of AN may be to include a structured, monitored activity programme in the treatment package.

Self-induced vomiting may form part of the clinical picture at presentation, or in some cases develops in response to increased anxiety around greater dietary intake and weight gain through treatment. Again when this feature is present at initial assessment, it may be something that has started on an occasional basis, gradually becoming more regular and established as the young person falls further into the trap of anorexia. Vomiting is almost always secretive, and often it is something that will not have crossed parents' minds. Indeed, they might appear quite affronted that you should suggest such a thing. Whilst it is undoubtedly hard for parents to imagine their child feeling so desperately unhappy having eaten what to everyone else might seem a normal family supper, even some very young patients engage in self-induced vomiting to rid themselves of unwanted food and calories. Thankfully though, there is a subset that says that they might have tried to make themselves sick, but couldn't do it, or found the experience so unpleasant that they don't do it. For some, the physical experience of loss of control that accompanies vomiting seems ironically to be the thing that prevents them from using this as a method of weight control.

Thus in terms of the core behaviours at presentation, dietary restriction, excessive exercising and self-induced vomiting are the most common. Other eating disorder behaviours, such as laxative misuse, diuretic and other substance misuse, are respectively uncommon and rare in children and younger adolescents. One other core behaviour warrants mention here – binge eating. As mentioned previously, DSM–IV distinguishes between restricting (AN-R) and binge-eating/purging (AN-BP) subtypes of AN. We have seen that younger patients can fall into either of those two subtypes primarily in relation to the presence or absence of self-induced vomiting. True binge eating (defined as eating objectively large amounts accompanied by a sense of loss of control over eating) is not often seen in early onset AN. At most children will describe occasionally overeating, but often these episodes do not constitute true binges, as the amounts eaten are rarely objectively large.

Summary and future directions

We have seen that there are significant problems and dissatisfactions with the currently available diagnostic and classification systems with regard to children and adolescents with AN. It seems important that proper attention is paid to pertinent elements of both diagnostic validity and clinical utility in relation to any future proposals around classifying childhood eating disturbances, and reviewing the diagnostic criteria. Additionally, although the importance of early identification is well recognized, it remains hard to act on this, and more research is needed into precursors of AN in young people. Such studies are difficult and costly to carry out, and regrettably relatively low down on research priority agendas. AN remains a serious illness that can develop in children well before puberty, and can have devastating effects. We need to continue to improve our means of identifying and describing this difficult disorder so that we can conduct the research needed to inform and improve available treatment.

REFERENCES

Agras, S., Brandt, H., Bulik, C. *et al.* (2004). Report on the National Institutes of Health Workshop on overcoming barriers to treatment research in anorexia nervosa. *International Journal of Eating Disorders*, **35**, 509–21.

American Psychiatric Association (1994). *Diagnostic and Statistical Manual of Mental Disorders*, 4th edition. Washington, DC: APA.

Bryant-Waugh, R. (2000). Overview of the eating disorders. In *Anorexia Nervosa and Related Eating Disorders in Childhood and Adolescence*, ed. Lask, B. & Bryant-Waugh, R. Hove, UK: Psychology Press, pp. 27–40.

Buchowski, K., Pardo, J., Ringel, R. & Guarda A. (2004). Inducible syncope in anorexia nervosa: two case reports. *International Journal of Eating Disorders*, **35**, 359–62.

Child Growth Foundation (1997). BMI charts. Available from Harlow Printing Ltd. *www. harlowprinting.co.uk*; *www.healthforallchildren.co.uk*.

Cole, T.J., Freeman, J.V. & Preece, M.A. (1995). Body mass index reference curves for the UK, 1990. *Archives of Diseases in Childhood*, **73**, 25–9.

Cooper, P., Watkins, B., Bryant-Waugh, R. & Lask, B. (2002). The nosological status of early onset anorexia nervosa. *Psychological Medicine*, **32**, 873–80.

Fairburn, C.G. & Harrison, P.J. (2003). Eating disorders. *Lancet*, **361**, 407–16.

Hebebrand, J., Casper, R., Treasure, T. & Schweiger, U. (2004). The need to revise the diagnostic criteria for anorexia nervosa. *Journal of Neural Transmission*, **111**, 827–40.

Holtkamp, K., Hebebrand, J. & Herpertz-Dahlman, B. (2004). The contribution of anxiety and food restriction on physical activity levels in acute AN. *International Journal of Eating Disorders*, **36**, 163–71.

Lask, B., Bryant-Waugh, R., Wright, F. *et al.* (2005). Family physician consultation patterns indicate high risk for early onset anorexia nervosa. *International Journal of Eating Disorders*, **38**, 269–72.

Manley, R., Smye, V. & Srikameswaran, S. (2001). Addressing complex ethical issues in the treatment of children and adolescents with eating disorders: application of a framework for ethical decision making. *European Eating Disorders Review*, **9**, 144–66.

NICE (National Institute of Clinical Excellence) (2004). *Eating Disorders: Core Interventions in the Treatment and Management of Anorexia Nervosa, Bulimia Nervosa and Related Eating Disorders*. CG 9. London: British Psychological Society and Gaskell Press.

Nicholls, D., Chater, R. & Lask, B. (2000). Children into DSM don't go: a comparison of classification systems for eating disorders in childhood and early adolescence. *International Journal of Eating Disorders*, **28**, 317–24.

Palmer, B. (2000). *Helping People with Eating Disorders: A Clinical Guide to Assessment and Treatment*. Chichester: John Wiley & Sons.

Palmer, B. (2003). Concepts of eating disorders. In *Handbook of Eating Disorders*, 2nd edition, ed. Treasure, J. Schmidt, U. & van Furth, E. Chichester: John Wiley & Sons, pp. 1–10.

Rosen, D. (2003). Eating disorders in children and young adolescents: etiology, classification, clinical features, and treatment. *Adolescent Medicine*, **14**, 49–59.

Royal College of Psychiatrists (2002). *Guidelines for the Nutritional Management of Anorexia Nervosa – Report of the Eating Disorders Special Interest Group (EDSIG)*. London: RCPsych.

Steiger, H. (2004). Eating disorders and the serotonin connection: state, trait and developmental effects. *Journal of Psychiatry and Neuroscience*, **29**, 20–9.

Tan, J., Hope, T. & Stewart, A. (2003). Competence to refuse treatment in AN. *International Journal of Law and Psychiatry*, **26**, 697–707.

Turner, H.M. & Bryant-Waugh, R. (2004). Eating disorder not otherwise specified (EDNOS): profiles of clients presenting at a community eating disorder service. *European Eating Disorders Review*, **12**, 18–26.

Western, D. & Harnden-Fischer, J. (2001). Personality profiles in eating disorders: Rethinking the distinction between Axis I and Axis II. *American Journal of Psychiatry*, **158**, 547–62.

World Health Organization (1993). *The ICD-10 Classification of Mental and Behavioural Disorders. Diagnostic Criteria for Research*. Geneva: WHO.

10

Eating disorders in boys

Brett McDermott

Mater Child & Youth Mental Health Service, South Brisbane, Queensland, Australia

Introduction

To the public and many clinicians eating disorders are synonymous with girls and young women. The experienced clinician knows this is not the case. This chapter will discuss eating disorders in boys. In the past this endeavour would have been hampered by a dearth of empirical studies. Fortunately, recent community and population-based studies have included boys in their sampling frame. However, the research literature on treatment and outcome in boys with eating disorders is far more limited, often to the point of no separate analysis of outcomes in the male subset of the sample.

Given that the strength of the current literature is community-based studies of putative modifiable determinants of eating disorders, such as body dissatisfaction, the chapter will begin with this area and then discuss eating disorder psychopathology and the prevalence of eating disorders diagnoses in boys. The chapter will conclude with treatment research available in this group. Past research that applied a developmental perspective to other psychopathology areas suggests gender differences across time should be expected. For example longitudinal research of depressive symptoms finds gender equality before 12 years of age (McGee et al., 1990), followed by elevated rates with earlier onset in adolescent girls (Kashani et al., 1987).

The key determinants in childhood eating disorders considered include psychological constructs such as body dissatisfaction and its influence on dieting and other weight loss strategies, biological factors such as height, weight, body mass index (BMI) and pubertal status, the experience of traumatic events including various forms of abuse and socio-cultural factors including family, peer and media influences.

Eating Disorders in Children and Adolescents, ed. Tony Jaffa and Brett McDermott. Published by Cambridge University Press. © Cambridge University Press 2007.

Boys and eating disorders risk factors

Several studies investigating body dissatisfaction have included boys. Truby & Paxton (2002) compared Australian boys and girls, average age 9 years, using a series of photographs of individuals of known BMI and varying body sizes. They reported that relative to girls, boys were less accurate at ascribing body size to pictures and were significantly less likely to want to be thinner, indeed were more likely to want to be larger. This gender differential in body satisfaction is a robust finding across studies. Replication studies of boys being less likely to want to be thinner or to have a lower score on a measure of body dissatisfaction include research on 9–10-year-old American 4th graders (Gustafson-Larson & Terry, 1992), a multiracial group of Australian 11–17-year-olds (Vincent & McCabe, 2000) and English 9-year-olds (Hill *et al.*, 1994). For younger children this differential may not be present. Musher-Eizenman (2005) reported no gender difference in 5-year-olds when they reported either their current or an ideal body shape. Further, the relationship between body dissatisfaction, when present, and subsequent eating psychopathology may be weaker in boys. Schur and colleagues (2000) reviewing children from age 6–14 years found body dissatisfaction was not a predictor of eating disorders scores in boys. Hill (Chapter 3, this volume) reviews the development of shape and weight concerns.

There has also been research on factors hypothesized to be related to body dissatisfaction. Field and colleagues (1999) reported that in both boys and girls the prevalence of a misconception of being overweight increased with age, however this phenomenon was less marked in boys.

One concomitant of body dissatisfaction is desire to change weight and behaviours to make this occur. Many researchers have reported the desire of many boys to put on weight (Hill *et al.*, 1994; Neumark-Sztainer *et al.*, 1999; Schur *et al.*, 2000; Truby & Paxton, 2002), to be taller (Gustafson-Larson & Terry, 1992) and to be more muscular (Neumark-Sztainer *et al.*, 1999). Smolak *et al.* (2001) reported adequate internal consistency and concurrent validity for a new factor, 'muscular look', in their adaptation of the Socio-cultural Attitudes Towards Appearance Questionnaire (SATAQ; Heinberg *et al.*, 1995) when the modified version was given to 6th and 7th grade white, middle-class boys. Increased desire amongst boys for muscularity is consistent with US findings of increased levels of anabolic steroid (Johnson *et al.*, 2000) and dietary supplements use in adolescent males (for more details see the review of Labre, 2002). Why boys, especially adolescent boys, aspire to a more muscular body appearance is probably multifactorial and possibly includes both a desire to avoid the stigma and bullying associated with being overweight, the perception that muscularity is related to attractiveness to potential partners and positive affirmation of a muscular physique from male peers. It should, however, be noted that the desire for weight gain and muscularity is not only a feature of boys. In a study of predominantly caucasian 9–12-year-old elementary school students from the San Francisco Bay area, a somewhat surprising finding was 37.9% of both girls and boys desired to gain weight (Schur et al., 2000). Further, Faigenbaum and colleagues (1998) reported approximately an equal number of middle-school male students (2.6%) and females (2.8%), average age 9–13 years, had used anabolic steroids.

One behavioural sequela of a desire to change body weight is dieting. Dieting is well recognized in children: 40% of 9–10-year-olds studied by Schur et al. (2000) 'very often or sometimes dieted', and in Field et al.'s sample (1999) 20% of aged 9 girls and 17% of boys were trying to lose weight. Across the child and adolescent developmental span fewer boys than girls report dieting (Gustafson-Larson & Terry, 1992; Edmonds & Hill, 1999; Field et al., 1999; Schur et al., 2000). Gender differences in the prevalence of dieting may diminish in younger children, for instance one study reported that primary school boys and girls reported similar levels of dieting (Thomas et al., 2000). In this sample low self-concept predicted later dieting in both boys and girls (Thomas et al., 2000). The 8–13-year-old boys in Schur et al.'s (2000) study were more likely to have heard of dieting from their father.

The relationship between the experience of abuse and eating disorder psychopathology in boys and girls has been investigated in several large population-based studies. Neumark-Sztainer et al. (2000) found that self-report of sexual abuse was an independent risk factor for disordered eating in a large (n = 9943) representative sample of boys attending Connecticut public schools. If a respondent had reported the experience of sexual abuse the odds ratio of experiencing subsequent disordered eating was higher in boys than in girls (4.88, CI 2.94–8.10 versus 1.99, CI 1.51–2.64). The odds ratio for increased experience of disordered eating in physically abused respondents was similar across both genders. In a sample of 81 247 9–12th graders from Minnesota, boys who experienced date violence or date rape were also more likely than girls to experience a range of eating-disorder-related behaviours, such as laxative abuse, self-induced vomiting, use of diet pills and bingeing (Ackard & Neumark-Stzainer, 2002). Emotional trauma and eating disorder symptoms in adolescent boys admitted to a mental health inpatient unit are discussed further by Brewerton (Chapter 13, this volume).

Biological factors, such as the changes in adrenal and gonadal hormones around puberty are described by Fornari and Dancyger (Chapter 5, this volume). These changes affect body morphology and thus weight, height and body mass index (BMI). The individual's interpretation of these changes may show subtle gender differences. For example, absolute height and weight measurements predicted eating disorder psychopathology in 6–14-year-old boys, whereas in girls of the same age relative measures such as weight and height percentiles were predictive (Gardner *et al.*, 2000). Whilst girls being more concerned with how body morphology changes place them relative to female peers has face validity, this finding needs to be replicated. Body mass index has often been reported as an important predictive factor. In a study of 9–11-year-olds increasing BMI was correlated with greater concerns about being overweight in both boys and girls (Gustafson-Larson & Terry, 1992). The latter finding was replicated in a stepwise regression analysis that showed increased BMI independently contributed to a range of dependent variables in boys including total eating disorder psychopathology scores on the ChEAT, dieting and desire to decrease body size (Muris *et al.*, 2005).

A developmental model is not complete without considering systemic factors which may influence the individual's trajectory. Most studies have considered the individual's perspective of their surroundings. Neumark-Sztainer *et al.* (2000) reported that grade 7, 9 and 11 Connecticut public school students' disordered eating patterns were associated with their perception of low family communication and parent caring. Several other studies have investigated the perception of peer and parent influence. Weight loss in 11–17-year-old boys was influenced by maternal encouragement (Vincent & McCabe, 2000). There is some evidence that eating patterns in boys are affected by peer and parental influences. Boys were more influenced than girls by negative peer commentary about weight and shape (Vincent & McCabe, 2000). Parent and peer factors were related to the higher eating disorders psychopathology scores and an increase in desired muscle size, and parent, peers and media influences were related to the desire to decrease weight (Muris *et al.*, 2005). Contrary results have also been reported: Schwartz *et al.* (1999) did not find a relationship between parent weight feedback and boys' body dissatisfaction in a young adult sample (mean age 20.26 years, SD 2.09). Further, adolescent boys, mean age 13.94 years (SD 1.14), did not report strong media pressure to achieve any particular body ideal (McCabe & Ricciardelli, 2001). There may also be gender differential effects in the conceptualization of food as a positive, by boys themselves and by the parents of boys. For example, compared with girls who are unwell, boys who are unwell are more likely to be treated with their favourite foods by their parents and to treat themselves with food (Edmunds & Hill, 1999). Tasks for future research include replicating this finding and determining the relative contribution of social, including media, reinforcement of parents treating boys with food versus the parents' own feelings that giving food treats to boys is more acceptable to themselves and/or will be received better by boys than girls.

Eating disorder psychopathology and diagnoses

Recently boys have been included in epidemiological studies of eating disorders. Using a modification of the Survey for Eating Disorders (Götestam & Agras, 1995) with 14- and 15-year-old Norwegian students, Ghaderi & Scott (2004) reported gender differences in lifetime prevalence of eating disorders. For all conditions female rates were higher than male: eating disorders 18.6% versus 6.5%, EDNOS 12.9% versus 4.8%, BN 3.6% versus 0.6% and AN 0.7% versus 0.2%. As with all study comparisons rates vary with the instrument used and the sampling framework. For instance in a community sample of Spanish 12–13-year-olds the eating disorder rate was 6.4% for girls vs. 0.6% in boys (Beato-Fernandez et al., 2004). The prevalence of boys with AN from a UK study of general practice was 4.2/100 000 (Turnbull et al., 1996). Some studies have published rates of boys diagnosed at eating disorders clinics: reported figures include 10% of individuals diagnosed with an eating disorder at a specialist eating disorders clinic were boys (Andersen, 1984) and 9.3% of a series of children with AN attending the Children's National Medical Center were boys (Robb & Dadson, 2002).

Gender differences in BN and BN symptoms have been reported. A Finnish epidemiological study of 14–16-year-old students reported boys less frequently meet diagnostic criteria for BN or report bulimic behaviours than girls, both pre- and post- the onset of puberty (Kaltiala-Heino et al., 1999). This is contrary to a similar study of 3175 US high school children that found binge eating in boys was greater than in girls (Childress et al., 1993). These results may demonstrate a developmental difference in binge eating given the younger US sample, may be due to employing different measures or may be true differences based on transcultural factors. Epidemiological findings are discussed in more detail by Nielsen (Chapter 7, this volume).

Eating disorder psychopathology has most usually been reported as the dependent variable in risk factor research. It has mainly featured the use of the ChEAT questionnaire (Maloney et al., 1988), a modification of the Eating Attitudes Test, or other questionnaires with established psychometric properties. Often descriptive psychopathology data on boys is not reported, for example, no details reported if no significant gender difference was found or only summary statements published such as gender being/not being significant in a multivariate model. Gardner *et al.* (2000) reported 1.6% of 6–14-year-old children scored in the indicative range for AN on the ChEAT. Schur *et al.* (2000) using the same instrument reported 4.8% of 8–13-year-olds were in the similar range. Neither group reported rates specifically by gender. In an older group of adolescent boys, attending grades 8–12 in Minnesota, a disordered eating pattern rate of 2% was identified using the drive for thinness and bulimia subscales of the EDI (Keel *et al.*, 1998).

It is known that boys engage in typical eating disorders weight loss behaviour. In the sample investigated by Field and colleagues, before 13 years of age the rate of vomiting and laxative use was less than 1% and no gender difference was reported; the rate significantly increased after 13 years (Field *et al.*, 1999). The literature on bingeing in boys is small and equivocal in findings. Most studies reported low symptom levels in boys and girls, with slightly higher rates in girls. Pinhas *et al.* (Chapter 11, this volume) report that more boys binge eat. However, if the investigated construct included the subjective sense of loss of control, girls were over-represented in reports of bingeing. Williams & Ricciardelli's 2003 analysis of characteristics of 14–16 year olds who binge reported fewer boys than girls scored 1 standard deviation above the norm on the bulimia scale of the Eating Disorders Inventory (Garner *et al.*, 1983). Boys and girls in this category, designated as a high binge eating symptoms group, had similar self-control styles (Williams & Ricciardelli, 2003). The high binge-eating symptom boys also scored lower on the positive masculinity subscale (Williams & Ricciardelli, 2003).

Treatment studies

In this volume, reviews of individual therapy (Hay & McDermott, Chapter 18, this volume) and family therapy (Lock & Couturier, Chapter 19, this volume) did not report any differential treatment effects for boys or young men. Very few treatment studies met the inclusion criteria of Robb & Dadson (2002) in their recent review. When studies were cited, small sample sizes allowed very limited conclusions. For example in the outcome study of Steinhausen *et al.* (2000) only 3 of 60 subjects were boys. Inferences may be possible from one larger study of 135 men with eating disorders of whom 22% had AN (Carlat *et al.*, 1997). However, only 40% of the original sample were available at one year follow-up. Again, limited conclusions can be made given potential bias in participant retention (Carlat *et al.*, 1997). Andersen & Holman (1997) make suggestions for treatment adaptations for males with eating disorders; they considered frequent therapy issues include sexual role and orientation issues, heightened stigma given community perception that eating disorders are not seen in males, difficulty in group settings if other sufferers are female and consideration of same sex therapist for some issues.

Conclusion

The research literature in clinical samples is dominated by studies of girls and women and this is to be expected given the much higher prevalence of eating disorders in these groups. Community-based studies are more likely to include boys and much of this chapter is based on this research. Female sample preponderance has also affected measurement development, for example, 'many body image measures address only the desire to be thinner' (Smolak *et al.*, 2001, p. 217). Developments of existing instruments, such as the adaptation of the SATAQ to include a 'muscular look' subscale are an advance.

Conclusions from the current literature highlight that boys do exhibit some of the psychological and biological factors that have been identified as eating disorders risk factors for girls. These factors include, in some boys, a desire to be thinner, a misconception of being overweight, dieting behaviour and a relationship between increasing BMI and the desire to be thinner. Most studies report that rates of body dissatisfaction and desire to be thinner are significantly higher in girls than same-age boys. Desire to be more muscular, whilst not restricted to boys, nevertheless is relatively more common in boys. This phenomenon in part explains the potentially dangerous illicit use of anabolic steroids and other substances in adolescent boys. One area of relative increase in boy samples is the strength of the relationship between sexual abuse and disordered eating, and date violence or date rape and subsequent purging and bingeing behaviour in boys. These behaviours in adolescent boys should raise clinical suspicions about possible exposure to sexually abusive experiences.

The treatment research concerning boys with eating disorders is currently very sparse. In the absence of empirical data current generic eating disorders practice guidelines should be followed. It is unlikely that an evidence-based treatment approach for boys and young men will be developed without multicentred trials that ensure adequate treatment sample sizes.

REFERENCES

Ackard, D. M. & Neumark-Sztainer, D. (2002). Date violence and date rape among adolescents: associations with disordered eating behaviours and psychological health. *Child Abuse and Neglect*, **26**, 455–73.

Andersen, A. (1984). Anorexia nervosa and bulimia in adolescent males. *Pediatric Annals*, **13**, 901–7.

Andersen, A.A. & Holman, J.E. (1997). Males with eating disorders: challenges for treatment and research. *Psychopharmacology Bulletin*, **33**, 391–7.

Beato-Fernandez, L., Rodriguez-Cano, T., Belmonte-Llario, A. & Martinez-Delgado, C. (2004). Risk factors for eating disorders in adolescents. A Spanish community-based longitudinal study. *European Journal of Child and Adolescent Psychiatry*, **13**, 287–94.

Carlat, D., Camargo, C. & Herzog, D. (1997). Eating disorders in males: a report of 135 patients. *American Journal of Psychiatry*, **154**, 1127–32.

Childress, A.C., Brewerton, T.D., Hodges, E.L. & Jarrell, M.P. (1993). The Kids' Eating Disorders Survey (KEDS): a study of middle school students. *Journal of the American Academy of Child and Adolescent Psychiatry*, **32**, 843–50.

Edmunds, H. & Hill, A.J. (1999). Dieting and the context of eating in young adolescent children. *International Journal of Eating Disorders*, **25**, 435–40.

Faigenbaum, A.D., Zaichkowsky, L.D., Gardner, D.E. & Micheli, L.J. (1998). Anabolic steroid use by male and female middle school students. *Pediatrics*, **101**, e6.

Field, A.E., Camargo, C.A., Barr Taylor, C. *et al.* (1999). Overweight, weight concerns and bulimic behaviours among girls and boys. *Journal of the Academy of Child and Adolescent Psychiatry*, **38**, 754–60.

Ghaderi, A. & Scott, B. (2004). The reliability and validity of the Swedish version of the Body Shape Questionnaire. *Scandinavian Journal of Psychology*, **45**, 319–24.

Gardner, R.M., Stark, K., Friedman, B.N. & Jackson, N.A. (2000). Predictors of eating disorder scores in children ages 6 through 14. A longitudinal study. *Journal of Psychosomatic Research*, **49**, 199–205.

Garner, D.M., Olmstead, M.P. & Polivy, J. (1983). Development and validation of a multidimensional eating disorder inventory for anorexia and bulimia. *International Journal of Eating Disorders*, **2**, 15–34.

Gotestam, K.G. & Agras, W.S. (1995). General population-based epidemiological study of eating disorders in Norway. *International Journal of Eating Disorders*, **18**, 119–26.

Gustafson-Larson, A.M. & Terry, R.D. (1992). Weight-related behaviours and concerns of fourth-grade children. *Journal of the American Dietetic Association*, **92**, 818–24.

Heinberg, L., Thompson, J.K. & Stormer, S. (1995). Development and validation of the Sociocultural Attitudes Towards Appearance Questionnaire. *International Journal of Eating Disorders*, **17**, 81–9.

Hill, A.J., Draper, E. & Stack, J. (1994). A weight on children's minds: body shape dissatisfactions at 9-years old. *International Journal of Obesity*, **18**, 383–9.

Johnson, L.D., O'Malley, P.M. & Bachman, J.G. (2000). *The Monitoring the Future National Survey Results on Adolescent Drug Use: Overview of Key Findings*. Rockville, MD: National Institute on Drug Abuse.

Kaltiala-Heino, R., Rissanen, A., Rimpela, M. & Rantanen, P. (1999). Bulimia and bulimic behaviour in middle adolescence: more common than thought. *Acta Psychiatrica Scandinavica*, **100**, 33–9.

Kashani, J.H., Beck, N.C., Hoeper, E.W. *et al.* (1984). Psychiatric disorders in a community sample of adolescents. *American Journal of Psychiatry*, **144**, 584–9. Erratum in: *American Journal of Psychiatry*, **144**(8), 1114.

Keel, P.K., Klump, K.L., Leon, G.R. & Fulkerson, J.A. (1998). Disordered eating from adolescent males from a school-based sample. *International Journal of Eating Disorders*, **23**, 125–32.

Labre, M.P. (2002). Adolescent boys and the muscular male body ideal. *Journal of Adolescent Health*, **30**, 233–42.

Maloney, M.J., McGuire, J. & Daniels, S.R. (1988). Reliability testing of the children's version of the Eating Attitudes Test. *Journal of the American Academy of Child and Adolescent Psychiatry*, **27**, 541–3.

McCabe, M.P. & Ricciardelli, L.A. (2001). Parent, peer and media influences on body image and strategies to both increase and decrease body size among adolescent boys and girls. *Adolescence*, **36**, 225–40.

McGee, R., Feehan, M., Williams, S., Partridge, F., Silva, P.A. & Kelly, J. (1990). DSM-III disorders in a large sample of adolescents. *Journal of the American Academy of Child and Adolescent Psychiatry*, **29**, 611–19.

Muris, P., Meesters, C., van de Blom, W. & Mayer, B. (2005). Biological, psychological, and sociocultural correlates of body change strategies and eating problems in adolescent boys and girls. *Eating Behavior*, **6**, 11–22.

Musher-Eizenman, D.R., Holub, S.C., Miller, A.B., Goldstein, S.E. & Edwards-Leeper, L. (2005). Body size stigmatization in preschool children: the role of control attributions. *Journal of Pediatric Psychology*, **29**, 613–20.

Neumark-Sztainer, D., Story, M., Falkner, N.H. *et al.* (1999). Sociodemographic and personal characteristics of adolescents engaged in weight loss and weight/muscle gain behaviours: Who is doing what? *Preventive Medicine*, **28**, 40–50.

Neumark-Sztainer, D., Story, M., Hannan, P.J., Beuhring, T. & Resnick, M.D. (2000). Disordered eating among adolescents: associations with sexual/physical abuse and other familial/psychosocial factors. *International Journal of Eating Disorders*, **28**, 248–58.

Robb, A.S. & Dadson, M.J. (2002). Eating disorders in males. *Child and Adolescent Psychiatric Clinics of North America*, **11**, 399–418.

Schur, E.A., Sanders, M. & Steiner, H. (2000). Body dissatisfaction and dieting in young children. *International Journal of Eating Disorders*, **27**, 74–82.

Schwartz, D.J., Phares, V., Tantleff-Dunn, S. & Thompson, J.K. (1999). Body image, psychological functioning and parental feedback regarding physical appearance. *International Journal of Eating Disorders*, **25**, 339–43.

Smolak, L., Levine, M.P. & Thompson, J.K. (2001). The use of the Sociocultural Attitudes Towards Appearance Questionnaire with middle school boys and girls. *International Journal of Eating Disorders*, **2**, 216–23.

Steinhausen, H.C., Seidel, R. & Winkler Metzke, C. (2000). Evaluation of treatment and intermediate and long-term outcome of adolescent eating disorders. *Psychological Medicine*, **30**, 1089–98.

Thomas, K., Ricciardelli, L.A. & Williams, R.J. (2000). Gender traits and self-concept as indicators of problem eating and body satisfaction among children. *Sex Roles*, **43**, 441–58.

Truby, H. & Paxton, S.J. (2002). Development of the Children's Body Image Scale. *British Journal of Clinical Psychology*, **41**, 185–203.

Turnbull, S., Ward, A., Treasure, J., Jick, H. & Derby, L. (1996). The demand for eating disorder care: an epidemiological study using the general practice research database. *British Journal of Psychiatry*, **169**, 705–12.

Vincent, M.A. & McCabe, M.P. (2000). Gender differences among adolescents in family, and peer influences on body dissatisfaction, weight loss and binge eating behaviours. *Journal of Youth and Adolescence*, **29**, 205–21.

Williams, R.J. & Ricciardelli, L.A. (2003). Negative perceptions about self-control and identification with gender-role stereotypes related to binge eating, problem drinking, and to co-morbidity among adolescents. *Journal of Adolescent Health*, **32**, 66–72.

11

Bingeing and bulimia nervosa in children and adolescents

Leora Pinhas, Debra K. Katzman, Gina Dimitropoulos and D. Blake Woodside

Toronto General Research Institute, Toronto, ON, Canada

Introduction

The identification of children and adolescents with bulimia nervosa (BN) or syndromes including binge-eating has been an area of development in recent years.

This chapter will review this increasingly important area, providing an overview of the nature of these phenomena, risk factors for their development and the medical complications of these disorders.

Definition

Bulimia nervosa was first described by Russell in 1979, appearing in the Diagnostic and Statistical Manual–III (DSM–III) in 1980. The current diagnostic criteria found in DSM–IV (American Psychiatric Association, 1994) include recurrent episodes of binge eating characterized by eating in a discrete period of time (2 hours or less) an amount that is larger than most people would eat under similar circumstances; a sense of loss of control over eating during a binge episode; as well as, recurrent inappropriate compensatory behaviours in order to prevent weight gain. These compensatory behaviours can include self-induced vomiting, misuse of laxatives, diuretics and other medications, fasting or excessive exercise. The binges and inappropriate compensatory behaviours must occur on average and least twice a week for 3 months. Self-evaluation is unduly influenced by body shape and weight, and the disturbance does not occur during episodes of anorexia nervosa (AN). Bulimia nervosa is typed as either purging, where self-induced vomiting or misuse of laxatives, diuretics and enemas are part of the presentation and non-purging, where these

Eating Disorders in Children and Adolescents, ed. Tony Jaffa and Brett McDermott. Published by Cambridge University Press. © Cambridge University Press 2007.

compensatory behaviours do not regularly occur and are replaced by behaviours such as exercising and fasting.

Bulimia nervosa occurs in 1% of the adolescent population and partial symptoms are thought to occur in 3–6% of the population (Patton *et al.*, 1999). The age of onset is commonly described as late adolescence, although there are reports of purging in prepubertal children (Morris *et al.*, 2003). Boys make up 10% of this population (Carlat & Carmango, 1991). Mortality rates range from 0–6% (Keel & Mitchell, 1997; Steinhausen, 1999). The diagnostic criteria for adolescents are identical to those in adults.

Binge eating disorder (BED), although first described in 1959 (Stunkard, 1959), only recently appeared in the DSM–IV (1994) and is listed under the category of eating disorder not otherwise specified (EDNOS). Research criteria in the DSM–IV include recurrent episodes of binge eating that are associated with three or more of the following: eating much more rapidly than normal, eating until uncomfortably full, eating large amounts of food when not feeling physically hungry, eating alone because of embarrassment over how much one is eating, or feeling disgusted with oneself, depressed or very guilty after overeating. Marked distress regarding eating is present. The binge eating occurs, on average, at least 2 days a week for 6 months. The binge eating is not associated with regular use of inappropriate compensatory behaviours to control weight and does not occur during the course of AN or BN.

There is a relative paucity of research into BED in children and adolescents. Recent community-based surveys suggest that BED occurs in 1–2% of children and adolescents between the ages of 10 and 19 (Johnson *et al.*, 2002). Binge eating disorder differs from AN and/or BN in that more males suffer from this disorder (Schneider, 2003). Approximately 36% of obese patients with BED are male (Striegel-Moore *et al.*, 1998).

A number of risk factors have been identified for both BN and BED. In a prospective study (Stice *et al.*, 1998), girls who dieted were at risk for developing BN. Retrospective studies in adolescents suggest that early menarche, early sexual experiences and increasing age are risk factors for developing BN in girls. In contrast, risks for developing BN in boys are very early or very late puberty and early sexual experiences (Kaltiala-Heino *et al.*, 2001).

In comparison to families of adults with eating disorders, there is relatively little empirical evidence regarding the functioning of families of children and adolescents with BN, and even less information regarding family factors in BED.

Family dysfunction is typically elevated in clinical samples of patients with BN assessed using standardized instruments of family functioning (McDermott *et al.*, 2002). Some studies have indicated that family dysfunction may be worse in families of patients with BN compared with AN (Fornari *et al.*, 1999); whereas others have found similar levels of family dysfunction in these two disorders (McDermott *et al.*, 2002).

In a recent study of monozygotic twin pairs discordant for lifetime BN, the twin developing BN reported less warmth but more overprotection by their mothers in childhood than did their non-BN twin (Wade *et al.*, 2001). Comparing families of adolescents with AN to families of adolescents with BN, Dare *et al.* (1994) reported increased conflict and criticism in families of adolescents with BN. Another characteristic feature of BN families may be parent–daughter discrepancy in perception of family dysfunction.

In terms of longitudinal studies of family function, Okon *et al.* (2003) asked 20 bulimic adolescent girls (mean age 17) to keep a daily experiences log for a week and to complete two measures of family functioning: the Family Environment Scale and the Conflict Behaviour Questionnaire. For adolescents who perceived their families as having high levels of conflict or low levels of emotional expressiveness, family stressors predicted bulimic symptoms occurring later the same day. However, this relationship was not present for adolescents who perceived their family functioning as within normal limits.

Studies in general population samples have also shed some light on the relationship between family functioning and disordered eating patterns characteristic of BED and BN. Neumark-Sztainer *et al.* (2000) reported increased risk of developing disordered eating among those who perceived parental communication, expectation and caring as low. In a nonclinical population sample, 'extreme weight control' behaviours, including vomiting and taking diet pills, laxatives or diuretics, were reported in 7% of adolescents. Such behaviours were associated with family factors including parental supervision/monitoring behaviours in boys, but not in girls. Protective family factors included: high parental expectations, connectedness with friends and adults outside the family (boys), maternal presence (in both sexes), family connectedness, positive family communication and high parental supervision and monitoring (in girls).

MacBrayer *et al.* (2001) found in their sample of 662 11–13-year-olds that negative teasing regarding weight and negative maternal modelling regarding food were both correlated with the development of bulimic symptomatology.

In summary, perceived family dysfunction appears to be elevated in families of children and adolescents with BN, as well as in children in general population samples displaying BN-like disordered eating behaviours. The cross-sectional design of most studies makes it difficult to ascertain whether family dysfunction is a result of a predisposing factor for ED symptoms. Parent–child disagreement on perceived family functioning is also a characteristic feature of BN. There is also evidence of significant heterogeneity within the BN population with respect to family functioning, with family stressors triggering ED symptoms only in a subset of patients with problematic family environments.

Course of illness

Little is known about the outcome of BN and BED in adolescence. Figures quoted for full recovery from BN in adolescence range from 33% at 2 years to an average of 48% after 5 years, 71.1% at 6 years and 69.9 % at 11 years (Fichter *et al.*, 1998; Keel *et al.*, 1999; Fairburn *et al.*, 2000).

The data on the age of onset remains inconclusive, but shorter duration of illness appears to positively affect outcome (Quadflieg & Fichter, 2003).

The course of recovery is not well elucidated, although in a 2-year follow-up of patients treated for BN, data suggested that behavioural symptoms of bingeing and purging remitted before the psychological symptom of fear of gaining weight. Obsession with weight and shape and disturbed body perception took the longer to remit and non-purging compensatory behaviours took the longest to remit (Clausen, 2004).

In retrospective studies on adults, BED appears to occur in two distinct patterns. In the first pattern, bingeing occurs prior to the onset of dieting (Raymond *et al.*, 1995) and in the second, the bingeing occurs after the onset of dieting (Marcus & Kalarchian, 2003). In the first group, weight problems begin at an age of about 12 years, bingeing occurs between 11–13 years and dieting at 14 to 17 years of age (Abbott *et al.*, 1998; Grilo & Masheb, 2000). This group appeared to have greater psychiatric disturbances including a history of BN and mood disturbances. In the second group, weight problems occur at a mean age of 19.6, dieting occurred at 20.4 years and binge eating at 28 years of age (Marcus *et al.*, 1995). Little is known about outcome. Fairburn *et al.* (2000) found that in a 5-year follow-up of adolescent and adult women, while only 8% received treatment, only 9% still met criteria for BED.

There is some crossover between diagnostic categories, including crossover from AN (Sullivan *et al.*, 1996), conversion to EDNOS (Fichter *et al.*, 1998) or, more rarely, crossover to AN (Keel & Mitchell, 1997).

Medical complications in bulimia nervosa and binge eating

Few clinical research studies have specifically focused on the medical complications of BED and BN in children and adolescents. The unique features of adolescents, and the developmental process of adolescence, are critical in understanding the medical complications of bingeing and BN (Brewerton, 2002). Like adults with BED and BN, children and adolescents utilize abnormal eating and weight-regulating behaviours (Mehler, 2003; Schneider, 2003). The interaction of these factors, coupled with the specific age of onset during adolescence, will influence the medical complications found in children and adolescents with BED and BN.

Common signs and symptoms

The signs and symptoms of children and adolescents with BED and BN are not always obvious, as these young people often appear physically healthy (Brewerton, 2002).

Russell's sign is the most characteristic sign of BN. Russell's sign is single or multiple abrasions, small lacerations or calluses on the dorsum of the hand overlying the metacarpophalangeal and interphalangeal joints, caused by repeated contact of the central incisors to the skin during induction of vomiting by stimulation of the gag reflex (Russell, 1979).

Other cutaneous findings associated with BN include petechial (usually on the face and neck) or conjunctival haemorrhages that appear soon after a vomiting episode (Gupta et al., 1987). Frequent vomiting and binge eating has been reported to cause hypertrophy of the salivary glands (Walsh, 1981). The prevalence in children and adolescents is unknown as is the exact aetiology. Tissue biopsies of these enlarged salivary glands have reported both normal and inflammatory tissue (Batsakis & McWhirter, 1972). The glandular enlargement is generally intermittent and typically bilateral painless and may occur within several days of excessive binge eating or vomiting. This is a medically benign condition, which resolves with the cessation of vomiting.

A wide array of oral and dental findings has been reported in adults with binge eating and BN. Clinicians should be aware of erythematous lesions or abrasion on the palate secondary to trauma by objects (toothbrush, cutlery, etc.) used to induce vomiting. There is evidence to suggest that the presence of dental enamel erosion is related to the duration and frequency of vomiting, which could explain why this is not a commonly reported physical sign in children and adolescents (McComb, 1993). Adolescents with binge eating and BN have a potential increased risk for dental caries due to excessive carbohydrate intake during binge eating.

Dehydration secondary to vomiting, laxative or diuretic use, and decreased fluid intake, will cause dry mouth and dry mucosa. Angular chelitis (dry and cracked lips with fissures at the angles of the mouth) may also be observed and suggest vitamin B deficiency due to dietary insufficiency (Gupta et al., 1987).

These young people may also experience significant weight fluctuations (5–10 lbs or 2.3–4.5 kg per week) as a result of their unpredictable eating and weight control behaviours.

Clinicians should also be aware that adolescents with BN may experience irregular menstrual periods, beyond the point in adolescent development where regular menstrual cycles should have been established (Gendall, 2000; Mehler, 2003; Le Grange, 2004). Finally, even though children and adolescents with BN may appear physically healthy and at a 'healthy weight' according to population norms, they may exhibit psychological signs of malnutrition – such as depression, irritability and obsessionality. This may be an indication that these children and adolescents are below a biologically determined set-point even at a weight considered to be 'normal'.

Every system in the body is affected by the dangerous weight control behaviours carried out by patients with BED and BN (Palla & Litt, 1988).

Fluids and electrolytes

Abnormalities of fluids and electrolytes, most commonly hypokalaemia, are found in children and adolescents with BN (Palla & Litt, 1988). This is the result of vomiting, laxative or diuretic abuse, water restriction, low salt intake and/or water-loading (Mitchell *et al.*, 1983; Mehler, 2003). Continual vomiting can cause hypokalaemic, hypochloraemic, metabolic alkalosis, and may be associated with cardiac arrythmias, muscular weakness and decreased gastro-intestinal motility. In one series, 27% of older adolescents and adults with BN developed a metabolic alkalosis (Mitchell *et al.*, 1983). Diuretic abuse may also result in hypochloraemic, metabolic alkalosis whereas acute diarrhoea associated with laxative use results in hyperchloraemic, metabolic acidosis. Vomiting or diuretic/laxative use can cause dehydration resulting in volume depletion causing dizziness, syncopy, weakness and confusion. Patients may develop hypotension, tachycardia, concentrated urine and increased blood urea nitrogen. Volume depletion induces hyperaldosteronism causing reflex fluid retention and peripheral oedema, particularly after an abrupt cessation of vomiting or the withdrawal of laxatives or diuretics (Mitchell *et al.*, 1983). This complication often makes it difficult for young people to discontinue their weight-control behaviours.

Cardiovascular complications

Cardiovascular abnormalities occur in adolescents with BN and cause significant morbidity and mortality. Generally, the cardiovascular instability is due to volume depletion or electrolyte imbalance. A case-control study of

Table 11.1. A Comparison of BN and BED

	Bulimia Nervosa	Binge Eating Disorder
Prevalence in adolescence	1%	1%
Age of onset	Late adolescence 18–19 years of age	Two peaks, 13–19 yrs of age or in adulthood mid to late twenties
Sex	1/10 are boys	1/3 of population are boys
Symptoms	Bingeing with compensatory behaviours such as purging or exercising	Bingeing without compensatory behaviours such as purging or exercising
Frequency of symptoms	Occurs minimum of twice a week for 3 months	Occurs minimum of twice a week for 6 months
Length of illness	Mean length of time to recover is 39 months	Unknown
Mortality	0–6%	Unknown
Weight	Can be underweight or normal weight or overweight	Majority are overweight or obese
Eating behaviour	Restriction predates bingeing/ purging	In younger age of onset bingeing predates dieting. In older age of onset dieting/restriction predates bingeing

electrocardiographic findings in adolescents with eating disorders reported no abnormalities in adolescents with BN (Panagiotopoulos, 2000). However, other studies have reported electrocardiographic abnormalities secondary to electrolyte disturbances, especially hypokalaemia (Palla & Litt, 1988).

In a study of patients with BN, 28% used syrup of ipecac to induce vomiting (Pope *et al.*, 1986). Ipecac contains the alkaloid emetine, a cardiotoxic substance that with repeated use can lead to irreversible cardiomyopathy (with sudden death). Ipecac has also been reported to cause hepatic toxicity (Tolstoi, 1990) and peripheral muscle weakness (Mitchell *et al.*, 1987).

Pulmonary complications

There is the potential for aspiration in those young people who vomit, leading to aspiration pneumonia. Young people who vomit are also at increased risk for primary pneumomediastinum, pneumothorax, subcutaneous emphysema and rib fractures (McAnarney *et al.*, 1983). Subcutaneous emphysema and pneumomediastinum, perhaps due to increased intrathoracic pressure, have been reported in an adolescent with self-induced vomiting (Overby & Litt, 1988).

Gastrointestinal complications

Gastrointestinal complications occur frequently and are a major source of morbidity for patients with BN. Binge eating can result in gastric dilatation, necrosis and perforation. Vomiting can lead to oesophageal and gastric irritation and bleeding, and gastro-oesophageal reflux (Mehler, 2003). Laxative abuse, primarily from stimulant laxatives, may lead to diarrhoea and fluid and electrolyte abnormalities. Long-term use of stimulant laxatives can result in hypofunctioning of the colon due to damage of the myenteric plexus. In addition, other long-term complications of stimulant laxative use include steatorrhoea, protein-losing gastroenteropathy, hypocalcaemia and hypomagnesaemia (Schneider, 2003).

Elevated serum amylase level has been found to be associated with frequent binge eating and vomiting behaviour (Mitchell et al., 1983). The elevated amylase is believed to be of salivary origin (Mitchell, 1987). Binge eating has been reported as a rare cause of acute pancreatitis.

Endocrine complications

Menstrual dysfunction, including oligomenorrhoea or amenorrhoea, is common in adolescents with BN. In a recent descriptive study of a large cohort of adolescents with eating disorders, more than a third of adolescents with BN reported menstrual irregularities (Le Grange et al., 2004). Patients with BN with irregular menses compared with those with regular menses were more likely to have a higher frequency of vomiting, a lower thyroxine (T_4) concentration, more cigarette smoking and lower fat intake. Patients with BN who have a history of AN or who have experienced oligomenorrhoea and amenorrhoea are at an increased risk for the development of osteopaenia (Schneider, 2003).

Neurologic consequences

To date, there have been no investigations using brain-imaging techniques in children and adolescents with binge eating or BN.

Conclusion

This chapter has attempted to provide a comprehensive review of the nature of BN and binge-eating symptoms in children and adolescents. Clinicians should have the same threshold of suspicion as to the presence of these conditions in children and adolescents as in adults. Many serious medical complications can occur with these disorders. Affected individuals should be carefully medically monitored.

REFERENCES

American Psychiatric Association (1994). *Diagnostic and Statistical Manual for Mental Disorders*, 4th edn. Washington, DC: APA.

Abbott, D.W., de Zwaan, M., Mussell, M.P. *et al.* (1998). Onset of binge eating and dieting in overweight women: Implications for etiology, associated features and treatment. *Journal of Psychosomatic Research*, **44**, 367–74.

Batsakis, J.G. & McWhirter, J.D. (1972). Non neoplastic diseases of the salivary glands. *American Journal of Gastroenterology*, **57**, 226–47.

Brewerton, T.D. (2002). Bulimia in children and adolescents. *Child and Adolescent Psychiatric Clinics of North America*, 237–56.

Carlat, D.J. & Carmango, C.A. Jr. (1991). Review of bulimia nervosa in males. *American Journal of Psychiatry*, **148**, 831–43.

Clausen, L. (2004). Time course of symptom remission in eating disorders. *International Journal of Eating Disorders*, **36**, 296–306.

Dare, C., Le Grange, D., Eisler, I. & Rutherford, J. (1994). Redefining the psychosomatic family: the pre-treatment family process in 26 eating disorder families. *International Journal of Eating Disorders*, **16**, 211–26.

Fairburn, C.G., Cooper, A.M., Doll, H.A., Norman, P. & O'Connor, M. (2000). The natural course of bulimia nervosa and binge eating in young women. *Archives of General Psychiatry*, **57**, 659–65.

Fichter, M.M., Quadflieg, N. & Gnutzmann, A. (1998). Binge eating disorder: treatment outcome over a 6-year course. *Journal of Psychosomatic Research*, **44**, 385–405.

Fornari, V., Wlodarczyk-Bisaga, K., Mathews, M., Sandberg, B., Mandel, F.S. & Katz, J.L. (1999). Perception of family functioning and depressive symptomatology in individuals with anorexia and bulimia nervosa. *Comprehensive Psychiatry*, **40**, 434–41.

Gendall, K.A., Bulik, C.M., Joyce, P.R., McIntosh, V.V. & Carter, F.A. (2000). Menstrual cycle irregularity in bulimia nervosa. Associated facts and changes with treatment. *Journal of Psychosomatic Research*, **49**, 409–15.

Grilo, C.M. & Masheb, R.M. (2000). Onset of dieting vs. binge eating in outpatients with binge eating disorder. *International Journal of Eating Disorders*, **24**, 404–9.

Gupta, M.A., Gupta, A.K. & Haberman, H.F. (1987). Dermatologic signs in anorexia nervosa and bulimia nervosa. *Archives of Dermatology*, **123**, 1386–90.

Johnson, W.G., Rohan, K.J. & Kirk, A.A. (2002). Prevalence and correlates of binge eating in White and African American adolescents. *Eating Behaviours*, **3**, 179–89.

Kaltiala-Heino, R., Rimpela, M., Rissanen, A. & Rantanen, P. (2001). Early puberty and early sexual activity are associated with bulimic-type eating pathology in middle adolescence. *Journal of Adolescent Health*, **28**, 346–52.

Keel, P.K. & Mitchell, J.E. (1997). Outcome in bulimia nervosa. *American Journal of Psychiatry*, **154**, 313–21.

Keel, P.K., Mitchell, J.E., Miller, K.B., Davis, T.L. & Crow, S.J. (1999). Long-term outcome of bulimia nervosa. *Archives of General Psychiatry*, **56**, 63–9.

Le Grange, D., Loeb, K.L., Van Orman, S. & Jellar, C.C. (2004). Bulimia nervosa in adolescents: a disorder in evolution? *Archives of Pediatric and Adolescent Medicine*, **158**, 478–82.

MacBrayer, E.K., Smith, G.I., McCarthy, D.M., Demos, S. & Simmons, J. (2004). The role of family of origin in food related experiences in bulimic symptomatology. *International Journal of Eating Disorders*, **30**, 149–60.

Marcus, M.D. & Kalarchian, M.A. (2003). Binge eating in children and adolescents. *International Journal of Eating Disorders*, **34** Suppl., S47–57.

Marcus, M.D., Moulton, M.M. & Greeno, C.G. (1995). Binge eating onset in obese patients with binge eating disorder. *Addictive Behaviours*, **20**, 747–55.

McAnarney, E.R., Greydanus, D.E., Campanella, V.A. & Hoekelman, R.A. (1983). Rib fractures and anorexia nervosa. *Journal of Adolescent Health Care*, **4**, 40–3.

McComb, R.J. (1993). Dental aspects of anorexia nervosa and bulimia nervosa. In *Medical Issues and the Eating Disorders: The Interface*, ed. Kaplan, A.S. & Garfinkel, P.E. New York: Brunner/Mazel.

McDermott, B.M., Batik, M., Roberts, L. & Gibbon, P. (2002). Parent and child report of family functioning in a clinical and child and adolescent eating disorders sample. *Australian and New Zealand Journal of Psychiatry*, **36**, 509–14.

Mehler, P.S. (2003). Bulimia nervosa. *New England Journal of Medicine*, **349**, 875–81.

Mitchell, J.E., Pyle, R.L., Eckert, E.D., Hatsukami, D. & Lentz, R. (1983). Electrolyte and other physiological abnormalities in patients with bulimia. *Psychological Medicine*, **13**, 273–8.

Mitchell, J.E., Seim, H.C., Colon, E. & Pomeroy, C. (1987). Medical complications and medical management of bulimia. *Annals of Internal Medicine*, **107**, 71–7.

Morris, A., Pinhas, L. & Katzman, D.K. (2003). Early-onset eating disorders. Canadian Pediatric Surveillance Program Annual Report, www.phac-aspc.gc.ca/publicat/cpsp-pcsp03/page6_e.html.

Neumark-Sztainer, D., Story, M., Hannan, P.J., Beuhring, T. & Resnick, M.D. (2000). Disordered eating among adolescents: associations with sexual, physical abuse and other familial/psychological factors. *International Journal of Eating Disorders*, **28**, 249–58.

Okon, D.M., Greene, A.L. & Smith, J.E. (2003). Family interactions predict intraindividual symptom variations. *International Journal of Eating Disorders*, **34**, 450–7.

Overby, K.J. & Litt, I.F. (1988). Mediastinal emphysema in an adolescent with anorexia nervosa and self-induced emesis. *Pediatrics*, **81**, 134–6.

Palla, B. & Litt, I.F. (1988). Medical complications of eating disorders in adolescents. *Pediatrics*, **81**, 613–23.

Panagiotopoulos, C., McCrindle, B.W., Hick, K. & Katzman, D.K. (2000). Electrocardiographic findings in adolescents with eating disorders. *Pediatrics*, **105**, 1100–5.

Patton, G.C., Selzer, R., Coffey, C., Carlin, J.B. & Wolfe, R. (1999). Onset of adolescent eating disorders: population based cohort study over 3 years. *British Medical Journal*, **318**, 765–8.

Pope, H.G. Jr, Hudson, J.I., Nixon, R.A. & Herridge, P.L. (1986). The epidemiology of ipecac abuse [letter]. *New England Journal of Medicine*, **314**, 245–6.

Quadflieg, N. & Fichter, M.M. (2003). The course and outcome of bulimia nervosa. *European Child and Adolescent Psychiatry*, **12**, Suppl. 1, 99–109.

Raymond, N.C., Mussell, M.P., Mitchell, J.E., de Zwaan, M. & Crosby, R.D. (1995). An age-matched comparison of subjects with binge eating disorder and bulimia nervosa. *International Journal of Eating Disorders*, **18**, 135–43.

Russell, G.F.M. (1979). Bulimia nervosa: an ominous variant of anorexia nervosa. *Psychological Medicine*, **9**, 429–48.

Schneider, M. (2003). Bulimia nervosa and binge eating disorder in adolescents. *Adolescent Medicine*, **14**, 119–31.

Steinhausen, H.C. (1999). Eating disorders. In *Risks and Outcome in Developmental Psychopathology*, ed. Steinhausen, H.C. & Verhulst, F. Oxford: Oxford University Press, pp. 210–30.

Stice, E., Killen, J.D., Hayward, C. & Taylor, C.B. (1998). Age of onset for binge eating and purging during late adolescence: a 4-year survival analysis. *Journal of Abnormal Psychology*, **107**, 671–5.

Striegel-Moore, R.H., Wilson, G.T., Wilfley, D.E., Elder, K.A. & Brownell, K.D. (1998). Binge eating in an obese community sample. *International Journal of Eating Disorders*, **23**, 27–37.

Stunkard, A.J. (1959). Eating patterns and obesity. *Psychiatric Quarterly*, **33**, 284–92.

Sullivan, P.F., Bulik, C.M., Carter, F.A., Gendall, K.A. & Joyce, P.R. (1996). The significance of a prior history of anorexia in bulimia nervosa. *International Journal of Eating Disorders*, **20**, 253–61.

Tolstoi, L.G. (1990). Ipecac-induced toxicity in eating disorders. *International Journal of Eating Disorders*, **9**, 371–5.

Wade, T.C., Treloar, S.A. & Martin, N.G. (2001). A comparison of family functioning, temperament, and childhood conditions in monozygotic twin pairs discordant for lifetime bulimia. *American Journal of Psychiatry*, **158**, 1155–7.

Walsh, B.T., Croft, C.B. & Katz, J.L. (1981). Anorexia nervosa and salivary gland enlargement. *International Journal of Psychiatry and Medicine*, **11**, 255–61.

12

Selective eating and other atypical eating problems

Dasha Nicholls[1] and Tony Jaffa[2]

[1]Great Ormond Street Hospital for Children NHS Trust, London, UK
[2]The Phoenix Centre, Fulbourn, Cambridge, UK

Introduction

This chapter describes the range of eating problems seen in middle childhood (latency) and early adolescence (prepubertal or early puberty) that do not fit within 'eating disorders' as a diagnostic category. The term 'atypical eating disorder' is, in our view, inadequate for the range of problems described here, since 'eating disorder' has come to mean something highly specific, namely eating disturbances associated with weight and shape concerns and a range of specific characteristic behaviours. Indeed, eating disorder definitions are so specific that many typical cases of anorexia nervosa seen in children and young adolescents would be classified as atypical, reflecting the developmental limitation of current definitions.

Equally, the term 'feeding disorder' is inadequate, since feeding disorders, both in name and in formal diagnostic criteria, refer to disorders starting in infancy and early childhood (usually before age 6) and which reflect a provider/child relationship in which the 'sufferer' has limited if any autonomy. It is beyond the scope of this chapter to discuss feeding disorders of infancy and early childhood in full – for a summary see Chatoor (2002) and Nicholls (2004). There is limited research evidence in the area of the eating problems we will describe and most of what is known is based on clinical experience. However, it is important to emphasize that the lack of research in the area does not reflect clinical severity – all the problems outlined below can present with severe physical, social and/or psychological impairment. Indeed it is often the most complex clinical cases that are hardest to classify.

Eating Disorders in Children and Adolescents, ed. Tony Jaffa and Brett McDermott. Published by Cambridge University Press. © Cambridge University Press 2007.

Problems of nosology

For feeding and eating, as for other everyday behaviours, the distinction between normal and abnormal is often not clear. While some eating behaviours could be considered clearly outside the normal range, for example self-induced vomiting, for the majority it is more a question of degree, necessitating agreement on when the threshold for 'abnormal' is reached and who defines this. A relative paucity of knowledge about normal feeding behaviours has led to reliance on parental report to determine 'disorder'. Good practice takes into account a combination of parental report, the subjective experience of the child and the observed behaviour of the child and of parent/child interaction, but even so the complex relationship between these perspectives makes operational criteria difficult to refine.

Our knowledge of problem eating behaviour in children is hampered as much by limited understanding of 'normal' eating behaviours as it is by a lack of large clinical samples. For example, information about typical length of mealtimes in infants and toddlers has only recently been established, from which a definition of slow eating was derived (Reau et al., 1996). Another example is picky or faddy eating, which occurs in over 20% of toddlers (Richman & Lansdown, 1988), and can be considered normal at a particular developmental stage. In a small number of children, particularly boys, the behaviour persists into middle childhood and adolescence. At some point the behaviour moves outside the bounds of normal development, but even then may be simply delayed, i.e. the child will eventually grow out of it, rather than deviant. As with many childhood disturbances of behaviour or emotion, categorical models are unhelpful, and a dimensional approach to problem definition preferable.

The dimensional nature of eating problems, lack of consensus about the perspective from which to describe eating problems, and the fact that mild eating problems are common but severe eating problems rare, mean that at this time there is no widely accepted theory-based or empirically derived classification system for the eating problems in childhood and early adolescence, and consequently very little empirical research in the field. Two papers merit mention in terms of attempting to improve nosology. Chatoor et al. (2002) have derived operational diagnostic criteria for six feeding disorders in infants and young children, based on clinical experience and empirical studies. They include: feeding disorder of state regulation, feeding disorder of reciprocity, infantile anorexia, sensory food aversions, feeding disorder associated with concurrent medical condition and post-traumatic feeding disorder. The potential value of this classification system to older children is unclear. Second, Crist & Napier-Phillips (2001) used a feeding screening questionnaire to empirically derive subtypes of feeding problem from control and clinically referred subjects. They identified five factors which accounted for 55% of the total variance for the combined clinical and normative groups: picky eaters, toddler refusal-general, toddler refusal-textured foods, older children refusal-general and stallers. This leaves a significant proportion of cases unclassified, but does have scientific merit.

The way in which feeding disorders and eating problems presenting clinically are categorized also depends on the profession to which they present. For example, speech and language therapists tend to consider the presence or absence of oromotor dysfunction a key factor (Wickendon, 2000), whilst symptom-based or attachment-based classifications predominate in the psychological literature. The terms we use below have arisen from clinical experience and from what literature exists.

From feeding to eating

One of many developmental tasks of childhood and early adolescence is managing the transition from feeding to eating. As with most developmental goals the task is multifaceted, and includes:

Selection of appropriate foods for age and developmental stage; broadening range of foods and achieving nutritional balance across the food groups

Physical handling of food, from swallowing and chewing through to using a knife and fork

Sensory integration – exposure to and tolerance of new sensory experiences in all domains, particularly taste and smell

Food hygiene and safety, linked to preparing and, later, buying food

Managing social aspects of eating, such as participating in meals, sharing, table manners, speed of eating, etc.

Developing regular eating patterns

Regulation of food intake including energy balance sufficient to sustain growth and development; accurate recognition of internal cues of hunger and satiety

Effective communication of needs (e.g. saying 'I'm upset' rather than 'my tummy hurts') and their accurate interpretation (e.g. parents recognizing when 'I'm not hungry' means 'I'm upset'). The older the child, the more the emphasis is on the child communicating effectively

Moving from dependence on caregivers to self-care, enabling separation

These continuous processes begin at birth and by adulthood a degree of independence around eating behaviour has usually been achieved. Whilst managing nutritional intake and energy balance can be a lifelong task, it is rare for adults to regress to earlier developmental stages typified by feeding except in circumstances of severe illness or disability. This process of transfer of responsibility for eating from carer to child is a careful balance of timing and encouragement – too much parental regulation and the child may rebel; too much autonomy for the child and he or she may not be able to cope. As such the transition from feeding to eating is highly susceptible to tension and conflict, particularly over issues of autonomy and control. It is also a point of communication between a child and his or her parent, and can be a means for communicating distress or anxiety.

Throughout childhood and adolescence, problems may arise in any of these developmental processes, either because the skills are never attained (primary problems) or through loss of skills previously gained (secondary problems). Each domain is susceptible to environmental influence, even those that may have a neurological basis such as dyspraxia. It is in the latter two components of feeding/eating transition, i.e. effective communication of needs and managing separation, where psychological problems most commonly arise. This may be in combination with difficulties of mastery in other aspects of the transition from feeding to eating or in other domains of everyday life. For each of the eating problems outlined below one or more of these components of the transition from feeding to eating has been affected, rendering the child dependent on others for adequate nutritional intake.

Aetiology

From the above, it is clear that understanding the development of feeding problems needs to take into account factors in the child, parental factors, factors within the child/parent relationship and parenting issues, within a bio-psycho-social framework. From the history, factors that may have been associated with onset can be identified, such as medical treatment; a traumatic incident such as choking, loss events or moves; a developmental problem; a medical condition; beliefs about feeding and parental roles; or any combination of these. Factors associated with onset can then be usefully differentiated from factors that appear to maintain the problem, such as continued medical problems/treatment causing discomfort, ongoing conflict and coercive cycles around feeding, etc.

Physical factors that have been identified as important in the aetiology of feeding problems include inefficient infant feeding due to poor sucking, which has been associated with subsequent growth, later feeding difficulties and maternal feeding practices (Ramsay *et al.*, 2002b). Taking fewer sucks per feed and a reduced volume of breast milk taken have also been reported in children aged 4–5 years described by parents as picky eaters when compared with control children (Jacobi *et al.*, 2003).

In terms of characteristics of the child, children with feeding difficulties are also more likely than controls to have their temperament described as difficult (propensity to distress), irregular (increased routine variability) and sober (propensity to negative emotionality) (Chatoor *et al.*, 2000), and are more likely to be reported as showing negative affect (Jacobi *et al.*, 2003).

Parental factors have also been suggested as important, although the findings are mixed. Particular concerns have been raised in children where maternal eating restraint and drive for thinness are prominent (Stice *et al.*, 1999). There is evidence that mothers with eating disorders are more likely to use food to reward and to express love, be concerned about their (female) child's weight and fail to express positive attitudes towards food and mealtimes in a way that may impact on enjoyment and discourage exploration of variety in the diet (Agras *et al.*, 1999; Waugh & Bulik, 1999). McDermott *et al.* (submitted manuscript) found that maternal depression and anxiety were factors in predicting whether children were picky eaters, whereas maternal depression was found not to affect feeding practices, infant feeding abilities or growth in a study looking at predictors of failure to thrive (Ramsay *et al.*, 2002). In a study of severe clinical feeding problems, parents rated the severity of feeding problems significantly higher than clinicians, and severity rating was correlated with parental self-report on the general health questionnaire (a measure of psychological well-being) (Nicholls & Avnon, in preparation). Quantifiable or observable items (e.g. weight, range of foods) showed greater reliability between parents and clinicians as descriptors of feeding problems than subjective measures (e.g. 'interest in food').

Finally, parent–child interaction is at the heart of the feeding process, and can contribute significantly regardless of whether additional factors, such as developmental delay, are also present. The classification of feeding problems proposed by Chatoor *et al.* (2002) includes at least two types where the difficulty is related to the dyadic nature of feeding, namely 'Feeding Disorder of Reciprocity (onset between 2 and 6 months of age)' and 'Infantile Anorexia (onset during the transition to spoon and self-feeding)'. In the former, Chatoor suggests, at a developmental period when regulation of food intake is closely linked to the infant's affective engagement, if caregiver and infant are not successfully engaged with each other, feeding and growth suffer. In infantile anorexia, the parent is thought to misinterpret the infant's cues and respond to the infant's emotional needs by offering food. The infant will then confuse hunger with emotional experiences and learn to eat or refuse to eat when bored, lonely, frustrated or angry (Chatoor *et al.*, 2000).

Selective eating

Extreme faddy eating that persists into middle childhood and adolescence has been termed selective eating (Bryant-Waugh, 2000), picky or choosy eating (Jacobi *et al.*, 2003) or perseverative feeding disorder (Harris & Booth, 1992). Variations in terminology make comparisons across the literature difficult, but all these descriptions describe children with two essential features: a highly limited range of foods (generally 10 foods or less) and extreme reluctance to try new foods. In terms of the developmental task of the transition to eating, in selective eating there are nutritional aspects not achieved, and since the preferred foods are often soft carbohydrate-based finger foods, the child may not have developed chewing skills or learnt to use a knife and fork. Difficulties in sensory integration may be a factor to a greater or lesser degree. In addition, this type of eating pattern has often led to exclusion from social norms around eating. Finally feeding as a point of parent–child communication has often become distorted by conflict and resistance. Each of these aspects needs to be considered in the assessment and management plan.

Many authors use the term food neophobia (fear of trying new foods) and picky eating interchangeably (Carruth & Skinner, 2000). Others such as Galloway and colleagues make a clear distinction between picky eating and neophobia, asserting from their study that whereas pickiness was predicted primarily by environmental or experiential factors subject to changes, neophobia was predicted by more enduring and dispositional factors (Galloway *et al.*, 2003). As noted above, picky eating is a common feature in toddlers and generally this is a phase that children 'grow out of', but for a minority of children food neophobic behaviours do not improve with maturity (Carruth & Skinner, 2000). Food neophobia is a dimensional trait which Pliner & Loewen (1997) conceptualize as a personality trait, embedded in other aspects of the child's temperament. Overall rates of food neophobia in the population are low (Koivisto & Sjoden, 1996), with males having higher rates than females, and reducing with age. Highly neophobic people can be influenced by strong modelling, but not generalize to non-modelled foods (Hobden & Pliner, 1995). Studies in adults have shown high neophobia to be positively correlated with trait anxiety and negatively correlated with novelty seeking. In children, Pliner

& Loewen (1997) found correlations between shyness and emotionality and reluctance to try unfamiliar foods.

Consistent with this, anxiety symptoms are sometimes, but not always, a feature of children and young adolescents with selective eating presenting to clinical services (Nicholls *et al.*, 2001). In selective eating, food neophobia is of such a marked degree that concern about the impact on the child's social activities or conflict as a result of the child's highly rigid eating patterns have arisen. Timimi *et al.* (1997) noted that whilst mealtimes are a battle-ground in families of younger selective eaters, many parents of older children with selective eating seemed to have given up trying to change their children's eating habits, and concern about the impact of restricted diet on physical health or social development is the presenting concern. In general gross measures of well-being (growth, pubertal development) are unaffected by a highly limited nutritional range, provided the child is not underweight (Nicholls *et al.*, 2001). However, Timimi *et al.* (1997), using a broader age range, and definition, found that 'a significant minority had poor growth or weight gain'.

Over a period of years children with selective eating develop an avoidance-reinforced anxiety associated with new foods. There may be anticipatory nausea (with sight or smell triggers), fear of vomiting (textures) or a fear of choking. Treatment is often required for the child to be able to broaden his/her food repertoire but inevitably the anxiety induced by treatment may itself result in exacerbation of the condition. If the child is not committed to change, the resultant anxiety may result in avoidance again. Motivational skills can be useful if the child is not committed to change, and otherwise suggesting they return at a later date may be appropriate. For those children who are ready to change, a cognitive-behaviour therapy model based on age-appropriate food records, relaxation and reward, led by the child, can be rapidly effective although the child's food range may remain somewhat limited. On follow-up, one mother described her much-recovered son as a 'normal fussy eater'. It is debatable whether progress is best measured psychologically or by counting foods.

There have been no long-term outcome studies looking at selective eating and little is known about the prevalence of selective eating in older children and adults. Interestingly, picky eating is the only type of early feeding problem that has been linked to later eating disorders, specifically anorexia nervosa (Marchi & Cohen, 1990). The similarity in terms of rigidity of eating pattern, anxiety and communication difficulties, and risk aversion would fit intuitively, although many subsequent studies have found no such link. The population in which selective eating is a common feature are children with autistic spectrum disorder (ASD) (Schreck *et al.*, 2004). Many children with ASD have, in common with many children with selective eating, increased sensitivity to texture and smell, a well-developed sense of disgust and difficulties with messy play. Assessment of children in whom selective eating has persisted or is extreme should include features of neurodevelopmental disorders which will be found in a proportion of clinical cases (Nicholls *et al.*, 2001).

Food avoidance emotional disorder (FAED)

This term is used to describe avoidance of food to a marked degree in the absence of the characteristic psychopathology of eating disorders in terms of weight and shape cognitions. The term was coined over 15 years ago (Higgs *et al.*, 1989) although few studies have emerged to clarify its nosological status other than to clearly distinguish it from anorexia nervosa (Cooper *et al.*, 2002). Clinically, this group would appear to be heterogeneous and to include patients for whom somatization is a prominent feature of their illness, with food avoidance one of the presenting symptoms. Others show many behaviours similar to 'true' eating disorders, but do not exhibit weight and shape concerns. The term FAED has mainly been used to describe cases presenting in middle childhood and early adolescence in which age group it may be more common than anorexia nervosa or bulimia nervosa. It excludes children who are chronically low in weight (restrictive eaters or failure to thrive), and those in whom the range of foods eaten is limited but weight is not generally compromised ('selective eating').

Presenting features include marked weight loss. Unlike patients with anorexia nervosa, children with FAED know that they are underweight, would like to be heavier, and may not know why they find this difficult to achieve. A child with FAED may give any number of reasons for not being able to eat: fear of being sick, 'not hungry', 'can't eat', 'hurts my tummy', etc. Comorbid obsessional anxiety or depression may be present, but often food avoidance exists as an isolated symptom. The anxiety related to eating can be as marked in FAED as in anorexia nervosa. The developmental issues affected are primarily around emotional communication and self-reliance.

These children are more likely to have other medically unexplained symptoms, and occasionally parents attribute weight loss to undiagnosed physical disorder. Addressing these concerns with a comprehensive physical assessment and an open mind is essential if a therapeutic alliance is to be successfully achieved. Inevitably some cases will actually have previously unidentified organic pathology, the commonest being inflammatory bowel diseases, food allergies and intracranial pathology (De Vile *et al.*, 1995). We have come to use the term FAED when food avoidance is marked and merits treatment intervention in its own right.

Treatment includes working with the child to find alternative ways of naming and identifying feelings, whilst supporting parents to support their child in his/her rehabilitation, alongside rigorous treatment of any comorbid psychological condition such as depression or anxiety disorder. The longterm course of FAED and its relationship with earlier feeding problems such as failure to thrive has not been established, although from clinical experience it is likely that a minority of children with FAED later develop anorexia nervosa.

Food phobias and obsessive-compulsive disorder

Phobias involving food occur in isolation (i.e. as simple phobias), or as part of a more generalized anxiety disorder. The overlap with other eating problems is evident, since food avoidance is a feature of most of the problems we describe. The nature of the specific fear will vary with, amongst other things, the child's developmental stage. Fears that are common are fear of vomiting (emetophobia), fear of contamination or poisoning, fear of choking or swallowing (functional dysphagia – discussed further below) and fear of the consequences of hypercholesterolaemia (Lifshitz, 1987). Common associated problems include depression, panic attacks, social anxiety, compulsions and difficulties with separation.

Food phobias are usually secondary events i.e. follow a period of normal eating for developmental stage. Clear trigger events may be identified in some but not all cases e.g. choking events, or in one case fear of cholesterol developed after the child saw his father die of a myocardial infarction. Presenting features include rigid eating patterns and associated conflict, restricted range of foods and, in more extreme cases, restricted quantity of food leading to weight loss. Factors influencing the extent to which obsessional rituals have taken hold include contextual factors such as familial responses to the child's anxiety. Singer *et al.* (1992) have described an approach to treatment, based on family involvement and anxiety management.

In some children, food phobias may be a feature of more pervasive anxiety disorder or obsessive-compulsive disorder (OCD). Obsessive-compulsive disorder can present as food-related obsessions in the absence of weight and shape concerns. For example, a child may develop obsessional fear about the content of food, or about the freshness of food, such that food intake is limited to those sources which are of 'known' safety in terms of cleanliness, and only certain family members are entrusted to prepare food. The association between anorexia nervosa and OCD is well recognized (Shafran *et al.*, 1995).

Functional dysphagia

Functional dysphagia is a term used to describe swallowing difficulties associated with a fear of choking. This symptom is found clinically in patients with FAED, selective eating, food refusal and sometimes anorexia nervosa. It is also found as an isolated symptom of acute onset, often following trauma. The validity of functional dysphagia as a separate diagnostic category needs clarification.

A range of interventions contribute to effective treatment. Psycho-education may for example take the form of showing the actual images of the barium swallow and explaining gastrointestinal anatomy. Graded exposure work with speech and language consultation may lead to trying different food textures, practice in chewing and swallowing increasingly large food items. Behavioural rewards are likely to be effective in combination with other interventions. Family therapy is used to look at beliefs, anxieties and expectations about food and fussy eating; to identify possible factors maintaining the problem; and to enlist family support for recovery, for instance by involving the family in practical aspects of meal time management. The effective use of anxiolytic medication has also been described (Koon, 1983). Treatment can take a number of months and may necessitate a period of inpatient treatment.

Psychogenic vomiting

Psychogenic vomiting is a distinct diagnostic category in the International Classification of Disease Version 10 (ICD–10), although little elaboration is provided other than to make the clear distinction between 'vomiting associated with other psychological disturbances' and vomiting as seen in bulimia nervosa. The diagnosis includes vomiting in association with dissociative disorders and in hypochondriacal disorder. The symptom may be anxiety related, although overt anxiety is not always evident. Assessment will determine whether the child has developed an extreme sensitivity to emetic triggers, for which children with a history of gastro-oesophageal reflux or vomiting associated with illness may be more at risk. Occasionally vomiting is of sufficient severity to inhibit all food intake, in which case the first step is to establish feeding, enterally if necessary, whilst anxiety management techniques in combination with family work aim for desensitization to oral feeding, using a non-confrontational approach and providing adequate emotional support to the child and family.

Food refusal

Food refusal as an isolated behaviour is an experience most parents encounter at some point during their child's development, hence 'the train is coming to the station' and other feeding games. Food refusal in older children is often associated with other defiant behaviours such as delaying eating by talking, trying to negotiate what food will be eaten, getting up from the table during meals, and refusing to eat much at a meal, but requesting food immediately afterwards. Much of the nutritional intake of these children is gained through snacking between meals. These behaviours mostly seem to reflect general disruptive behaviour, rather than possible oral motor difficulties (Crist & Napier-Phillips, 2001).

Occasionally food refusal is severe and extreme, associated with other refusal behaviours and poor functioning. Pervasive refusal syndrome (Lask et al., 1991) is a term used to describe 'profound and pervasive refusal to eat, walk, talk or engage in self care'. This rare condition has been conceptualized as both an extreme post-traumatic stress reaction in cases of evident or suspected abuse (Lask et al., 1991), and as a form of learned helplessness (Nunn & Thompson, 1996). The term pervasive refusal, though evocative and easily recognized by anyone who has met these children, may itself be problematic in the development of a therapeutic alliance.

Priorities for future research

The eating problems described herein are of uncertain nosological status and linked to this is a lack of systematic research in the area. Priority areas for future research include epidemiological studies of childhood problem eating behaviours to enable a better understanding of the range of normal eating in childhood and early adolescence. From this a dimensional approach to defining problems eating could be derived.

Also needed are longitudinal prospective clinical studies to clarify the course of problem eating, explore links with earlier feeding and later eating pathology and to determine the extent to which developmental pathways converge or diverge with maturity.

Service issues

As is the case for anorexia nervosa, services for those with atypical eating problems are generally deficient. This reflects the mistaken perception that these conditions are rare and not serious. There may also be differing views as to whether they are best managed by generic versus specialist services. Our own belief is that these problems should be managed by practitioners who not only have the required skills and training but also who see a sufficient volume of such cases to maintain these. It is perhaps of secondary importance whether they are located in specialist teams or in special interest sections of generic teams. A further dilemma is whether management should be by psychiatric or paediatric services. As above our own view is that it is the skill rather than the discipline which is important, though, perhaps reflecting our own professional backgrounds, our bias is towards child mental health services taking primary responsibility with adequate liaison with paediatricians where necessary.

REFERENCES

Agras, S., Hammer, L. & McNicholas, F. (1999). A prospective study of the influence of eating-disordered mothers on their children. *International Journal of Eating Disorders*, **25**, 253–62.

Bryant-Waugh, R. (2000). Overview of the Eating Disorders. In *Anorexia Nervosa and Related Eating Disorders in Childhood and Adolescence*, 2nd edition, ed. Lask, B. & Bryant-Waugh, B. Hove, East Sussex: Psychology Press, pp. 27–40.

Carruth, B.R. & Skinner, J.D. (2000). Revisiting the picky eater phenomenon: neophobic behaviors of young children. *Journal of the American College of Nutrition*, **19**, 771–80.

Chatoor, I. (2002). Feeding disorders in infants and toddlers: diagnosis and treatment. *Child and Adolescent Psychiatric Clinics of North America*, **11**, 163–83.

Chatoor, I., Ganiban, J., Hirsch, R., Borman-Spurrell, E. & Mrazek, D.A. (2000b). Maternal characteristics and toddler temperament in infantile anorexia. *Journal of the American Academy of Child and Adolescent Psychiatry*, **39**, 743–51.

Cooper, P.J., Watkins, B., Bryant-Waugh, R. & Lask, B. (2002). The nosological status of early onset anorexia nervosa. *Psychological Medicine*, **32**, 873–80.

Crist, W. & Napier-Phillips, A. (2001). Mealtime behaviors of young children: a comparison of normative and clinical data. *Journal of Developmental and Behavioral Pediatrics*, **22**, 279–86.

De Vile, C.J., Sufraz, R., Lask, B. & Stanhope, R. (1995). Occult intracranial tumours masquerading as early onset anorexia nervosa. *British Medical Journal*, **311**, 1359–60.

Galloway, A.T., Lee, Y. & Birch, L.L. (2003). Predictors and consequences of food neophobia and pickiness in young girls. *Journal of the American Dietetic Association*, **103**, 692–8.

Harris, G. & Booth, I.W. (1992). The nature and management of eating problems in pre-school children. In *Feeding Problems and Eating Disorders in Children and Adolescents. Monographs in Clinical Pediatrics No. 5*, ed. Cooper, P.J. & Stein, A. Chur: Harwood Academic Publishers, pp. 61–85.

Higgs, J.F., Goodyer, I.M. & Birch, J. (1989). Anorexia nervosa and food avoidance emotional disorder. *Archives of Disease in Childhood*, **64**, 346–51.

Hobden, K. & Pliner, P. (1995). Effects of a model on food neophobia in humans. *Appetite*, **25**, 101–13.

Jacobi, C., Agras, W.S., Bryson, S. & Hammer, L.D. (2003). Behavioral validation, precursors, and concomitants of picky eating in childhood. *Journal of the American Academy of Child and Adolescent Psychiatry*, **42**, 76–84.

Koivisto, U.K. & Sjoden, P.O. (1996). Food and general neophobia in Swedish families: parent-child comparisons and relationships with serving specific foods. *Appetite*, **26**, 107–18.

Koon, R. (1983). Conversion dysphagia in children. *Psychosomatics*, **24**, 182–4.

Lask, B., Britten, C., Kroll, L., Magagna, J. & Tranter, M. (1991). Pervasive refusal in children. *Archives of Disease in Childhood*, **66**, 866–9.

Lifshitz, F. (1987). Nutritional dwarfing in adolescents. *Growth, Genetics and Hormones*, **3**, 1–5.

Marchi, M. & Cohen, P. (1990). Early childhood eating behaviors and adolescent eating disorders. *Journal of the American Academy of Child and Adolescent Psychiatry*, **29**, 112–17.

Nicholls, D. (2004). Feeding disorders in infancy and early childhood. In *Clinical Handbook of Eating Disorders*, ed. Brewerton, T.D. New York: Marcel Dekker, pp. 47–69.

Nicholls, D., Christie, D., Randall, L. & Lask, B. (2001). Selective eating: symptom, disorder or normal variant? *Clinical Child Psychology and Psychiatry*, **6**, 257–70.

Nunn, K.P. & Thompson, S. (1996). The pervasive refusal syndrome: learned helplessness and hopelessness. *Clinical Child Psychology and Psychiatry*, **1**, 121–32.

Pliner, P. & Loewen, E.R. (1997). Temperament and food neophobia in children and their mothers. *Appetite*, **28**, 239–54.

Ramsay, M., Gisel, E.G., McCusker, J., Bellavance, F. & Platt, R. (2002a). Infant sucking ability, non-organic failure to thrive, maternal characteristics, and feeding practices: a prospective cohort study. *Developmental Medicine and Child Neurology*, **44**, 405–14.

Reau, N.R., Senturia, Y.D., Lebailly, S.A. & Christoffel, K.K. (1996). Infant and toddler feeding patterns and problems: normative data and a new direction. Pediatric Practice Research Group. *Journal of Developmental and Behavioural Pediatrics*, **17**, 149–53.

Richman, N. & Lansdown, R. (1988). *Problems of Preschool Children*. Chichester: John Wiley and Sons.

Schreck, K.A., Williams, K. & Smith, A.F. (2004). A comparison of eating behaviors between children with and without autism. *Journal of Autism and Developmental Disorders*, **34**, 433–8.

Shafran, R., Bryant-Waugh, R., Lask, B. & Arscott, K. (1995). Obsessive-compulsive symptoms in children with eating disorders: a preliminary investigation. *Eating Disorders: The Journal of Treatment and Prevention*, **3**, 304–10.

Singer, L. T., Ambuel, B., Wade, S. & Jaffe, A. C. (1992). Cognitive-behavioral treatment of health-impairing food phobias in children. *Journal of the American Academy of Child and Adolescent Psychiatry*, **31**, 847–52.

Stice, E., Agras, W. S. & Hammer, L. D. (1999). Risk factors for the emergence of childhood eating disturbances: a five-year prospective study. *International Journal of Eating Disorders*, **25**, 375–87.

Timimi, S., Douglas, J. & Tsiftsopoulou, K. (1997). Selective eaters: a retrospective case note study. *Child: Care, Health and Development*, **23**, 265–78.

Waugh, E. & Bulik, C. M. (1999). Offspring of women with eating disorders. *International Journal of Eating Disorders*, **25**, 123–33.

Wickendon, M. (2000). The development and disruption of feeding skills: how speech and language therapists can help. In *Feeding Problems in Children: A Practical Guide*, ed. Southall, A. & Schwartz, A. Abingdon, Oxon: Radcliffe Medical Press, pp. 3–23.

13

Comorbid anxiety and depression and the role of trauma in children and adolescents with eating disorders

Timothy D. Brewerton

Medical University of South Carolina, Charleston, SC, USA

Introduction

In many cases it is not the eating disorder (ED) symptom or sign per se that brings the child or adolescent with an ED into treatment, but instead it is a related yet serious comorbid problem or condition which merits medical and/or psychiatric attention, e.g. suicide attempt, depression and/or anxiety. Even when the ED is established at presentation the recognition of comorbid anxious and depressive symptoms in children and adolescents is of paramount importance for successful treatment and outcome. The presence or absence of comorbidity may affect long-term prognosis.

Anxiety

In a study of 2525 Australian teenagers Patton *et al.* (1997) found psychiatric comorbidity to be the clearest factor associated with extreme dieting with 62% of extreme dieters reporting high levels of both anxiety and depression.

Bulik *et al.* (1997) looked at the prevalence and age of onset of anxiety disorders in 68 women with anorexia nervosa (AN), 116 women with bulimia nervosa (BN), 56 women with major depression (MD) with no ED and 98 randomly selected controls (RC). Comorbid anxiety disorders were common in all three patient groups (AN, 60%; BN, 57%; MD, 48%). In those cases with comorbid anxiety, 90% of AN women, 94% of BN women and 71% of MD women had anxiety disorders preceding the current primary condition ($P \leq$ 0.01). It is of note, however, that panic disorder tended to develop after the onset of AN, BN or MD rather than preceding these conditions. In multivariate

Eating Disorders in Children and Adolescents, ed. Tony Jaffa and Brett McDermott. Published by Cambridge University Press. © Cambridge University Press 2007.

logistic regressions, the odds ratios (OR) for overanxious disorder (OD) (OR = 13.4) and obsessive-compulsive disorder (OCD) (OR = 11.8) were significantly elevated for AN. The ORs for OD and social phobia (SP) were significantly elevated for BN (OR OD = 4.9; OR SP = 15.5) and MD (OR OD = 6.1; OR SP = 6.4). It appears from these data that certain anxiety disorders are nonspecific risk factors for later mood and EDs, and others may represent more specific antecedent risk factors. Although this is a study of adults, the fact that the onset of OD is exclusively during childhood and the onsets of social phobia and OCD are usually during childhood is relevant to this discussion.

Separation anxiety disorder (SAD) is probably the most common anxiety disorder presenting during childhood and may increase the risk of subsequent anxiety and mood disorders. Bailly-Lambin & Bailly (1999) assessed current and lifetime psychiatric disorders and psychopathological profiles using structured interviews and self-report questionnaires in 81 young patients with AN or BN according to DSM–III–R criteria. Results revealed that approximately 20% of patients with AN and BN had a past history of childhood SAD. This subgroup had significantly higher rates of associated anxiety and mood disorders compared to those without childhood SAD.

In another French study of 63 patients with DSM–IV-defined AN or BN, Godart et al. (2000) assessed the lifetime prevalence of seven anxiety disorders, including childhood SAD, and the age of onset of anxiety disorders relative to that of EDs. Seventy-one percent of BN subjects and 83% of AN subjects had at least one lifetime diagnosis of an anxiety disorder. The most frequent anxiety disorder diagnosis was social phobia (59% of BN; 55% of AN), which has been found in other studies (Lilenfeld, 2004). Notably, the comorbid anxiety disorder was found to predate the onset of the ED in 88% of subjects with BN and 75% of subjects with AN. Anxiety disorders during childhood and/or adolescence may therefore function as important risk factors in the development of EDs.

These same investigators (Flament et al., 2001) found that the great majority of AN and BN subjects had significant and measurable impairments in social and occupational domains. Further, these were predicted by a history of childhood SAD, social avoidance symptoms, as well as a higher number of lifetime anxiety disorders. Their results further underscore the importance of early recognition and treatment of comorbid anxiety disorders and symptoms in children and adolescents with EDs in order to improve social adaptation and global psychopathological outcome.

Moorhead et al. (2003) reported results from a 22-year longitudinal community study which investigated early predictors for developing EDs by young adulthood. Twenty-one women identified at age 27 with lifetime full or partial

EDs were compared with 47 women with no ED history on predictive factors from three broad domains. The women with EDs had more serious health problems before age 5 and mother-reported anxiety and depression at age 9. At 15, mothers also described them as having more behaviour problems.

In a prospective 10-year study, Herpertz-Dahlmann *et al.* (2001) evaluated 39 inpatients with adolescent-onset AN at 3, 7 and 10 years after discharge and compared them with 39 matched controls using structured interviews. The authors found that while 69% of the original subjects were fully recovered from their AN at the 10-year follow-up, 51% of the former AN patients currently had an axis I psychiatric disorder and 23% met the full criteria for a personality disorder. Apart from the ED, anxiety disorders and avoidant-dependent and obsessive-compulsive personality disorders were the most common diagnoses. Furthermore, at each time point there were significant associations between psychiatric comorbidity and the outcome of the ED and between outcome and psychosocial adaptation.

In one of the best prospective studies, Johnson *et al.* (2002) used data from a community-based longitudinal investigation to determine whether adolescents with EDs are at elevated risk for physical and mental disorders during early adulthood. Structured interviews were administered to a representative community sample of 717 adolescents and their mothers in 1983, 1985–86 and 1991–93. Follow-up of adolescents diagnosed with EDs revealed that by early adulthood they had elevated rates of anxiety disorders and other medical and psychiatric conditions, including depressive disorders, cardiovascular symptoms, chronic fatigue, chronic pain, limitations in activities due to poor health, infectious diseases, insomnia, neurological symptoms and suicide attempts. Impressively, these findings were substantiated even after age, sex, socio-economic status (SES), co-occurring psychiatric disorders, adolescent health problems, body mass index (BMI) and worries about health during adulthood were controlled for statistically. Only 22% of the adolescents with current EDs had received psychiatric treatment within the past year. These results leave no doubt that EDs during adolescence are likely associated with an elevated risk for a broad range of physical and mental health problems during early adulthood, including anxiety and mood disorders. For further discussion on longitudinal perspectives, outcome and prognosis see Steinhausen (Chapter 22, this volume).

Depression

Some of the studies mentioned above in regard to anxiety also indicate high rates of depressive symptoms in association with EDs, but these will not be repeated here. Devaud *et al.* (1998) measured the prevalence of EDs and behavioural–mental problems in a national representative sample of 1084 15- to 20-year-old adolescent girls in Switzerland. These female students completed a self-administered questionnaire focusing on eating behaviour and body image. Those girls who indicated high levels of weight and body image concern or problematic eating behaviour reported significantly more mood problems (P < 0.05), suicidal behaviours (P < 0.05) and violent and aggressive behaviours (P < 0.05). No relationship was found between ED and substance use. Associations with acting-out behaviours were greater among subjects with high rates of problematic eating behaviour, whereas associations with mood disorders were stronger among subjects with high rates of weight and body image concerns.

In a sample of 1000 adolescents age 15–19 years from northeastern Italy, Miotto *et al.* (2003) investigated the links between EDs and suicidal tendencies by means of self-report measures. More females than males reported abnormal eating patterns suggesting EDs. However, both males and females reporting suicidal ideation had significantly higher scores on ED measures, and this was not accounted for by age, SES or BMI.

Perez *et al.* (2004) noted that very few studies have investigated the specific associations of major depression (MD) versus dysthymia with EDs. They studied 937 adolescents who were repeatedly assessed for mood disorders until the age of 24. Statistical analyses revealed that dysthymia was a more powerful correlate with (and possible risk factor for) BN than MD, even after controlling for other mood disorders and a history of MD and dysthymia.

Trauma and eating disorder comorbidity

The role of various forms of child abuse and neglect, especially childhood sexual abuse (CSA), has been a major focus of investigation (Brewerton, 2004; Wonderlich *et al.*, 1997). Recent reviews conclude that CSA is a significant, albeit nonspecific, risk factor for the development of EDs, particularly those with bulimic features that present in association with psychiatric comorbidity (Molinari, 2001; Smolak & Murnen, 2002).

In a review of available studies, Wonderlich *et al.* (1997) confirmed a strong relationship between CSA and BN with comorbidity. There was no relationship found between CSA and the severity of BN or with a diagnosis of AN. Since traumatic experiences and subsequent post-traumatic stress disorder (PTSD) are associated with an array of psychiatric disorders similar to those found in association with bulimic EDs (Brady *et al.*, 2000), and bulimic EDs are linked with trauma and PTSD (Dansky *et al.*, 1997; Brewerton *et al.*, 1999), then it is reasonable that trauma and PTSD may mediate the association between psychiatric comorbidity and bulimic EDs (Brewerton, 2002, 2004). Data from the National Women's Study reveal that the number of comorbid diagnoses is highly correlated with rates of childhood rape as well as any type of direct crime victimization, such as rape, molestation and aggravated assault (Brewerton, 2004). Significantly, two-thirds of all rapes in the USA occur during childhood and adolescence before the age of 18. This link between BN, CSA and comorbidity has been confirmed in other large data sets, including the Virginia Twin Registry, which has the advantage of controlling for genetic factors (Kendler *et al.*, 2000).

There have been a number of other studies done in children and adolescents that confirm these interrelationships between child abuse and subsequent bulimic ED features and comorbidity. In a well-controlled investigation, Wonderlich *et al.* (2000) studied 20 sexually abused girls and 20 age-matched non-abused control girls ages 10–15 years, who completed several psychometric instruments. Abused subjects had significantly higher rates of weight dissatisfaction, purging and dieting behaviour compared with control subjects. In addition, abused children ate significantly less when emotionally upset, were less likely to exhibit perfectionistic tendencies, and were more likely to desire thinner body types than control children.

In a large study of over 5000 students in grades 9–12, Perkins & Luster (1999) reported that sexual victimization was linked with weight regulation in adolescent girls. This relationship was completely independent of physical victimization. Sexual abuse was also linked with both more extreme forms and multiple forms of weight regulation in girls, including purging.

Sherwood *et al.* (2002) reported results from the administration of a 225-item questionnaire to 5163 7th, 9th and 11th grade female public school students intended to examine factors associated with EDs among girls involved in weight-related sports (those in which it is important to stay a certain weight). Eating disorder symptoms were found in almost one-third of girls involved in both weight-related and nonweight-related sports. However, after controlling for grade, race and SES, girls in weight-related sports were 51% more likely to have ED symptoms than girls in nonweight-related sports. Girls in weight-related sports who had EDs had more physical abuse (OR = 3.29) and sexual abuse (OR = 3.87) than girls in weight-related sports without EDs.

Other published reports in youth demonstrate significant associations between binge–purge behaviours and sexual or physical abuse. This has been shown in large national samples of adolescents in both the USA

(Ackard *et al.*, 2001; Thompson *et al.*, 2001; Ackard & Neumark-Sztainer, 2003) and Sweden (Edgardh & Ormstad, 2000). These links have also been shown to persist in sexually abused children long past the time of abuse (Swanston *et al.*, 1997). Some interesting data have emerged that support the association between EDs, victimization and comorbidity in males, including boys, an area that has often been overlooked in prior studies. Lipschitz *et al.* (1999) reported that inpatient adolescent males with PTSD were more likely to have comorbid EDs as well as somatization and other anxiety disorders.

In a study of a representative sample of 9943 students in grades 7, 9 and 11 in Connecticut, Neumark-Sztainer *et al.* (2000) reported significantly more disordered eating among those with physical or sexual abuse and low levels of family communication, parental caring and expectations. The associations between abuse and disordered eating persisted after controlling for psychosocial and familial factors. The OR for the occurrence of disordered eating following sexual abuse was 4.88 for boys and 1.99 for girls, while the OR following physical abuse was 1.95 for boys and 2.0 for girls. Ackard & Neumark-Sztainer (2002) studied the prevalence of rape and violence during dating in adolescents and the links between these events and disordered eating behaviours and psychopathology in 81 247 high school boys and girls (1998 Minnesota Student Survey). The investigators found that both date rape and violence were related to elevated rates of disordered eating behaviours in boys and girls. Date rape and/or violence were also linked with suicidal thoughts and attempts, as well as lower scores on measures of emotional well-being and self-esteem. Even after accounting for age and race, adolescents who reported both date violence and rape were more likely to use laxatives (OR: boys = 28.22; girls = 5.76), vomit (OR: boys = 21.46; girls = 4.74), use diet pills (OR: boys = 16.33; girls = 5.08), binge eat (OR: boys = 5.80; girls = 2.15) and have suicidal thoughts or attempts (OR: boys = 6.66; girls = 5.78) than their nonabused peers.

Ackard & Neumark-Sztainer (2003) used these same data to examine the relationship between multiple forms of sexual abuse, disordered eating and psychological health. After controlling for both race and grade, boys with multiple forms of abuse had statistically significant ORs for bingeing (OR = 5.6), fasting (OR = 2.3), vomiting (OR = 24.2), laxative abuse (OR = 29.2), diet pill abuse (OR = 17.3) and thinking about/attempting suicide (OR = 9.5). Girls with multiple forms of abuse had significant ORs for bingeing (OR = 2.2), fasting (OR = 2.3), vomiting (OR = 4.1), laxative abuse (OR = 5.1), diet pill abuse (OR = 4.3) and thinking about/attempting suicide (OR = 6.12). Interestingly, boys and girls with multiple forms of sexual abuse reported similar rates of bingeing (42.6% vs. 41.1%), taking diet pills

(22.3% vs. 26.5%) and vomiting (18.7% vs. 23.3%), but boys had greater rates of laxative abuse than girls (22.4% vs. 7.4%).

Ackard et al. (2003) investigated the prevalence of dating violence in a nationally representative sample of 3533 high school students in grades 9 through 12 (Commonwealth Fund Survey of the Health of Adolescent Boys and Girls). They reported that dating violence for both boys and girls was associated with dieting, binge eating, purging, alcohol consumption, drug use, cigarette smoking, depression, poor self-esteem and suicidal thoughts. Boys and girls who experienced both sexual and physical abuse endorsed higher rates of dieting (boys: 50.0% vs. 22.5%; girls: 70.4% vs. 56.4%) and binge–purge behaviour (boys: 48.4% vs. 4.7%; girls: 47.4% vs. 13.7%) than their nonabused peers. These differences persisted after controlling for race, SES and BMI. Notably, 100% of boys with sexual abuse and 95% of boys with both sexual and physical abuse reported bingeing and purging several times per week compared with 57% of nonabused boys.

Using a comprehensive survey of 9042 Connecticut students (7th, 9th and 11th grades), Fonseca et al. (2002) examined several familial factors, including sexual abuse, in relationship to extreme weight control measures. Extreme dieters, who purposely vomited, took diet pills, laxatives or diuretics in order to lose weight, were compared with adolescents who reported none of these behaviours. Risk factors for boys included a history of sexual abuse (OR = 2.8, P < 0.001) and high levels of parental supervision/monitoring. For girls, the only significant risk factor besides BMI (OR = 2.17, P < 0.002) was a sexual abuse history (OR = 1.45, P < 0.001).

Data supporting a role for various forms of childhood maltreatment as a risk factor for BED have also emerged in the literature. Grilo & Masheb (2001) showed higher rates of childhood psychological, physical and sexual maltreatment in outpatients with BED. Eighty-three per cent of BED patients reported some form of child abuse, including 59% reporting emotional abuse, 36% physical abuse, 30% sexual abuse, 69% emotional neglect and 49% physical neglect. Another study identified other forms of victimization, like bullying and discrimination, as risk factors for BED (Striegel-Moore et al., 2002). Unfortunately, these studies did not report on rates of PTSD in these patients.

Other investigators have expanded the spectrum of abuse that may contribute to the development of EDs, including neglect (Johnson et al., 2002), childhood emotional abuse (Kent et al., 1999; Kent & Waller, 2000), an adverse family background (Kinzl et al., 1997), extreme food deprivation (Favaro et al., 2000), sexual harassment over the internet (Gati et al., 2002) and Munchausen's syndrome by proxy (Vanelli, 2002).

Finally, there are several reports that have examined the role of mediating variables between prior child abuse and the development of BN, all of which have important implications of treatment. This research has revealed that impulsivity as well as core beliefs involving shame, self-esteem and perceived control are mediating variables that should be taken into account for treatment (Andrews, 1997; Waller, 1998; Waller *et al.*, 2001; Wonderlich *et al.*, 2001; Murray & Waller, 2002).

Summary and conclusions

This chapter examines our present knowledge regarding the most common comorbid psychiatric conditions seen in association with eating disorders in children and adolescents. There are several major points. (1) Significant symptoms of comorbid disorders, particularly anxiety and/or depression, occur more often than not in the majority of ED cases (Brewerton, 2002, 2004; Lilenfeld, 2004). (2) Comorbid disorders may be primary or secondary to EDs. In the majority of cases anxiety disorders are the most common primary conditions, i.e. appear first. (3) Studies of comorbidity in the EDs must be interpreted with caution given the well-recognized role of semi-starvation as a cause of psychiatric symptoms (Keys *et al.*, 1950). These may include depressed and/or labile mood, neurovegetative symptoms, obsessive thinking and com-pulsive behaviours. Even when comorbid syndromes or symptoms are clearly of primary origin, the presence of dieting, weight loss and other eating-disordered behaviours can markedly exacerbate such conditions, especially anxiety and depression (Keys *et al.*, 1950; Lilenfeld, 2004). (4) The occurrence of childhood abuse and/or neglect is strongly associated with higher rates of comorbidity in association with disturbed eating characterized by bulimic symptoms, especially purging. (5) The boundaries between diagnoses are clearly not rigid, and there is a strong overlap between comorbid conditions, such as mood and anxiety disorders, especially during childhood and adoles-cence. Like the EDs in children and adolescents, such conditions often fail to meet full DSM–IV or ICD–10 criteria for a full-fledged diagnosis. However, this does not suggest that such symptoms are not clinically significant.

REFERENCES

Ackard, D. M. & Neumark-Sztainer, D. (2002). Date violence and date rape among adolescents: associations with disordered eating behaviors and psychological health. *Child Abuse and Neglect*, **26**, 455–73.

Ackard, D.M. & Neumark-Sztainer, D. (2003). Multiple sexual victimizations among adolescent boys and girls: Prevalence and associations with eating behaviors and psychological health. *Journal of Child Sexual Abuse*, **12**, 17–37.

Ackard, D.M., Neumark-Sztainer, D., Hannan, P.J., French, S. & Story, M. (2001). Binge and purge behavior among adolescents: associations with sexual and physical abuse in a nationally representative sample: the Commonwealth Fund survey. *Child Abuse and Neglect*, **25**, 771–85.

Ackard, D.M., Neumark-Sztainer, D. & Hannan, P. (2003). Dating violence among a nationally representative sample of adolescent girls and boys: associations with behavioral and mental health. *Journal of Gender-Specific Medicine*, **6**, 39–48.

Andrews, B. (1997). Bodily shame in relation to abuse in childhood and bulimia: a preliminary investigation. *British Journal of Clinical Psychology*, **36**, 41–9.

Bailly-Lambin, I. & Bailly, D. (1999). Separation anxiety disorder and eating disorders. *Encephale*, **25**, 226–31.

Brady, K., Killeen, T.K., Brewerton, T.D. & Sylverini, S. (2000). Comorbidity of psychiatric disorders and posttraumatic stress disorder. *Journal of Clinical Psychiatry*, **61** Suppl. 7, 22–32.

Brewerton, T.D. (2002). Bulimia in children and adolescents. *Child Adolescent Psychiatry Clinics of North America*, **11**, 237–56.

Brewerton, T.D. (2004). Treatment principles of eating disorder patients with comorbidity: relationship to victimization and PTSD. In *Clinical Handbook of Eating Disorders: An Integrated Approach*, ed. Brewerton, T.D. New York: Marcel Dekker, pp. 509–45.

Brewerton, T.D., Dansky, B.S., Kilpatrick, D.G. & O'Neil, P.M. (1999). Bulimia nervosa, PTSD and "forgetting": Results from the National Women's Study. In *Trauma and Memory*, ed. Williams, L.M. & Banyard, V.L. Durham, UK: Sage Publications, pp. 127–38.

Bulik, C.M., Sullivan, P.F., Fear, J.L. & Joyce, P.R. (1997). Eating disorders and antecedent anxiety disorders: a controlled study. *Acta Psychiatrica Scandinavica*, **96**, 101–7.

Dansky, B.S., Brewerton, T.D., O'Neil, P.M. & Kilpatrick, D.G. (1997). The National Women's Study: Relationship of crime victimization and PTSD to bulimia nervosa. *International Journal of Eating Disorders*, **21**, 213–28.

Devaud, C., Jeannin, A., Narring, F., Ferron, C. & Michaud, P.A. (1998). Eating disorders among female adolescents in Switzerland: prevalence and associations with mental and behavioral disorders. *International Journal of Eating Disorders*, **24**, 207–16.

Edgardh, K. & Ormstad, K. (2000). Prevalence and characteristics of sexual abuse in a national sample of Swedish seventeen-year-old boys and girls. *Acta Paediatrica*, **89**, 310–19.

Favaro, A., Rodella, F.C. & Santonastaso, P. (2000). Binge eating and eating attitudes among Nazi concentration camp survivors. *Psychological Medicine*, **30**, 463–6.

Flament, M.F., Godart, N.T., Fermanian, J. & Jeammet, P. (2001). Predictive factors of social disability in patients with eating disorders. *Eating and Weight Disorders*, **6**, 99–106.

Fonseca, H., Ireland, M. & Resnick, M.D. (2002). Familial correlates of extreme weight control behaviors among adolescents. *International Journal of Eating Disorders*, **32**, 441–8.

Gati, A., Tenyi, T., Tury, F. & Wildmann, M. (2002). Anorexia nervosa following sexual harassment on the internet: a case report. *International Journal of Eating Disorders*, **31**, 474–7.

Godart, N.T., Flament, M.F., Lecrubier, Y. & Jeammet, P. (2000). Anxiety disorders in anorexia nervosa and bulimia nervosa: co-morbidity and chronology of appearance. *European Psychiatry: the Journal of the Association of European Psychiatrists*, **15**, 38–45.

Grilo, C.M. & Masheb, R.M. (2001). Childhood psychological, physical, and sexual maltreatment in outpatients with binge eating disorder: frequency and associations with gender, obesity, and eating-related psychopathology. *Obesity Research*, **9**, 320–5.

Herpertz-Dahlmann, B., Muller, B., Herpertz, S., Heussen, N., Hebebrand, J. & Remschmidt, H. (2001). Prospective 10-year follow-up in adolescent anorexia nervosa–course, outcome, psychiatric comorbidity, and psychosocial adaptation. *Journal of Child Psychology, Psychiatry and Allied Disciplines*, **42**, 603–12.

Johnson, J.G., Cohen, P., Kasen, S. & Brook, J.S. (2002). Eating disorders during adolescence and the risk for physical and mental disorders during early adulthood. *Archives of General Psychiatry*, **59**, 545–52.

Kendler, K.S., Bulik, C.M., Silberg, J. *et al.* (2000). Childhood sexual abuse and adult psychiatric and substance use disorders in women: an epidemiological and cotwin control analysis. *Archives of General Psychiatry*, **57**, 953–9.

Kent, A. & Waller, G. (2000). Childhood emotional abuse and eating psychopathology. *Clinical Psychology Review*, **20**, 887–903.

Kent, A., Waller, G. & Dagnan, D. (1999). A greater role of emotional than physical or sexual abuse in predicting disordered eating attitudes: the role of mediating variables. *International Journal of Eating Disorders*, **25**, 159–67.

Keys, A., Brozek, J., Henschel, A., Mickelsen, O. & Taylor, H.L. (1950). *The Biology of Human Starvation*. Minneapolis, MN: University of Minnesota Press.

Kinzl, J.F., Mangweth, B., Traweger, C.M. & Biebl, W. (1997). Eating-disordered behavior in males: the impact of adverse childhood experiences. *International Journal of Eating Disorders*, **22**, 131–8.

Lilenfeld, L.R.R. (2004). Psychiatric comorbidity associated with anorexia nervosa, bulimia nervosa, and binge eating disorder. In *Clinical Handbook of Eating Disorders: An Integrated Approach*, ed. Brewerton, T.D. New York: Marcel Dekker, pp. 183–207.

Lipschitz, D.S., Winegar, R.K., Hartnick, E., Foote, B. & Southwick, S.M. (1999). Posttraumatic stress disorder in hospitalized adolescents: psychiatric comorbidity and clinical correlates. *Journal of the American Academy of Child and Adolescent Psychiatry*, **38**, 385–92.

Miotto, P., De Coppi, M., Frezza, M. & Preti, A. (2003). Eating disorders and suicide risk factors in adolescents: an Italian community-based study. *Journal of Nervous and Mental Disease*, **191**, 437–43.

Molinari, E. (2001). Eating disorders and sexual abuse. *Eating and Weight Disorders*, **6**, 68–80.

Moorhead, D.J., Stashwick, C.K., Reinherz, H.Z., Giaconia, R.M., Streigel-Moore, R.M. & Paradis, A.D. (2003). Child and adolescent predictors for eating disorders in a community population of young adult women. *International Journal of Eating Disorders*, **33**, 1–9.

Murray, C. & Waller, G. (2002). Reported sexual abuse and bulimic psychopathology among nonclinical women: the mediating role of shame. *International Journal of Eating Disorders*, **32**, 186–91.

Neumark-Sztainer, D., Story, M., Hannan, P.J., Beuhring, T. & Resnick, M.D. (2000). Disordered eating among adolescents: associations with sexual/physical abuse and other familial/psychosocial factors. *International Journal of Eating Disorders*, **28**, 249–58.

Patton, G.C., Carlin, J.B., Shao, Q. *et al.* (1997). Adolescent dieting: healthy weight control or borderline eating disorder? *Journal of Child Psychology, Psychiatry and Allied Disciplines*, **38**, 299–306.

Perez, M., Joiner, T.E., Jr. & Lewinsohn, P.M. (2004). Is major depressive disorder or dysthymia more strongly associated with bulimia nervosa? *International Journal of Eating Disorders*, **36**, 55–61.

Perkins, D.F. & Luster, T. (1999). The relationship between sexual abuse and purging: findings from community-wide surveys of female adolescents. *Child Abuse and Neglect*, **23**, 371–82.

Rabe-Jablonska, J.J. & Sobow, T.M. (2000). The links between body dysmorphic disorder and eating disorders. *European Psychiatry: the Journal of the Association of European Psychiatrists*, **15**, 302–5.

Sherwood, N.E., Neumark-Sztainer, D., Story, M., Beuhring, T. & Resnick, M.D. (2002). Weight-related sports involvement in girls: who is at risk for disordered eating? *American Journal of Health Promotion*, **16**, 341–4.

Smolak, L. & Murnen, S.K. (2002). A meta-analytic examination of the relationship between child sexual abuse and eating disorders. *International Journal of Eating Disorders*, **31**, 136–50.

Striegel-Moore, R.H., Dohm, F.A., Pike, K.M., Wilfley, D.E. & Fairburn, C.G. (2002). Abuse, bullying, and discrimination as risk factors for binge eating disorder. *American Journal of Psychiatry*, **159**, 1902–7.

Swanston, H.Y., Tebbutt, J.S., O'Toole, B.I. & Oates, R.K. (1997). Sexually abused children 5 years after presentation: a case-control study. *Pediatrics*, **100**, 600–8.

Thompson, K.M., Wonderlich, S.A., Crosby, R.D. & Mitchell, J.E. (2001). Sexual victimization and adolescent weight regulation practices: a test across three community based samples. *Child Abuse and Neglect*, **25**, 291–305.

Vanelli, M. (2002). Munchausen's syndrome by proxy web-mediated in a child with factitious hyperglycemia. *Journal of Pediatrics*, **141**, 839.

Waller, G., Meyer, C., Ohanian, V., Elliott, P., Dickson, C. & Sellings, J. (2001). The psychopathology of bulimic women who report childhood sexual abuse: the mediating role of core beliefs. *Journal of Nervous and Mental Disease*, **189**, 700–8.

Waller, G. (1998). Perceived control in eating disorders: relationship with reported sexual abuse. *International Journal of Eating Disorders*, **23**, 213–16.

Wonderlich, S.A., Brewerton, T.D., Jocic, Z., Dansky, B.S. & Abbott, D.W. (1997). The relationship of childhood sexual abuse and eating disorders: a review. *Journal of the American Academy of Child and Adolescent Psychiatry*, **36**, 1107–15.

Wonderlich, S., Crosby, R., Mitchell, J. *et al.* (2001). Pathways mediating sexual abuse and eating disturbance in children. *International Journal of Eating Disorders*, **29**, 270–9.

Wonderlich, S.A., Crosby, R.D., Mitchell, J.E. *et al.* (2000). Relationship of childhood sexual abuse and eating disturbance in children. *Journal of the American Academy of Child and Adolescent Psychiatry*, **39**, 1277–83.

Wonderlich, S.A., Crosby, R.D., Mitchell, J.E. *et al.* (2001). Eating disturbance and sexual trauma in childhood and adulthood. *International Journal of Eating Disorders*, **30**, 401–12.

14

Eating disorders in children with disabilities and chronic illness

Peter B. Sullivan

John Radcliffe Hospital, Oxford, UK

Eating, nutrition and growth

Good health demands good nutrition and in the child it is reflected in normal growth. Children who cannot or do not eat properly often become unwell and do not grow. This becomes a source of great concern and anxiety for their parents. Several chronic illnesses in children impair normal feeding; this chapter aims to describe the interrelationship between eating and disease in children with reference to some common conditions. The effects of childhood eating disorders on parents and families will also be considered.

The physiology of feeding

Understanding feeding problems in children rests on detailed knowledge of oral-motor function, the neurophysiology of feeding and child development and behaviour. The development of oral-motor skills reflects general neurological maturation and requires the coordination of the movement of at least 31 pairs of striated muscles in the mouth, pharynx and oesophagus by 5 cranial nerves, the brainstem and the cerebral cortex (Bosma, 1986). The control centre for swallowing, the nucleus tractus solitarius and the adjacent ventral medial reticular formation around the nucleus ambiguous, receive input from rostral brainstem centres, cerebellum, basal ganglia and higher cortical centres.

The swallowing process occurs in four phases: oral preparatory, oral, pharyngeal and oesophageal. The first two phases are under voluntary control, with the pharyngeal phase partly voluntary, and mostly involuntary, whilst the oesophageal phase is entirely involuntary.

Eating Disorders in Children and Adolescents, ed. Tony Jaffa and Brett McDermott. Published by Cambridge University Press. © Cambridge University Press 2007.

Transitional feeding, weaning and associated problems

In the neonate feeding begins as a result of a range of reflexes (gag, phasic bite, tongue protrusion, rooting, suckling and swallowing reflexes) and it later becomes a voluntary act with only the pharyngeal and oesophageal parts of the swallow remaining under reflex control. Transitional feeding from a predominantly sucking mode of feeding to mature solid food eating begins between 3 and 6 months of age. Growth in the upper digestive tract occurs as the mandible grows downwards and forwards and the hyoid bone and larynx move downwards. The sucking pads are gradually absorbed. All of these changes contribute to an enlargement of the buccal cavity which allows food to be manipulated between the tongue and the buccal wall. The gradual eruption of teeth allows the infant to progress towards eating harder and lumpier foods. So growth and maturation play a role in feeding development, but learning from experience is also crucial. An important aspect of learning is sensation and sensory feedback. This involves proprioception, touch, pressure, temperature and taste. Other important factors contributing to learning are gross and fine motor development, the methods of food presentation and cognitive development.

Weaning failure

Weaning is the process whereby an infant becomes accustomed to an intake of solid food in preference to milk. This transitional phase may be associated with disorganization of feeding and infants are often seen to be agitated or unsettled at this stage. During this critical period infants are vulnerable to develop feeding difficulties. Feeding is a reciprocal process that depends not only on the abilities and characteristics of the infant but also on those of their parent. Avoidance by parents of encouraging the infant to make the transition from milk to solids at this time may make the process considerably more difficult at a later time.

Infant feeding problems

There has been remarkably little research on the development of infant feeding problems. Seminal studies by Dahl and colleagues in Sweden on 50 infants meeting strict diagnostic criteria, however, have helped to identify the characteristics and consequences of infant feeding problems (Dahl & Sundelin, 1986; Dahl et al., 1986; Dahl, 1987; Dahl & Kristiansson, 1987). Feeding problems in this group had been ongoing for a mean duration of 5 months. The commonest problems were refusal to eat (56%), colic (18%) and vomiting

(16%). The majority (86%) of infants were underweight and 14% were malnourished ($>$ 2 SD below mean weight for age). Physical disorder (e.g. gastro-oesophageal reflux) was present in only 14% but in 6% this was a serious organic disease (e.g. congenital heart disease – see below). Follow-up studies at 2 years showed that over a third of the refusal-to-eat group had a persistent feeding problem (Dahl, 1987).

Oral-motor impairment

Oral-motor impairment may occur as a result of structural lesions (e.g. cleft lip and palate, macroglossia, Pierre–Robin syndrome, oesophageal atresia) or functional lesions (e.g. cerebral palsy, bulbar and pseudobulbar palsies, myopathies). In order to attain optimum oral-motor skill a child must have the ability to move oral and facial structures independently of the rest of the body. Poor control of posture, uncoordinated movements of the upper limbs, lack of independent mobility, visual, hearing and communication problems all contribute to feeding difficulties in disabled children.

Cerebral palsy

Severe disability is common in the graduates from neonatal intensive care units; the EPICure study group evaluated children who were born at 25 or fewer completed weeks of gestation at the time when they reached a median age of 30 months and 49% were disabled with 23% meeting the criteria for severe disability (Wood et al., 2000). Epidemiological studies have shown that these are the children who will encounter feeding difficulties. The North American Growth in Cerebral Palsy Project is a population-based study that evaluated the growth and nutritional status in children with moderate to severe cerebral palsy and found the majority (58%) had reported feeding problems (Fung et al., 2002). The Oxford Feeding Study examined 440 children with cerebral palsy and feeding problems and found that 89% required assistance with feedings and there were other concerns such as frequent choking (56%), stressful and prolonged feeding (43%) and vomiting (22%) (Sullivan et al., 2000). Oral motor dysfunction is the primary cause of feeding difficulties in children with disabilities. Prolonged feeding times, drooling, coughing and choking with feeds and gagging are all signs of oral-motor dysfunction. In one study of 271 children with cerebral palsy, the median length of time caregivers spent feeding per day was 2.5 hours, with 28% (72/261) spending more than three hours a day on this activity alone (Sullivan et al., 2000).

Enteral feeding via gastrostomy tube is increasingly being used in disabled children with oral-motor dysfunction and feeding problems to provide nutrition. Moreover, tube feeding is more likely to be initiated in those children with severe disability (Sullivan et al., 2002) and reports from various groups have indicated that both growth and nutritional status improve following enteral feeding (Patrick et al., 1986; Sanders et al. 1990; Corwin et al., 1996). In a systematic review of gastrostomy feeding in disabled children, however, Samson-Fang and colleagues concluded that there is considerable uncertainty about its safety and efficacy (Samson-Fang et al., 2003). Since then a longitudinal, prospective, multicentre cohort study designed to measure the outcomes of gastrostomy tube feeding in children with cerebral palsy has been reported (Sullivan et al., 2005). In this study, statistically significant and clinic-ally important increases in weight gain and subcutaneous fat deposition were demonstrated following gastrostomy feeding. Fifty-seven children with cere-bral palsy (28 female; median age 4 years 4 months, range 5 months to 17 years) and undernutrition were assessed prior to gastrostomy placement and at 6 and 12 months afterwards. The main reason for referral for gastrostomy tube insertion was their nutritional status for the preceding 12 months. Outcome measures included growth/anthropometry and nutritional intake, general health and complications of gastrostomy feeding.

At baseline, half of the children were more than 3 standard deviations below the average weight for their age and sex, when compared with the standards for normal children. Weight increased substantially over the study period; the median weight z score increased from −3.0 pre-gastrostomy placement to −2.2 at 6 months and −1.6 at 12 months. Weight gain was accompanied by significant increases in skin fold thickness indicating deposition of subcutane-ous fat. Minor complications (e.g. gastrostomy site infection) were common, but serious complications following gastrostomy tube insertion were rare. Almost all parents reported a significant improvement in their child's health following this intervention accompanied by a significant reduction in time spent feeding. An improvement in the quality of life in carers of children with cerebral palsy associated with the introduction of gastrostomy tube feeds has been demonstrated in a prospective cohort study aimed to evaluate the impact of gastrostomy-tube feeding on caregiver Quality of Life in carers of children with cerebral palsy (Sullivan et al., 2004). The Short Form 36 was used to measure Quality of Life in caregivers of the same children described above at 6 and 12 months after insertion of a gastrostomy tube. Responses were cali-brated against a normative dataset, the Oxford Healthy Life Survey III (OHLS). Six months after gastrostomy feeding was started, substantial rises in average

Table 14.1. Summary statistics for Short Form 36 domain scores and physical and mental component summaries pre and post gastrostomy placement (GS) plus P values for comparison with OHLS population norms (Sullivan et al., 2004)

Domain	OHLS mean	Baseline			6 months post GS		12 months post GS		
		n	Mean	P value[a]	n	Mean	n	Mean	P value[a]
Physical functioning	87.99	50	83.50	0.1	35	87.43	40	86.25	0.5
Role physical[b]	87.17	48	73.44	0.003	34	81.25	38	80.59	0.1
Role emotional[c]	85.75	48	68.06	0.0003	35	75.71	40	73.54	0.007
Social functioning	82.77	48	63.54	0.0003	35	71.07	39	76.60	0.1
Mental health	71.92	50	58.5	<0.0001	37	65.95	40	68.38	0.2
Energy/vitality	58.04	49	41.58	<0.0001	36	46.01	40	51.56	0.076
Pain	78.80	50	78.25	0.9	36	81.60	40	74.38	0.2
General health perception	71.06	49	67.96	0.3	36	67.42	38	72.89	0.5
Physical component summary	50.00	47	48.77	0.4	31	50.61	35	49.60	0.8
Mental component summary	50.00	47	40.10	0.0001	31	43.99	35	46.37	0.079

Notes:

[a] Single sample t-test, OHLS mean *vs.* observed mean.

[b] Role limitations due to physical problems.

[c] Role limitations due to emotional problems.

domain scores were observed for mental health, role limitations due to emotional problems, physical functioning, social functioning and energy/ vitality (Table 14.1). At 12 months after gastrostomy placement, caregivers reported significant improvements in social functioning, mental health, energy/vitality and in general health perception when compared with results at baseline. Moreover, the values obtained for these domains at 12 months were not significantly different from the OHLS reference standard. Interestingly, the greatest improvements seen were observed within six months of insertion of a gastrostomy feeding tube.

Chronic disease

This section will examine in detail the feeding problems associated with selected chronic childhood diseases. As a preliminary it is important to recognize that chronic disease in any organ system in a child can be associated with poor feeding. Thus, anorexia is a consequence of chronic inflammatory diseases such as inflammatory bowel disease and of the metabolic derangement that accompanies chronic renal failure. Dysphagia secondary to the oesophagitis caused by gastro-oesophageal reflux is a common cause of poor feeding (Field *et al.*, 2003). Infants with bronchopulmonary dysplasia (BPD) can also experience significant feeding difficulty, possibly secondary to tachypnoea interfering with suck coordination.

Congenital heart disease

Children with congenital or acquired cardiac disease frequently require supportive regimes with regard to feeding in order to maintain weight, resulting in altered experiences for both the child and family. Difficulties with feeding are common in children with congenital heart disease (CHD). Both decreased energy intake and increased energy requirements in this group contribute to malnutrition (Cameron *et al.*, 1995; Mitchell *et al.*, 1995). Cameron *et al.* (1995), for example, investigated nutritional status in 160 hospitalized children with congenital heart disease and showed that acute and chronic malnutrition occurred in 33% and 64% of the patients respectively.

For most parents feeding of infants and children with CHD poses significant difficulties, is time consuming and is associated with considerable anxiety (Thommessen *et al.*, 1992; Imms, 2000). Moreover, having a child with congenital cardiac disease producing difficulty in feeding has a strong negative impact on the whole family. The feeding pattern of children with CHD is characterized by a large variation in caloric intake. When heart failure is mild the infant commonly overfeeds, and fluid and sodium overload disturb cardiac haemodynamics, leading to decompensation of heart failure and decreased intake (Varan *et al.*, 1999). The magnitude of the growth disturbance is generally related to the anatomical lesion but children with cyanotic heart disease accompanied by pulmonary hypertension are the most severely affected in terms of nutrition and growth. Anorexia also accompanies malnutrition and further compromises the patient's condition. Dyspnoea and tachypnoea in patients with congestive heart failure lead to propensity for fatigue and decreased intake. Heart disease causes an increase in cardiac and respiratory work. Decreased intake caused by anorexia combined with increased respiratory effort results in a greater nutrient deficit. The malnutrition associated with CHD varies in severity from mild undernutrition to failure-to-thrive and can significantly affect the outcome of surgery increasing morbidity and mortality. Children with heart disease may need as much as 50% more calories than normal children in order to achieve normal growth. A combination of these factors predisposes the infant to malnutrition and growth failure.

Adequate nutrition is thus crucial to the management of children and infants with cardiac disease. Maintenance of an adequate caloric intake, in order to achieve sustained growth, is often not possible without nutritional support. Such support can come in the form of caloric supplementation (Jackson & Poskitt, 1991) or continuous enteral feeding (Vanderhoof *et al.*, 1982) with or without percutaneous endoscopic gastrostomy tubes (Hofner *et al.*, 2000; Ciotti *et al.*, 2002).

Cystic fibrosis

Good nutritional care is also an essential part of the management of the child with cystic fibrosis (CF) and is one of the major factors contributing to the improved longevity of such children. Energy requirements vary but can be in excess of 150% of the daily recommended value for the normal child and this may pose a significant challenge to parents as they try to meet these requirements. A number of studies have highlighted that children with CF are at risk of developing behaviour problems during mealtimes (Jelalian *et al.*, 1998; Stark *et al.*, 2000; Duff *et al.*, 2003). Behavioural therapy has been shown by meta-analysis of several studies to be as effective as oral supplementation and enteral and parenteral feeding in improving weight gain in young people with CF (Jelalian *et al.*, 1998). Duff *et al.* (2003) used the Behavioural Paediatric Feeding Assessment Scale (BPFAS) to study feeding behaviour problems in children with CF in the UK. In children aged 5–12 years there were significantly more problematic disruptive child behaviours and inappropriate parental responses in the CF group than in the control group. Typical disruptive child behaviours observed during mealtimes in this study included no enjoyment of eating, poor appetite, reluctance to come to mealtimes, preferring to drink rather than eat, eating snack food but not eating at mealtimes and trying to negotiate foods to be eaten. Duff et al. (2003) report that these behaviours seem to lead to frustration and unhappiness for parents and result in ineffectual and counter-productive strategies (e.g. coaxing) during mealtimes. In view of the fact that there is a high prevalence of feeding behaviour problems in pre-pubertal children with CF it is important that preventive and reactive interventions, tailored to the child's developmental age, continue throughout childhood.

Type 1 Diabetes

Adolescent girls with type 1 diabetes encounter several difficulties which may affect their disease. Early puberty is associated with decreased insulin sensitivity during the growth spurt and sexual maturation (Bloch et al., 1987); in the later stages of puberty (as growth diminishes), however, insulin sensitivity increases. The adolescent years are often characterized by deterioration in the metabolic control of diabetes and it is not uncommon for adolescent girls particularly to be overweight. These changes coincide with the peak period of risk for the development of eating disorders. The cycle of weight loss and then weight gain that accompanies the onset and treatment of diabetes may increase body dissatisfaction and the drive for thinness in vulnerable adolescent females. Management strategies which impose dietary restraint and an intentional disregard of the natural promptings of hunger and satiety may activate dietary dysregulation and disturbed eating patterns. Early studies in this area have been confounded by their small size and conflicting results but more recent research has confirmed the risks for the development of eating disorders in young women with type 1 diabetes. Engström et al. (1999) studied 89 adolescent females (aged 14–18 years) with type 1 diabetes and compared them with age-matched healthy controls. They used the Eating Disorder Inventory, a Likert-type self-report questionnaire which tracks symptoms associated with eating disorders and showed highly significant differences between the diabetes group and the control group on the Drive for Thinness subscale. Fifteen diabetic girls (16.9%) scored above the cut-off level for disturbed eating behaviour compared with 2 control girls (2.2%) ($P < 0.01$). The commonest abnormality encountered in this study was binge eating and purging behaviour (self-induced vomiting or insulin omission). These observations were confirmed and extended in another study by Jones *et al.* (2000) who studied 356 diabetic females (aged 12–19 years) and 1098 age-matched controls. Using DSM–IV criteria they found that eating disorders were twice as common (OR 2.4) in those with type 1 diabetes. Moreover, diabetics with eating disorders had higher HbA_{1c} concentrations than those without eating disorders. It is not surprising, therefore, that patients with type 1 diabetes and eating disorders have more long-term diabetic complications. Such patients have been shown to have an increased prevalence of retinopathy, microalbuminuria and painful neuropathy when compared with those diabetics without an eating disorder (Steel *et al.*, 1987; Rydall *et al.*, 1997). Some young women utilize their insulin-dependency as a potent means of weight control and induce urinary calories wasting either by insulin omission or under-dosing (Bryden *et al.*, 1999; Engström *et al.*, 1999). Such behaviour is more likely to occur in those who also have an eating disorder (Jones *et al.*, 2000). The importance of this is that insulin omission worsens glycaemic control, increases the risk of microvascular complications and in adolescents has been identified as the primary cause of recurrent diabetic ketoacidosis (Glasgow *et al.*, 1991). Family relationships play an important part in the development of eating disorders in adolescent girls with diabetes. In eating-disturbed diabetic girls, Maharaj *et al.* (1998) have identified an association (not necessarily causal) between dysfunctional family environments characterized by poor communication, mistrust of parents' responsiveness to their needs and consequently greater feelings of anger and hopelessness. Moreover, eating disturbances in girls with diabetes are significantly associated with heightened weight and shape concerns in their mothers (Maharaj *et al.*, 1998). Figure 14.1 provides a model of the interaction between type 1 diabetes and eating disorders.

Neurodevelopmental disorders

Developmental disorders characterized by communication difficulties are often accompanied by eating problems. Two conditions, autism and Rett syndrome, will suffice as examples.

Autism is a developmental disorder characterized by severe deficits in social interaction and communication along with stereotypic behaviour patterns. The unusual eating patterns and feeding difficulties of children with autism (which is more common in boys) has long been recognized. They often have an extremely limited food repertoire occasionally with apparent craving for certain foods. Research in this area is limited but Williams *et al.* (2000)

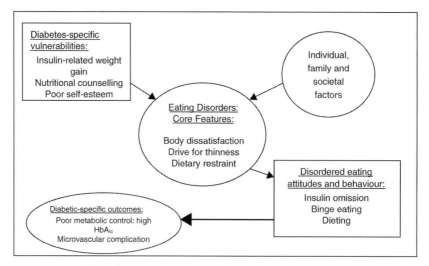

Figure 14.1. Model of the interaction between type 1 diabetes and eating disorders (reproduced with permission from Dr Denis Daneman, 2002).

undertook a parent survey of the eating habits of 340 autistic children. Two-thirds of respondents considered their child to be a 'picky' eater. The commonest behavioural problems reported were unwillingness to try new foods, mouthing objects and rituals surrounding eating. Other problems were licking objects, smelling and throwing food and pica. According to Kinnell (1985), 60% of his series of 70 autistic patients exhibited pica.

Rett syndrome may be confused with autism but arises from a mutation in the transcription regulating gene MECP2 on the X chromosome; it occurs almost exclusively in girls. Feeding problems are common in Rett syndrome in which there are characteristic oropharyngeal abnormalities (Morton *et al.*, 1997b; Isaacs *et al.*, 2003). Videofluoroscopic studies of feeding in girls with Rett syndrome have shown reduced movements of the mid and posterior tongue, with premature spillover of food and liquid from the mouth into the pharynx and laryngeal penetration of liquids and solid food during swallowing (Morton *et al.*, 1997a; Motil *et al.*, 1999). Air swallowing has also been noted as a problem in these patients (Morton *et al.*, 2000).

Conclusion

Much of the interaction between an infant and its parents surrounds feeding and thus early feeding experience is important to the psychological development of the child. This fundamental aspect of life is reflected in the interconnectedness of the words 'nourish', 'nurture' and 'nurse'. Feeding thus plays a central role in the life of the child not only in relation to their growth but also in its contribution to their social integration. Problems with feeding can cause a major disruption to normal growth and development. In addition, they can pose additional complications for the child coping with a chronic disease. To protect the child from the adverse effects of these complications requires great patience and skill on the part of parents and clinicians alike.

REFERENCES

Bloch, C. A., Clemons, P. & Sperling, M. A. (1987). Puberty decreases insulin sensitivity. *Journal of Pediatrics*, **110**, 481–7.

Bosma, J. F. (1986). Development of feeding. *Clinical Nutrition*, **5**, 210–18.

Bryden, K. S., Neil, A., Mayou, R. A., Peveler, R. C., Fairburn, C. G. & Dunger, D. B. (1999). Eating habits, body weight, and insulin misuse. A longitudinal study of teenagers and young adults with type 1 diabetes. *Diabetes Care*, **22**, 1956–60.

Cameron, J. W., Rosenthal, A. & Olson, A. D. (1995). Malnutrition in hospitalized children with congenital heart disease. *Archives of Pediatric and Adolescent Medicine*, **149**, 1098–102.

Ciotti, G., Holzer, R., Pozzi, M. & Dalzell, M. (2002). Nutritional support via percutaneous endoscopic gastrostomy in children with cardiac disease experiencing difficulties with feeding. *Cardiology in the Young*, **12**, 537–41.

Corwin, D. S., Isaacs, J. S., Georgeson, K. E., Bartolucci, A. A., Cloud, H. H. & Craig, C. B. (1996). Weight and length increases in children after gastrostomy placement. *Journal of the American Dietetic Association*, **96**, 874–9.

Dahl, M. (1987). Early feeding problems in an affluent society. III. Follow-up at two years: natural course, health, behaviour and development. *Acta Paediatrica Scandinavica*, **76**, 872–80.

Dahl, M., Eklund, G. & Sundelin, C. (1986). Early feeding problems in an affluent society. II. Determinants. *Acta Paediatrica Scandinavica*, **75**, 380–7.

Dahl, M. & Kristiansson, B. (1987). Early feeding problems in an affluent society. IV. Impact on growth up to two years of age. *Acta Paediatrica Scandinavica*, **76**, 881–8.

Dahl, M. & Sundelin, C. (1986). Early feeding problems in an affluent society. I. Categories and clinical signs. *Acta Paediatrica Scandinavica*, **75**, 370–9.

Daneman, D. (2002). Eating disorders in adolescent girls and young adult women with type 1 diabetes. *Diabetes Spectrum*, **15**, 84–5.

Duff, A. J., Wolfe, S. P., Dickson, C., Conway, S. P. & Brownlee, K. G. (2003). Feeding behavior problems in children with cystic fibrosis in the UK: prevalence and comparison with healthy controls. *Journal of Pediatric Gastroenterology and Nutrition*, **36**, 443–7.

Engstrom, I., Kroon, M., Arvidsson, C. G. *et al.* (1999). Eating disorders in adolescent girls with insulin-dependent diabetes mellitus: a population-based case-control study. *Acta Paediatrica*, **88**, 175–80.

Field, D., Garland, M. & Williams, K. (2003). Correlates of specific childhood feeding problems. *Journal of Paediatrics and Child Health*, **39**, 299–304.

Fung, E.B., Samson-Fang, L., Stallings, V.A. *et al.* (2002). Feeding dysfunction is associated with poor growth and health status in children with cerebral palsy. *Journal of the American Dietetic Association*, **102**, 3–73.

Gewolb, I.H., Bosma, J.F., Taciak, V.L. & Vice, F.L. (2001). Abnormal developmental patterns of suck and swallow rhythms during feeding in preterm infants with bronchopulmonary dysplasia. *Developmental Medicine and Child Neurology*, **43**, 454–9.

Glasgow, A.M., Weissberg-Benchell, J., Tynan, W.D. *et al.* (1991). Readmissions of children with diabetes mellitus to a children's hospital. *Pediatrics*, **88**, 98–104.

Hofner, G., Behrens, R., Koch, A., Singer, H. & Hofbeck, M. (2000). Enteral nutritional support by percutaneous endoscopic gastrostomy in children with congenital heart disease. *Pediatric Cardiology*, **21**, 341–6.

Imms, C. (2000). Impact on parents of feeding young children with congenital or acquired cardiac disease. *Cardiology in the Young*, **10**, 574–81.

Isaacs, J.S., Murdock, M., Lane, J. & Percy, A.K. (2003). Eating difficulties in girls with Rett syndrome compared with other developmental disabilities. *Journal of the American Dietetic Association*, **103**, 224–30.

Jackson, M. & Poskitt, E.M. (1991). The effects of high-energy feeding on energy balance and growth in infants with congenital heart disease and failure to thrive. *British Journal of Nutrition*, **65**, 2–43.

Jelalian, E., Stark, L.J., Reynolds, L. & Seifer, R. (1998). Nutrition intervention for weight gain in cystic fibrosis: a meta analysis. *Journal of Pediatrics*, **132**, 486–92.

Jones, J.M., Lawson, M.L., Daneman, D., Olmsted, M.P. & Rodin, G. (2000). Eating disorders in adolescent females with and without type 1 diabetes: cross sectional study. *British Medical Journal*, **320**, 1563–6.

Kinnell, H.G. (1985). Pica as a feature of autism. *British Journal of Psychiatry*, **147**, 80–2.

Maharaj, S.I., Rodin, G.M., Olmsted, M.P. & Daneman, D. (1998). Eating disturbances, diabetes and the family: an empirical study. *Journal of Psychosomatic Research*, **44**, 479–90.

Mitchell, I.M., Logan, R.W., Pollock, J.C. & Jamieson, M.P. (1995). Nutritional status of children with congenital heart disease. *British Heart Journal*, **73**, 277–83.

Morton, R.E., Bonas, R., Minford, J., Kerr, A. & Ellis, R.E. (1997a). Feeding ability in Rett syndrome. *Developmental Medicine and Child Neurology*, **39**, 331–5.

Morton, R.E., Bonas, R., Minford, J., Tarrant, S.C. & Ellis, R.E. (1997b). Respiration patterns during feeding in Rett syndrome. *Developmental Medicine and Child Neurology*, **39**, 607–13.

Morton, R.E., Pinnington, L. & Ellis, R.E. (2000). Air swallowing in Rett syndrome. *Developmental Medicine and Child Neurology*, **42**, 271–5.

Motil, K.J., Schultz, R.J., Browning, K., Trautwein, L. & Glaze, D.G. (1999). Oropharyngeal dysfunction and gastroesophageal dysmotility are present in girls and women with Rett syndrome. *Journal of Pediatric Gastroenterology and Nutrition*, **29**, 31–7.

Patrick, J., Boland, M., Stoski, D. & Murray, G.E. (1986). Rapid correction of wasting in children with cerebral palsy. *Developmental Medicine and Child Neurology*, **28**, 734–9.

Rydall, A.C., Rodin, G.M., Olmsted, M.P., Devenyi, R.G. & Daneman, D. (1997). Disordered eating behavior and microvascular complications in young women with insulin-dependent diabetes mellitus. *New England Journal of Medicine*, **336**, 1849–54.

Samson-Fang, L., Butler, C. & O'Donnell, M. (2003). Effects of gastrostomy feeding in children with cerebral palsy: an AACPDM evidence report. *Developmental Medicine and Child Neurology*, **45**, 415–26.

Samson-Fang, L., Fung, E., Stallings, V.A. (2002). Relationship of nutritional status to health and societal participation in children with cerebral palsy. *Journal of Pediatrics*, **141**, 637–43.

Sanders, K.D., Cox, K., Cannon, R. *et al.* (1990). Growth response to enteral feeding by children with cerebral palsy. *Journal of Parenteral and Enteral Nutrition*, **14**, 23–6.

Stark, L.J., Jelalian, E., Powers, S.W. *et al.* (2000). Parent and child mealtime behavior in families of children with cystic fibrosis. *Journal of Pediatrics*, **136**, 195–200.

Steel, J.M., Young, R.J., Lloyd, G.G. & Clarke, B.F. (1987). Clinically apparent eating disorders in young diabetic women: associations with painful neuropathy and other complications. *British Medical Journal (Clinical Research Edition)*, **294**, 859–62.

Sullivan, P.B., Lambert, B., Rose, M. *et al.* (2000). Prevalence and severity of feeding and nutritional problems in children with neurological impairment: Oxford Feeding Study. *Developmental Medicine and Child Neurology*, **42**, 10–80.

Sullivan, P.B., Juszczak, E., Lambert, B.R. *et al.* (2002). Impact of feeding problems on nutritional intake and growth: Oxford Feeding Study II. *Developmental Medicine and Child Neurology*, **44**, 461–7.

Sullivan, P.B., Juszczak, E., Bachlet, A.M. *et al.* (2004). Impact of gastrostomy tube feeding on the quality of life of carers of children with cerebral palsy. *Developmental Medicine and Child Neurology*, **46**, 796–800.

Sullivan, P.B., Juszczak, E., Bachlet, A.M. *et al.* (2005). Gastrostomy tube feeding in children with cerebral palsy: a prospective, longitudinal study. *Developmental Medicine and Child Neurology*, **47**, 77–85.

Thommessen, M., Heiberg, A. & Kase, B.F. (1992). Feeding problems in children with congenital heart disease: the impact on energy intake and growth outcome. *European Journal of Clinical Nutrition*, **46**, 457–64.

Vanderhoof, J.A., Hofschire, P.J., Baluff, M.A. *et al.* (1982). Continuous enteral feedings. An important adjunct to the management of complex congenital heart disease. *American Journal of Disease in Childhood*, **136**, 825–7.

Varan, B., Tokel, K. & Yilmaz, G. (1999). Malnutrition and growth failure in cyanotic and acyanotic congenital heart disease with and without pulmonary hypertension. *Archives of Disease in Childhood*, **81**, 49–52.

Williams, P.G., Dalrymple, N. & Neal, J. (2000). Eating habits of children with autism. *Pediatric Nursing*, **26**, 259–64.

Wood, N.S., Marlow, N., Costeloe, K., Gibson, A.T. & Wilkinson, A.R. (2000). Neurologic and developmental disability after extremely preterm birth. EPICure Study Group. *New England Journal of Medicine*, **343**, 378–84.

15

Childhood obesity

Caroline Braet

Ghent University, Ghent, Belgium

Childhood obesity: conceptualization

International guidelines for defining overweight status and obesity in children and adolescents were published recently (Cole *et al.*, 2000). Weight standards were expressed as 'BMI-percentiles' for children and will become the gold standard for determining the degree of obesity. Utilizing these guidelines the prevalence of obesity among children has never before reached such epidemic proportions as today (Dietz, 1998). When overweight status is defined by the NHES as the 85th percentile of BMI (Frederiks *et al.*, 2000) approximately 26–31% of American children and about 14–22% of European children are overweight. When defined by the 95th percentile of BMI, about 9–13% of American children are obese (Flegal & Troiano, 2000).

When trying to categorize a particular child, overweight status can also be expressed in terms of percentage of the current weight to the 'standard BMI'. The latter is comparable to the 50th percentile. A deviation of more than 20% is considered as overweight. Child obesity represents a range of forms with on the one hand moderately obese children (20–40% overweight), obese children (40–60% overweight) and severely obese children (>60% overweight).

Paediatric obesity increases the risk of adult obesity (Whitaker *et al.*, 1997) and long-standing obesity is associated with health risks in adults (Mossberg, 1989). Furthermore, childhood obesity is associated with health complications, including elevated blood pressure, hyperinsulinaemia and glucose intolerance, and respiratory abnormalities (Dietz, 1998; Freedman *et al.*, 1999). The effects of childhood obesity on morbidity and mortality suggest that effective prevention and intervention for childhood obesity is essential. Childhood obesity is also characterized by psychological problems which are important to take into

Eating Disorders in Children and Adolescents, ed. Tony Jaffa and Brett McDermott. Published by Cambridge University Press. © Cambridge University Press 2007.

consideration. It is noteworthy that obese children presenting for treatment of obesity display a higher prevalence of psychological problems than obese children not seeking treatment (Braet *et al.*, 1997). Obese people are, on the basis of their appearance, stigmatized as being unattractive, stupid, lazy or unfriendly (Strauss *et al.*, 1985). Obese people are often considered as being completely responsible for their condition (Bray, 1986), which provokes antipathy from others. As a consequence, obese youngsters often have fewer friends which in turn can interfere with the development of their social skills (Dietz, 1998). The psychological burden for children with enduring obesity is significant and can lead to social isolation and depression (Banis *et al.*, 1988; Rössner, 1998). The adverse consequences of obesity can affect developmental trajectories. For example, once they become young adults, obese people seem to receive less higher education, earn less money and are less likely to marry (Gortmaker *et al.*, 1993; Stunkard & Sobal, 1995).

Aetiology of childhood obesity

There is a clear consensus about the aetiology of obesity. The mechanism for its development in children is the same as that for adults. Obesity refers to an excess accumulation of body fat as a result of an imbalance between energy intake and energy expenditure (Bouchard *et al.*, 1998). When the energy intake exceeds the physical requirements, the excess energy is in some people converted into fat, which may in time produce fat reserves and lead to obesity.

The causes of a disturbed balance in overweight people are multifactorial, with changes in energy intake and expenditure related to both subtle and obvious movements in societal behavioural habits. US studies show a positive correlation between television viewing and overweight status (Dietz & Gortmaker, 1985). Energy expenditure has been reduced by an increase in sedentary activities, a decrease in the need to expend energy in daily routines and an increase in the use of cars and other forms of transport. On a related level, the safety of the environment can encourage or discourage a child from being physically active (Sallis *et al.*, 1995). Furthermore, food is now more attractive, promoted and simply obtained. Energy-dense foods are plentiful and relatively inexpensive. These factors may be more pertinent for families living in lower socio-economic strata, where financial constraints may favour the purchase of less expensive yet more fattening foods.

To attribute obesity solely to eating habits or low levels of exercise would be a gross generalization. Studies of twins and adopted children have demonstrated a genetic 'susceptibility' to obesity. Genetic factors have recently received much attention in medical literature and the lay press after the discovery of the leptin gene. Numerous genes have been reported, together explaining 30% of the variance of the overweight status (Bouchard *et al.*, 1990; Bouchard, 1995). The risk of developing obesity increases with the number of these genes present. This partial clarification of the genetic factors that influence the development of overweight status has so far not led to therapeutic options although leptin has been used successfully in selected cases. In view of the diversity of the genetic factors, it is not very likely that this will change in the near future.

As the geneticist Bouchard indicates, even a genetic predisposition to obesity is only translated to the real thing in a situation of personal overfeeding for some time. This is hopeful for the future treatment of childhood obesity: it suggests the usefulness of searching, together with the patient, for a balance between energy intake and energy expenditure and in this way preventing further overfeeding.

Berkowitz *et al.* (1993) observed symptoms of binge eating in about 30% of adolescent obese girls who sought weight reduction. Similar findings were found by Decaluwé *et al.* (2003). The clear differences between obese children with and without binge eating suggest the need for specific interventions for obese binge eaters.

Schlundt *et al.* (1991) demonstrated that obese people can display at least five different eating behaviours over a period of 2 weeks, i.e. healthy eating habits, strict food restraint, dietary behaviour alternated with binge eating, emotional eating and unrestricted overeating. Thus, eating behaviour appears more complex than initially thought and each of these eating patterns is now the subject of further research. The heterogeneity between the obese and within individuals over time clearly has implications for treatment; for example distinguishing between obese people who do/do not suffer from binge eating or who are/are not on a diet.

There seems to be a specific paradoxical relationship between overeating and dieting. The boundary model of Herman & Polivy (1980) has been proposed as an explanatory model for this. It suggests that attempts to maintain a low calorie diet almost inevitably lead to relapse in the form of uncontrolled binge-eating. In this model, it is assumed that frequent dieting shifts biological thresholds with respect to hunger and satiety which become determined by cognitive processes. However, these processes are vulnerable to breakdown. According to this model overweight people who diet will paradoxically have more problems with 'overeating'. Although this model has face validity when considering bulimia nervosa (Jansen, 1993), it is assumed that it can also explain the eating problems of some obese people (Fairburn & Wilson, 1993).

In addition to dieting and binge-eating, a range of other problematic eating behaviours are observed in the obese. Behavioural analysis suggests that obese people have bad eating habits such as eating in the car, in front of the television, at work or when feeling alone. Consequently, too many situations are associated with 'eating', which could explain the susceptibility of obese children to external food factors. The treatment consequence of such analysis is the use of techniques derived from self-regulation exercises, such as restriction of the number of eating situations.

There is a need for further investigation into the role of parents and the family in the development and maintenance of bad eating habits in children. Food is often used by parents to reinforce desired or undesired behaviour. It appears that parents rewarding their children with sweets increases the attractiveness of sweets in general (Birch, 1987). Parents may also adopt a stance of encouraging their children to eat (Johnson & Birch, 1994) reinforcing eating 'more' and for 'longer', and eating all that is on the plate.

Finally, delay of the fulfilment of one's needs, tolerance of hunger and dealing with frustrations are self-regulation skills that are gradually acquired through education and learning. Within this context, overeating and overly frequent eating may also be considered as behaviour deficits, that is, not yet having learned good eating habits. In some obese children, the lack of control over food may be situated within a general lack of self-regulation skills. The parents of these children often find it difficult to set clear limits and to make concrete arrangements with their child. In such cases, treatment of the child's obesity necessarily implies attention to parenting skills.

Treatment of childhood obesity

For many decades 'dieting' has been considered the ultimate solution to the problem of excess weight. Unfortunately, time and again weight is regained after the dietary treatment period and indeed the weight regained may be greater than that lost (Wilson, 1994). Moreover, going on a diet may have harmful side effects, such as an increased risk of developing binge eating and disorders in the regulation of the basal metabolism (Garner & Wooley, 1991). Wilson (1994) concluded that there is currently no treatment method for obese adults with an adequate evidence base and that there are only a few 'promising' treatment goals which include: (1) aiming at weight management instead of weight loss, with a maximum of 10% weight loss allowed; (2) establishing a healthy lifestyle, which implies a more favourable prognosis with respect to the prevention of diseases; and (3) the prevention of becoming overweight, e.g. through early intervention in obese children. Jelalian & Saelens (1999) reviewed 61 studies of obesity treatment, 41 of which met their criteria for good research. They concluded that effective treatments for obese children must always occur within a behavioural-therapy framework.

Illustrations of childhood obesity treatment within a behavioural framework are described by Epstein *et al.* (1998) and by Goldfried *et al.* (2002). On the basis of experience and research, they suggested dividing food products into three categories: to be eaten without limit (green), to be eaten in moderation (orange) and forbidden (red). All programmes stimulate the child to adopt a healthy lifestyle by following strictly the guidelines as prescribed by the National Institute for Food (http://www.nutrition.gov). They suggest a regime of breakfast between 7 and 8 a.m., a morning snack at 10 a.m., lunch between 12 and 1 p.m., an afternoon snack at 4 p.m., dinner around 6 p.m. and if so desired a final snack at 8 p.m. Other between-meal snacks are discouraged. This programme aims to obtain the weight goal of 10% weight loss. In this approach, food is classified within a food pyramid, with eating varied and healthy food as the major principle. Attention is paid to what is still allowed, such as vegetables and fruit. Snacks, soft drinks and fatty calorie-dense food are not forbidden but can be consumed only in limited portions. Whole families following these principles probably increases the chance of long-term compliance (Braet *et al.*, 1999).

In most obesity treatments, reduction of caloric intake is the most significant contribution to negative energy balance. Increased physical activity, however, also contributes, and may accelerate weight loss and improve maintenance of lost weight. Epstein & Wing (1987) suggest initiating an exercise programme in which mainly aerobic exercises of moderate intensity are planned, such as cycling, swimming, walking, jogging, rope-skipping or rowing. These activities are planned in an exercise scheme, which encourage children to undertake physical exercise for approximately 20 minutes a day.

How can children adopt new eating and exercise habits? Interesting results are provided by Epstein *et al.* (1990) who demonstrated the importance of behavioural techniques like self-monitoring (e.g. using a food diary), contracting (e.g. eating breakfast, no soft drinks during meals) and rewarding the child for sticking to the contract. Stimulus control is another important technique: children are advised to reduce the number of places where they eat, preferably to only one place, for example the kitchen, even if special treats are occasionally provided. Other good eating habits to be encouraged include eating slowly, chewing properly, avoiding reading while eating, waiting for a moment before deciding on a second helping, tasting nothing in advance and avoiding lingering at the table. It is, of course, important if these are to be established that they are practised regularly. Programmes such as those described, incorporating dietary advice and physical activity regimes in a behavioural-therapeutic approach can prove effective. Weight loss of 5% to 20% is reported (Epstein & Wing, 1987; Braet *et al.*, 1997).

The age of the child is important in considering whether treatment is indicated. Approximately 80% of children who are obese at age 10 will remain so (Whitaker *et al.*, 1997). Based on these findings and applying an 'early intervention' perspective, obese children between the ages of 7 and 10 are indicated as ideal candidates for treatment. It is advisable that obese 5–7-year-olds are monitored, though active intervention with this group may not be warranted given the higher chance of spontaneous recovery. In deciding whether to intervene the following components appear to be important: the weight of the parents, economic class and current eating habits (Whitaker *et al.*, 1997). In particular, children from lower socio-economic groups with at least one obese parent were 'high risk' children. In contrast, if both parents have normal weight and they already encourage their obese child to eat healthy food a positive prognosis can be made.

Although the previous guidelines described the goals for treating childhood obesity in terms of regulating body weight, it is also important to pay attention to the psychological sequelae of obesity. Common themes in discourse with obese children include harassment by others or their feelings of guilt and shame. Furthermore, the therapist should help the child in learning to accept that their weight is a problem. To this end the therapist can do exercises that enhance the self-image of the child (Braet, 2000). Therefore, it is also the goal of the treatment that the child will continue to enjoy eating without gaining weight and moreover will become proud of being able to control their weight.

The role played by the parents and the family

Targeting parents in a behavioural treatment of childhood obesity enhances the results (Jelalian & Saelens, 1999). Generalizing change is important, thus parents are asked to continue at home what has been dealt with in therapy and to help their child in the completion of therapy tasks. Our own experience is based on this latter approach. A recently completed long-term follow-up study of children treated for obesity, conducted at our university, indicated that the children that had followed an educational behavioural-therapeutic group programme were still 17% below their initial obese weight level 4 years later (effect size: 1.07), whereas the group of children that received advice only once, showed a 6% decrease of their initial obese weight level, or an effect size of 0.25 (Braet & Van Winckel, 2000).

There are different ways to involve parents in the treatment. In our approach, at the end of each session, one parent is invited to go through the contract together with the therapist. In doing so, it is examined whether the goals of the contract can be implemented, for instance whether the house can be organized so that the child is not constantly stimulated to eat and whether they can put more healthy than unhealthy purchases on the shopping list. They are further encouraged to cycle together with their child, to plan a walk on Sundays or to try out a new healthy recipe. In this way parents are assisted in setting clear and realistic rules, being consistent, monitoring treatment contracts and in giving helpful feedback to their child. This often restores peace and quiet in the family, since there are fewer conflicts about when they should eat, and about what should or should not be eaten and there is no longer requirement for discussions and doubts about how to implement a weight-control programme. If a child cannot live up to their contract, the parents do not blame the child for this, but they do record it in the child's diary. This is then discussed during the next treatment session. Parents can also be helped with improving their problem-solving skills.

Where parents, grandparents or other family members are not willing or able to give up old habits a more individual treatment may be necessary. While there will still need to be involvement of the family this will be in separate sessions which do not include the obese child. It is advisable to take a non-accusatory, empathizing attitude, and to look for possible solutions to problems in a cooperative atmosphere.

Where parents are finding it difficult to support or cooperate with treatment it may be helpful to discuss with them their thoughts about their child, about the treatment programme and about their attributions on the causes of childhood obesity. Their convictions may relate to 'it is all a matter of our genes' or 'I want to be a good mother'. Some parents give up early. Others are poorly informed about good eating habits or may report family conflicts. In such cases involvement of multidisciplinary colleagues may be important. Information about good eating habits can be given by means of leaflets or cooking evenings and is preferably organized with the help of a dietician. In case there are family conflicts, a family therapist or cotherapist may be required.

Children have a right to treatment for their obesity no matter how difficult it is to engage them or their parents in treatment. Where a family or a child threatens to drop out of treatment it is advisable that the therapists be proactive and contact the family to examine whether the obstacles that are hindering treatment can be eliminated.

Problems in the treatment of childhood obesity

There is considerable interindividual variation in response to interventions such that not all children achieve the recommended weight loss of 10%. Follow-up research indicates that only 1 out of 3 obese children achieves a weight loss of 20% of their overweight level (Epstein *et al.*, 1990; Braet & Van Winckel, 2000). With current interventions, most obese children will stay overweight for the rest of their lives. Moreover, approximately 15% of obese children keep gaining weight. This increases to 30% when the long-term evaluations are included (Braet & Van Winckel, 2000). Further research is required to identify intake interview predictors of a positive or negative therapy outcome. One predictor of a long-term favourable outcome is initial weight loss, measured 3 months after the intake (Braet *et al.*, 1997).

Treatment in childhood profits from the fact that children are still growing and this growth requires energy. However, in fully grown adolescents this energy expenditure diminishes and weight control is much more difficult to instigate. As Jelalian & Saelens (1999) noted, 'Much of the adolescent treatment fails to demonstrate short- or long-term success. There is much to be gained from examining how to adapt successful adult and/or child obesity programs for adolescents'. Also for those fitting a specific genetic profile or for those who fail to respond to behavioural treatment, new interventions need to be considered. Further advances may lead from pharmacological interventions, surgery or inpatient treatment. However, at present there is debate about the effectiveness of these interventions (Braet *et al.*, 2004).

Parents and obese children should be clear that the child has a lifelong predisposition to obesity (Bouchard, 1995). This is exacerbated by the current food excess in developed countries. More research is planned to investigate whether weight regain can be prevented if the treatment programme is followed by individualized booster sessions in which the children learn maintenance strategies or relapse prevention techniques. Recently, Latner *et al.* (2000) argued that continuous care of indefinite duration may be necessary to achieve long-term treatment effects in most obese people. Although progress has been made in treating obesity in childhood, new developments are needed to improve long-term weight regulation.

REFERENCES

Banis, H. T., Varni, J. W., Wallander, J. L. *et al.* (1988). Psychological and social adjustment of obese children and their families. *Child Care Health Development*, **14**, 157–73.

Berkowitz, R., Stunkard, A. J. & Stallings, V. A. (1993). Binge eating disorder in obese adolescent girls. In *Prevention and Treatment of Childhood Obesity*, ed. Williams, L. C. & Kimm, S. Y. S. *Annals of the New York Academy of Sciences*, **699**, 200–6.

Birch, L. L. (1987). The acquisition of food acceptance patterns in children. In *Eating Habits. Food, Physiology and Learned Behaviour*, ed. Boakes, R. A., Popplewell, D. A. & Burton, M. J. *Volume V.* New York: John Wiley, pp. 107–31.

Bouchard, C. (1995). Genetic influences on body weight and shape. In *Eating Disorders and Obesity. A Comprehensive Handbook*, ed. Brownell, K. D. & Fairburn, C. New York: Guilford Press, pp. 21–6.

Bouchard, C., Tremblay, A., Després, J. P. *et al.* (1990). The response to long-term overfeeding in identical twins. *New England Journal of Medicine*, **21**, 1477–82.

Bouchard, C., Pérusse, L., Rice, T. & Rao, D. C. (1998). The genetics of human obesity. In *Handbook of Obesity*, ed. Bray, G. A., Bouchard, C. & James, W. P. T. New York: Marcel Dekker, pp. 157–90.

Braet, C. (1999). Treatment of obese children: a new rationale. *Clinical Child Psychology and Psychiatry*, **4**, 579–91.

Braet, C. (2000). Action techniques for boosting self-esteem in obese children. In *A Theoretical and Practical Guide to Action and Drama Techniques*, ed. Verhofstadt-Denève, L. London: Jessica Kingsley Publishers, pp. 233–54.

Braet, C., Mervielde, I. & Vandereycken, W. (1997). Psychological aspects of childhood obesity. A controlled study in a clinical and non-clinical example. *Journal of Pediatric Psychology*, **22**, 59–71.

Braet, C., Van Winckel, M. & Van Leeuwen, K. (1997). Follow-up results of different treatment programs for obese children. *Acta Paediatrica*, **86**, 397–402.

Braet, C. & Van Winckel, M. (2000). Long-term follow-up of a cognitive behavioral treatment program for obese children. *Behavior Therapy*, **31**, 55–74.

Braet, C., Tanghe, A., Decaluwé, V., Moens, E. & Rosseel, Y. (2004). Inpatient treatment for children with obesity: weight loss, psychosocial well being, and eating behavior. *Journal of Pediatric Psychology*, **29**, 519–29.

Bray, G. A. (1986). Effects of obesity on health and happiness. In *Handbook of Eating Disorders: Physiology, Psychology, and Treatment of Obesity*, ed. Brownell, K. D. & Foreyt, J. P. New York: Basic Books, pp. 3–44.

Cole, T. J., Bellizzi, M. C., Flegal, K. M. & Dietz, W. H. (2000). Establishing a standard definition for child overweight and obesity worldwide: international survey. *Britisch Medical Journal*, **320**, 1–6.

Decaluwé V., Braet, C. & Fairburn, C. (2003). Binge eating in obese children and adolescents. *International Journal of Eating Disorders*, **33**, 78–94.

Dietz, W. H. (1998). Health consequences of obesity in youth: childhood predictors of adult disease. *Pediatrics*, **101** (suppl), 518–25.

Dietz, W. H. & Gortmaker, S. L. (1985). Do we fatten our children at the TV set? Obesity and television viewing in children and adolescents. *Pediatrics*, **75**, 807–12.

Epstein, L. H. & Wing, R. R. (1987). Behavioral treatment of childhood obesity. *Psychological Bulletin*, **101**, 331–42.

Epstein, L. H., Valoski, A., Wing, R. R. & McCurley, J. (1990). Ten-year outcomes of behavioral family-based treatment for childhood obesity. *Health Psychology*, **13**, 373–83.

Epstein, L. H., Myers, M. D., Raynor, H. A. & Saelens, B. E. (1998). Treatment of pediatric obesity. *Pediatrics*, **101**, 554–70.

Fairburn, C. G. & Wilson, G. T. (1993). *Binge Eating: Nature, Assessment and Treatment*. New York: Guilford Press.

Fairburn, C. G., Welch, S. L., Doll, H. A., Davies, B. A. & O'Connor, M. E. (1997). Risk factors for bulimia nervosa: a community-based case control study. *Archives of General Psychiatry*, **54**, 509–17.

Flegal, K. M. & Troiano, R. P. (2000). Changes in the distribution of body mass index of adults and children in the US population. *International Journal of Obesity*, **24**, 807–18.

Frederiks, A. M., van Buuren, S., Wit, J. M. & Verloove-Vanhorick, S. P. (2000). Body index measurements in 1996–1997 compared with 1980. *Archives of Disease in Childhood*, **82**, 107–12.

Freedman, D. S., Dietz, W. H., Srinivasan, S. R. & Berenson, G. S. (1999). The relation of overweight to cardiovascular risk factors among children and adolescents: the Bogalusa Heart Study. *Pediatrics*, **103**, 1175–82.

Garner, D. M. & Wooley, S. C. (1991). Confronting the failure of behavioral and dietary treatments for obesity. *Clinical Psychological Review*, **11**, 729–80.

Goldfried, G. S., Raynor, H. A. & Epstein, L. H. (2002). Treatment of pediatric obesity. In *Handbook of Obesity Treatment*, ed. Wadden, T. A. & Stunkard, A. J. New York: Guilford Press, pp. 532–55.

Gortmaker, S. L., Must, A., Perrin, J. M., Sobol, A. M. & Dietz, W. H. (1993). Social and economic consequences of overweight in adolescence and young adulthood. *New England Journal of Medicine*, **329**, 1008–12.

Herman, C. P. & Polivy, J. (1980). Restrained eating. In *Obesity*, ed. Stunkard, A. J. Philadelphia: W. B. Saunders, pp. 208–25.

Jansen, A. (1993). *Bulimia nervosa effectief behandelen. Een handleiding voor therapeuten*. Lisse: Swets & Zeitlinger.

Jelalian, E. & Saelens, B. E. (1999). Empirically supported treatments in pediatric psychology: pediatric obesity. *Journal of Pediatric Psychology*, **24**, 223–48.

Johnson, S. L. & Birch, L. L. (1994). Parents' and children's adiposity and eating style. *Pediatrics*, **94**, 653–61.

Latner, J. D., Stunkard, A. J., Wilson, G. T., Jackson, M. L., Zelitch, D. S. & Labouvie, E. (2000). Effective long-term treatment of obesity: a continuing care model. *International Journal of Obesity*, **24**, 893–8.

Mossberg, H. O. (1989). 40-year follow-up of overweight children. *Lancet*, **2**, 491–3.

Rodin, J. & Slochower, Y. (1976). Externality in the non-obese: effects of environmental responsiveness on weight. *Journal of Personality and Social Psychology*, **33**, 338–44.

Rössner, S. (1998). Childhood obesity and adult consequences. *Acta Paediatrica*, **87**, 1–5.

Sallis, J. F., Broyles, S. L. & Frankspohrer, G. (1995). Childs home-environment in relation to the mothers adiposity. *International Journal of Obesity*, **19**, 190–7.

Schlundt, D. G., Taylor, D., Hill, J. O. *et al.* (1991). A behavioral taxonomy of obese female participants in a weight loss program. *American Journal of Clinical Nutrition*, **109**, 1151–8.

Strauss, C. C., Smith, K., Frame, C. & Forehand, R. (1985). Personal and interpersonal characteristics associated with childhood obesity. *Journal of Pediatric Psychology*, **10**, 337–43.

Stunkard, A. J. & Sobal, J. (1995). Psychological consequences of obesity. *Eating Disorders and Obesity*, **23**, 83–8.

Whitaker, R. C., Wright, J. A., Pepe, M. S., Seidel, K. D. & Dietz, W. H. (1997). Predicting obesity in young adulthood from childhood and parental obesity. *New England Journal of Medicine*, **337**, 869–73.

Wilson, G. T. (1994). Behavioral treatment of obesity: thirty years and counting. *Advances in Behaviour Research and Therapy*, **16**, 31–75.

Part IV

Evidence-based care

16

Assessment and treatment of acute medical complications during the refeeding process

Carl Laird Birmingham

University of British Columbia, Vancouver, BC, Canada

Introduction

This chapter explains the refeeding syndrome, how to prevent it and how to treat it should it occur. Next, the causes, differential diagnosis and treatment of serious acute medical syndromes that occur during refeeding are explained. Finally, the indications for paediatric consultation are listed.

The refeeding syndrome: acute nutritional management

The refeeding syndrome is a combination of signs and symptoms that can result from feeding a malnourished patient (Golden & Meyer, 2004). It may occur along a spectrum that ranges from none, to the sudden onset of congestive heart failure. Typically, signs and symptoms will include oedema and aching bones and muscles.

Deficiency states in anorexia nervosa

It is important to consider what deficiencies are likely to exist at the beginning of the refeeding process in children and adolescents. This is particularly true of children and adolescents because growth and development increase nutritional requirements. As most patients with anorexia nervosa have had unhealthy eating habits for many months or years (Golden *et al.*, 2003), their stores of nutrients are likely to be severely depleted. However, it is difficult to know which nutrients will be deficient because the pattern of food intake may have been significantly disrupted by purging. Furthermore, patients may take

Eating Disorders in Children and Adolescents, ed. Tony Jaffa and Brett McDermott. Published by Cambridge University Press. © Cambridge University Press 2007.

vitamin or mineral supplements in an attempt to compensate for nutritional deficiencies. A further complication is that baseline nutrient stores in the normal human body vary greatly from nutrient to nutrient. For example, it is usual to have a 17-year store of selenium and vitamin A, but only a 3–5-year store of vitamin B12. In addition, some deficiencies may cause other deficiencies, as in the case of thiamine deficiency, which can be caused by magnesium or phosphate deficiencies because both of these are required for thiamine metabolism. It is worth noting that a magnesium deficiency usually causes a potassium deficiency, often a calcium deficiency and sometimes a phosphorus deficiency.

Some of the most serious complications of the refeeding syndrome, such as congestive heart failure, result from deficiency states. Before refeeding begins the malnourished patient typically has a low metabolic rate, low serum insulin, reduced or absent glycogen stores in the liver and depleted stores of various vitamins and minerals. Paradoxically, blood levels of nutrients are usually normal and there are usually no symptoms or signs of nutrient deficiency. This is because the serum levels and function of many nutrients adjust to remain within normal limits while tissue stores are falling. The deficiencies that occur during refeeding result from a dramatic increase in the use of nutrients caused by the increased caloric intake — in essence the rapid use of nutrients uncovers the deficient stores. Physiologically, refeeding results in a rapid rise in the resting metabolic rate. This means that there must be a gradual increase in the meal plan in the first week or two for weight gain to occur. Serum levels of insulin rise in response to the increased glucose load, which results in the movement of glucose, potassium and phosphorus into the cells where they are necessary for nutritional recovery. This often causes a rapid drop of serum potassium and serum phosphorus (Ornstein *et al.*, 2003). Similarly, as insulin moves glucose into cells from the blood, the blood sugar level falls. The body normally stabilizes the falling glucose by releasing more from liver glycogen stores in response to the secretion of glucagon from the pancreas. But the serum glucose cannot respond if the glycogen stores in the liver are depleted. Thus, paradoxically, postprandial hypoglycaemia can occur in early refeeding. Finally, nutrient stores are further depleted as nutrients are used to repair and rebuild the body.

Prevention and management of the refeeding syndrome

To reduce the risk of refeeding, it is advisable to begin correcting deficiencies before feeding, to commence feeding slowly and to increase the rate gradually. Serious complications of refeeding are more likely to occur in those patients who have low serum levels of vitamins or minerals before refeeding, those who binge and purge compared with those who restrict, those with more severe malnutrition and those who are treated with rapid refeeding. Begin feeding at a slower rate and monitor serum potassium, phosphorus and magnesium more frequently and longer in those who binge and purge and those with severe malnutrition. Twelve steps for the successful refeeding of malnourished children and adolescents are as follows.

1. Consult a dietician who has experience in treating eating disorders.

2. A. Take a dietary history. A nutrition history may help indicate possible deficiencies. For example, a vegetarian-like diet is often associated with iron, zinc, magnesium and B12 deficiencies.

    B. Determine whether nutrient deficiencies are present before refeeding begins. Measure serum potassium, bicarbonate, sodium, chloride, creatinine, blood urea nitrogen, albumen, aspartate transaminase, alkaline phosphatase, ferritin, red blood cell folate, B12, magnesium, phosphorus, calcium and zinc.

3. Correct the baseline deficiencies.

4. Begin feeding with one-third to one-half the estimated caloric requirement. This often means beginning with 800–1200 calories a day. There are a number of variables that might theoretically increase the caloric requirement for refeeding. For example, cigarette smoking increases energy expenditure, occult exercise is common, purging may continue despite close observation and the level of anxiety may be high. However, the best predictor of caloric requirement remains the past caloric requirement for refeeding. If that information is not available the rate of feeding should simply be gradually increased.

5. Route of feeding: the vast majority of patients can be fed orally if there is a programme of meal support. Meal support varies between programmes but always includes healthcare professionals providing distraction and behavioural support while eating with the patients. Often, the meal support person will determine how much of a liquid supplement is needed to replace uneaten food.

6. Hypoglycaemia can occur in early refeeding. It usually occurs an hour or two after meals but may occur at other times, depending on many factors including exercise, stress and caloric intake. The blood sugar should be measured fasting and 2 hours after meals for at least 2 days after feeding begins. As well, it should be measured if symptoms of confusion, dizziness or tiredness occur. A blood sugar level of less than 2.5 mm/l is diagnostic of hypoglycaemia. Similar symptoms occur with a rapid drop in blood sugar independent of the blood sugar level. If hypoglycaemia is diagnosed intravenous glucose should be given at a rate sufficient to maintain a normal

blood sugar until the blood sugar level can be maintained without it. It usually takes 2 weeks of refeeding to re-establish adequate liver glycogen to prevent hypoglycaemia.

7. Thiamine must be supplemented parenterally before intravenous glucose is given. Thiamine (100 mg) should be administered intramuscularly or intravenously in addition to 100 mg orally a day for 5 days. Intravenous glucose can precipitate Wernicke's encephalopathy in malnutrition.

8. If meal support is not available, and particularly on medical wards, tube feeding or a combination of tube feeding and oral feeding should be used. A soft feeding tube is recommended, the position should be confirmed by X-ray and a pump that has an auto-shutoff device with a pressure sensor should be used. The caloric density of the feed, the rate of feeding and timing of feeding can be adjusted to improve compliance.

9. Parenteral nutrition is rarely necessary for feeding and adds additional risks. The central line may cause infection, pneumothorax or thrombosis. Patients may tamper with the line itself, the intravenous site, or even disconnect it to drain the feeding solution. Disconnecting the line can lead to air embolism.

10. Percutaneous endoscopic gastrostomy (PEG) tubes are used very rarely. These feeding tubes can be implanted from the skin into the upper bowel by gastroenterologists or surgeons. Although in many ways they are similar to nasogastric tubes they are much more acceptable to some patients and may allow them to be treated as outpatients.

11. Supplements: routinely give a multivitamin daily, thiamine 100 mg for the first 5 days, zinc gluconate 100 mg daily for 2 months, potassium 20 mm three times a day and phosphorus 500 mg three times a day. If hypomagnesaemia should occur supplement with intravenous magnesium 20 mm in 250 cc normal saline over 4 hours a day for 5 days (do not give magnesium in renal insufficiency). Intramuscular magnesium is painful and oral magnesium is poorly absorbed and therefore causes diarrhoea.

12. Monitoring: measure serum potassium, magnesium and phosphorus daily for 5 days and then 3 times a week. Although a drop in the level of these minerals is more likely to occur in the first week it may occur during the first 3 weeks or longer.

Acute medical complications of refeeding

A variety of serious physical complaints have been reported upon refeeding malnourished patients (Table 16.1). A discussion of these follows.

Table 16.1. Causes of serious physical complaints that occur during refeeding

	Loss of consciousness	Seizure	Confusion	Chest pain	Shortness of breath	Palpitations	Abdominal pain	Rapid onset weakness	Hematemesis
Overdose	***	**	***					***	
Drug withdrawal	***	***	***					***	
Hypoglycaemia	***	**	***					***	
Hyponatraemia		**	***					***	
Hypomagnesaemia		**	***		*	**		***	
Hypocalcaemia		*	*						
Hypophosphataemia					**				
Severe alkalosis		*							
Wernicke's parotitis			***						
Bacterial infection			**	**			**	**	
Arrhythmia	**	*	*			***			
Heart failure					**	*		*	
Aspiration				**	**				
Mallory–Weiss tear				**			**		
Renal stone							**		
SMA							**		

Table 16.1. (*cont.*)

	Loss of consciousness	Seizure	Confusion	Chest pain	Shortness of breath	Palpitations	Abdominal pain	Rapid onset weakness	Hematemesis
Pancreatitis							*		
Oesophageal rupture				*			*		
Common causes	Postural hypotension, vasovagal	Withdrawal, overdose	Severe malnutrition, hypoglycaemia, drug toxicity	Chest wall pain, oesophagitis	Hypophosphataemia	Purging, hypokalaemia, hypomagnesaemia	Constipation, intestinal dysmotility	Hypomagnesaemia, hypokalaemia	Tear of oropharynx, Mallory–Weiss tear

Notes:

***Common,

**occasional,

*rare.

Seizures

Causes

Common: metabolic causes: hypophosphataemia, hypoglycaemia, hyponatraemia, hypomagnesaemia, decreased cerebral perfusion due to arrhythmia, hypotension or vasovagal episode, drug toxicity (e.g. bupropion), drug overdose, drug withdrawal including alcohol withdrawal; rarely hypocalcaemia.

Differential diagnosis

Pseudo seizure — a markedly elevated serum prolactin level can be used to rule out a pseudo seizure; however, about one-third of patients with pseudo seizures also have seizures.

Comment

The history from a witness and consideration of predisposing factors, like benzodiazepine use, are important. Seizures are common during benzodiazepine withdrawal. Hypoglycaemia occurs because the liver has no glycogen left to form glucose when the blood glucose level drops. Hyponatraemia can cause seizures, usually when the serum sodium is less than 120 mm/L. Hypomagnesaemia can cause seizures, usually when the serum magnesium is less than 0.45 mm/L. Drug toxicity can occur, especially when the patient gets prescriptions from multiple physicians. Seizures that are due to alcohol withdrawal usually occur 1 to 3 days after cessation of alcohol intake. Cardiac monitoring may be necessary to determine whether seizures are due to arrhythmias.

Treatment

The treatment of seizures is not different in eating disorders. Determining the cause of the seizures and treatment of that cause is most important. Standard drug treatment and dosages for seizures can be used. Although the BMI is very low and the lean body mass is low, the apparent volume of distribution of drugs appears remarkably normal and kidney and liver function are usually normal.

Loss of consciousness

Causes

Common: hypophosphataemia, hypoglycaemia, hypotension, vasovagal episode. Occasional: seizure, arrhythmia, hyponatraemia. Less common: drug overdose, drug toxicity.

Differential diagnosis

Functional amnesia, being interpreted as loss of consciousness, and drug toxicity causing the serotonergic syndrome, the malignant neuroleptic syndrome or an acute dystonia. Impairment of memory can be tested for. Drug toxicities must be considered for diagnosis to be made. Although acute dystonia may result in an inability to communicate the patient's memory is not impaired during the event.

Comment

Hypoglycaemia occurs after eating because glucagon cannot normalize the falling sugar if the liver stores of glycogen are depleted. Hyponatraemia can cause a loss of consciousness, especially if the serum sodium is less than 115 mm/L. However, a rapid increase or decrease in serum sodium can cause loss of consciousness due to a shift in the fluid within the brain. This is because the skull cannot change size while the brain cells swell or shrink — like a grape to a raisin — depending on the salinity of the blood. The most severe dangerous complication of rapidly correcting low serum sodium in the malnourished is central pontine myelolysis, which usually results in death. Drug overdoses are common in eating disorders. The overdose is usually from a stockpile of medications that the patient has had prescribed. Arrhythmias and hypoglycaemia can occur during treatment of the overdose.

Treatment

The treatment of loss of consciousness is supporting airway, breathing and circulation, treating the underlying cause and general supportive treatment.

Confusion

Causes

Common: severe malnutrition, hypoglycaemia, hypophosphataemia, hyponatraemia, hypomagnesaemia, Wernicke's encephalopathy. Occasional: bacterial infection. Rare: postictal, drug withdrawal, drug toxicity (e.g. malignant neuroleptic syndrome, serotonergic syndrome), drug overdose, alcohol withdrawal, hypothermia (Patchell et al., 1994).

Differential diagnosis

Confusion has a broad differential diagnosis that is best approached by looking for focal neurological findings and using the differential diagnosis of a decreased level of consciousness above.

Comment

The confusion caused by severe malnutrition is proportional to the severity of the malnutrition. It progresses slowly and it reverses within a week or two of refeeding. The confusion caused by hypoglycaemia usually occurs an hour or two after eating. It clears within minutes of glucose administration (e.g. orange juice). Wernicke's encephalopathy is caused by inadequate active thiamine. Because thiamine requires phosphorus and magnesium to function in humans, a deficiency in either of these minerals can precipitate Wernicke's encephalopathy without a deficiency of thiamine itself. The treatment of Wernicke's encephalopathy is an emergency. If thiamine is administered soon after the confusion (and phosphorus and magnesium are normal or corrected), difficulty walking and gaze abnormalities will reverse within hours. Without treatment a permanent short-term memory deficit will result. Bacterial infection is often occult in anorexia nervosa because there is a delay in an elevation of body temperature and white count above normal. The white count and temperature are usually low in anorexia nervosa on admission. The most common sites of infection in anorexia nervosa are the chest, the urinary tract and phlebotomy or intravenous sites.

Treatment

Check the blood sugar by measuring serum glucose, chemstrips are less accurate for the measurement of a low blood sugar. Search for occult infection, examine the eye movements and carefully review the medication history. Treat the cause.

Chest pain

Causes

Common: chest wall pain, heartburn, oesophagitis, oesophageal spasm, atypical angina, panic attack. Occasional: rib fracture, angina, aspiration pneumonia. Rare: pleurisy, pericarditis, oesophageal rupture (Birmingham *et al.*, 2003b).

Differential diagnosis

Chest wall pain is the most common cause of chest pain in eating disorders. It is similar to aches and pains experienced in other parts of the body. It occurs in the chest wall (not deep), although it may have been present for days. Episodes of worsening usually last only a few seconds, and it may be reproduced or worsened by pressure on the chest wall over the site of the complaint, movement or deep breathing. The pain of oesophagitis usually accompanies a history of worsening heartburn. Oesophageal spasm is quite different from heartburn but very similar to angina pectorus. The pain of oesophageal spasm is usually a pressure felt in the mid-chest that may radiate to the arms and neck. However, unlike angina that is precipitated by exercise, relieved by rest and lasts a few minutes to half an hour, oesophageal spasm is not changed by exertion, is not relieved by rest and usually lasts many hours or days. A rib fracture is characterized by marked point tenderness at the site of the fracture.

Comment
A careful history is the most useful way to determine the cause of chest pain.

Treatment
Treat the underlying cause. Chest wall pain requires reassurance and analgesics. The pain of oesophagitis usually responds to a proton pump inhibitor but may require the addition of an antireflux medication. The acute pain of oesophageal spasm decreases with nitroglycerine and calcium channel blockers but will require the same treatment as oesophagitis to clear long term. Several patients with anorexia nervosa have died of coronary artery disease when young; however, atherosclerosis appears to progress more rapidly only in relation to the duration of amenorrhea, not the duration of anorexia nervosa. Thus, angina or atypical angina should be investigated with an exercise test if amenorrhea has been present for more than 10 years.

Shortness of breath
Causes
Common: aspiration pneumonia, respiratory muscle weakness. Occasional: congestive heart failure (usually due to hypophosphataemia), empyema. Rare: lung abscess, hypomagnesaemia, arrhythmia, oesophageal rupture (Birmingham & Tan, 2003; Coxson et al., 2004).

Differential diagnosis
The most common causes of acute shortness of breath in anorexia nervosa are aspiration and congestive heart failure.

Comment
Pulmonary aspiration most commonly occurs in a sedated patient during tube feeding. The chest X-ray may remain normal for 24 hours or more after aspiration. Acute congestive heart failure is most often caused by hypophosphataemia. If the phosphate level in the blood drops to less than half the lower

limit of normal, congestive heart failure may occur. Elevation of fever and white count may be delayed in bacterial pneumonia, empyema and lung abscess. Respiratory muscle weakness is caused by the generalized muscle wasting seen in malnutrition. Because it is due to smooth muscle wasting it may take many months or years to recover after refeeding.

Treatment

Treat the underlying cause. Congestive heart failure should be treated in an intensive care unit because it is frequently progressive and unresponsive to standard treatments unless phosphorus is adequately repleted. Blood gases should be measured in patients with aspiration pneumonia because severe hypoxia may not be clinically apparent. The immune response to bacterial infections is abnormal in anorexia nervosa; this is likely due to an impairment of white blood cell motility. The optimal dose of an antibiotic chosen on the basis of antibiotic sensitivities and administered intravenously is necessary.

Palpitations

Causes

Common: sinus tachycardia, autonomic dysfunction, paroxysmal atrial tachycardia. Occasional: premature ventricular contractions. Rare: ventricular tachycardia, torsades de pointes (Galetta et al., 2003).

Differential diagnosis

A history of the palpitations is key: how often, what time of day, sudden or slow onset, sudden or slow offset, rapid or slow, regular or irregular, associated symptoms. The most common cause of reported palpitations is a sinus tachycardia. This often occurs after purging or exercise.

Comment

Premature ventricular beats that come from the left ventricle that are frequent, or that are in runs, warrant assessment. The medications used by the patient should be reviewed to determine cardiotoxicity and interactions. The serum electrolytes, magnesium and phosphorus should be measured and corrected if necessary. A resting electrocardiogram should be inspected with special attention to a prolongation of the QTc interval to longer than 440 ms or markedly prolonged compared with previous tracings. Autonomic dysfunction is frequent in anorexia nervosa without refeeding. Clinically there may be marked fluctuations in heart rate and blood pressure over the day that are unexplained by activity or purging. There is an increase in the variability of the interval between heart beats on special analysis of the cardiac tracing (e.g. spectral analysis of the Holter monitor). There is growing evidence that arrhythmias are more likely to occur during times of change in heart rate variability.

Treatment

There are no controlled trials of antiarrhythmics in anorexia nervosa. However, as cardiologists usually have little experience with the treatment of arrhythmias in young women and less with young women with eating disorders, they may be inherently disinclined to treat arrhythmias. I have used long-term low-dose metoprolol with good results in a few patients who have frequent arrhythmias.

Abdominal pain

Causes

Common: constipation, delayed gastric emptying, oesophagitis. Occasional: urinary tract infection, renal colic, superior mesenteric artery syndrome. Rare: pancreatitis, oesophageal rupture.

Differential diagnosis

Abdominal pain occurs frequently in most patients with eating disorders. This can cause a relative lack of concern on the part of the physician and patient with consequent under-reporting of symptoms by the patient and under-investigation by the physician. This is particularly the case for pancreatitis. Another reason for missed diagnoses is a lack of familiarity with the clinical presentation of the superior mesenteric artery (SMA) syndrome.

Comment

Superior mesenteric artery syndrome is caused by a partial obstruction of the small bowel by the superior mesenteric artery at the level of the third part of the duodenum. This occurs because of a disappearance of the normal padding (intra-abdominal fat) in severe malnutrition. Thus if a patient has nausea and vomiting after eating when they are severely malnourished the diagnosis should be considered and a CT scan can be used to investigate. Pancreatitis may be overlooked because the symptoms of abdominal pain, nausea and vomiting may be regarded as consistent with the eating disorder. Although the serum amylase may be elevated in pancreatitis and in patients with eating disorders, the serum lipase is only elevated in pancreatitis and an ultrasound or CT scan of the pancreas can help make the diagnosis.

Treatment

Treatment is specific to cause.

Haematemesis

Causes

Common: traumatic laceration of the throat. Occasional: Mallory–Weiss tear. Rare: ulcer.

Differential diagnosis

The most common cause of haematemesis in eating disorders is mouth or throat mucosal laceration caused by vomiting or the instrument used to induce vomiting.

Comment

A traumatic laceration results in the vomiting of a small amount of blood coincident with pain in the mouth or throat. A Mallory–Weiss tear is a laceration in the lower oesophagus due to repeated purging. This should be suspected if the patient had purged forcefully many times before bright red blood was vomited. Haematemesis may continue if the patient continues to vomit at that time and may reoccur if there are episodes of purging in the next day or two. The diagnosis of an ulcer is made more difficult because in young patients the symptoms of ulcer disease may be absent or atypical.

Treatment

No treatment is necessary for a traumatic laceration of the mouth or throat. However, patients are often very concerned about vomiting blood and a careful explanation may serve as a disincentive to purge. Similarly, Mallory–Weiss tears need no investigation or treatment unless they are recurrent or the volume of blood vomited is large. The diagnosis and treatment of an ulcer is not different in eating disorders.

Fever

Causes

Common: skin infection at the site of a wound or intravenous site, pneumonia. Occasional: renal infection, parotitis. Rare: empyema, lung abscess, osteomyelitus, pancreatitis, oesophageal rupture (Birmingham *et al.*, 2003a).

Differential diagnosis

A wound site will have signs of inflammation. If the area was the site of self-injurious behaviour the patient may not bring it to the physician's attention. Chest X-ray evidence of pneumonia may be delayed by a day or two if the patient is volume depleted (dehydrated). Tenderness is usually present in the flanks with pyelonephritis, but there are often no signs on examination in cystitis. Parotitis may be difficult to distinguish if the patient has had large tender glands all along.

Comment

Patients with anorexia nervosa have a normal response to viral infections and indeed seem to get fewer of them. There is no evidence that they have more frequent bacterial infections either. However, there is evidence that they have a delayed fever and elevation of white cells and are prone to more severe bacterial infections because of an impairment of white blood cell movement to the site of infection. Therefore, an increase in temperature or white cell count, even within normal limits, should be regarded as possible evidence of infection. Pneumonia, empyema and lung abscess may be advanced at the time of diagnosis. Renal infection may be overlooked due to diminished concern about abdominal pain in a patient who has frequent and varied abdominal pains. Bacterial infection of the parotid gland almost always occurs in malnourished and dehydrated patients and is usually caused by *Staphylococcus aureus*. The parotid will be very tender and there may be pus at the site of Stensen's duct just above the second molar on the side of the infection.

Treatment

Treatment of fever is not different except that magnesium and zinc deficiencies can impair healing and should be corrected, and occult purging or noncompliance should be considered.

Rapid onset of weakness

Causes

Common: hypokalaemia, hypomagnesaemia. Occasional: hypophosphataemia, overdose, hypoglycaemia. Rare: bacterial infection.

Differential diagnosis

Hypokalaemia and hypomagnesaemia cause proximal weakness. The patient will have weakness holding her arms up to comb her hair and/or climbing stairs. Hypophosphataemia usually presents with shortness of breath due to pulmonary oedema caused by weakness of the heart.

Comment

Phosphate is necessary for producing adenosine triphosphate (ATP), the chemical that provides energy for everything in the body including the heart. Patients may overdose on drugs brought in by visitors or their own stocks even when hospitalized. The weakness due to hypoglycaemia is usually overshadowed by marked confusion. If a bacterial infection presents with the rapid onset of weakness this usually means there is a gram-negative bacterial septicaemia that is usually caused by a kidney infection.

Treatment

Treat the underlying condition. Remember that hypomagnesaemia usually causes renal wastage of potassium, so these two often occur together and both will respond to magnesium repletion.

Bed sores

Causes

Common: emaciation, decreased level of consciousness, sleeping on a hard surface, oversedation. Occasional: self-injurious behaviour, decreased skin perfusion due to hypothermia, severe anaemia, volume depletion, habitual exercise. Rare: neuropathy.

Differential diagnosis

Most bed sores occur due to an impaired level of consciousness due to sedation in a patient lying on a regular mattress. The sore will occur over the point of greatest pressure. Self-injurious behaviour causing a 'bed sore' usually occurs in a patient who has a history of self-injurious behaviour. Any factor that causes abnormalities of the skin or skin perfusion by blood, such as skin eruption, hypothermia, anaemia and volume depletion, will predispose to bed sores.

Comment

The response to bacterial infection may be impaired (see 'Fever', above).

Treatment

Prevent bed sores! Any patient with anorexia nervosa who has a decreased level of consciousness is likely to develop complications including bed sores, aspiration pneumonia, pressure neuropathies of the ulnar, radial and lateral peroneal nerves, urinary tract infections, infectious parotitis and skin infections. Increased nursing care, regular turning of the patient in bed, frequent physical examination of the skin, chest, mouth, intravascular volume are warranted. If a bed sore does occur, do not assume the bed sore is solely due to pressure. Continued covert exercise, self-injurious behaviour or impaired skin perfusion should be considered. Culture the wound even if it does not look infected, including anaerobic culture. Consult a dermatologist early. The care of bed sores is specialized and inadequate treatment can cause prolonged pain and delay discharge from hospital by weeks.

When should mental health professionals consult a paediatrician?

Finally, it is my observation and personal opinion that mental health professionals should consult paediatricians more often than they do when caring for children and adolescents with eating disorders. These young people often consider medical complications more motivating than psychological ones. This is especially so if the medical complications are managed by a paediatrician. Thus, a paediatric consultation may bring additional benefits. The need for a paediatric consultation depends on many factors, including the medical expertise of the mental health professional, the state of health of the child and concurrent treatment outside the eating disorders programme. The following recommendations should be used only as a guide to the need for paediatric consultation.

1. All patients should have a complete assessment by a consultant paediatrician when they begin a programme.
2. All patients should have a family paediatrician or family doctor who sees them regularly (at least every 2 months) during treatment.
3. All patients should be assessed by a paediatrician before and during refeeding.
4. A paediatric consultation should be sought for any major medical complication such as a seizure, shortness of breath or rapid onset of weakness.

REFERENCES

Birmingham, C.L. & Tan, A.O. (2003). Respiratory muscle weakness and anorexia nervosa. *International Journal of Eating Disorders*, **33**, 230–3.

Birmingham, C.L., Hodgson, D.M., Fung, J. *et al.* (2003a). Reduced febrile response to bacterial infection in anorexia nervosa patients. *International Journal of Eating Disorders*, **34**, 269–72.

Birmingham, C.L., Lear, S.A., Kenyon, J. *et al.* (2003b). Coronary atherosclerosis in anorexia nervosa. *International Journal of Eating Disorders*, **34**, 375–7.

Coxson, H.O., Chan, I.H., Mayo, J.R. *et al.* (2004). Early emphysema in patients with anorexia nervosa. *American Journal of Respiratory and Critical Care Medicine*, **170**, 748–52.

Galetta, F., Franzoni, F., Prattichizzo, F. *et al.* (2003). Heart rate variability and left ventricular diastolic function in anorexia nervosa. *Journal of Adolescent Health*, **32**, 416–21.

Golden, N.H., Katzman, D.K., Kreipe, R.E. *et al.* (2003). Eating disorders in adolescents: position paper of the Society for Adolescent Medicine. *Journal of Adolescent Health*, **33**, 496–503.

Golden, N.H. & Meyer, W. (2004). Nutritional rehabilitation of anorexia nervosa. Goals and dangers. *International Journal of Adolescent Medicine and Health*, **16**, 131–44.

Ornstein, R.M., Golden, N.H., Jacobson, M.S. & Shenker, I.R. (2003). Hypophosphatemia during nutritional rehabilitation in anorexia nervosa: implications for refeeding and monitoring. *Journal of Adolescent Health*, **32**, 83–8.

Patchell, R.A., Fellows, H.A. & Humphries, L.L. (1994). Neurologic complications of anorexia nervosa. *Acta Neurologica Scandinavica*, **89**, 111–16.

17

Assessment and treatment of chronic medical complications

Richard E. Kreipe

Golisano Children's Hospital at Strong,
Rochester, NY, USA

Approach to young patients with chronic medical complications

Patients with chronic medical complications associated with an eating disorder (ED) often elicit negative countertransference from medical care providers (Franko & Rolfe, 1996). Common reactions by professionals include frustration with treating conditions that patients 'bring on themselves' or anger at a patient's resistance to treatment or intentional falsification of body weight during weigh-ins. What makes these conditions especially vexing is that they often occur in extremely bright, talented young people who seem to be unaware of the harm that they are doing to themselves. As noted by Strober (2004), the chronically ill patient requires a unique approach to care, one that minimizes the risk of iatrogenic effects of too-rapid weight restoration or failure to be aware of potentially negative effects of countertransference 'by integrating clinical experience, empirical psychological findings and a conceptual understanding of developmental and phenomenologic aspects of the illness'.

Given the tendency for younger patients with chronic medical complications to resist efforts to change, it is worthwhile for practitioners to apply the biopsychosocial approach in a manner that optimizes the likelihood that patients will cooperate with treatment recommendations. Promising in this regard is the use of motivational interviewing, closely linked with readiness-to-change. Although Wilson & Schlam (2004) question the theoretical underpinnings of motivational interviewing in EDs, Hasler et al. (2004) found that diagnostic subtype, age, illness duration and previous treatments were not associated with motivational stages, but that emotional involvement, specific behavioural change processes and beginning ongoing treatment were correlated with more advanced stages of change. In addition, Vitousek et al. (1998)

Eating Disorders in Children and Adolescents, ed. Tony Jaffa and Brett McDermott. Published by Cambridge University Press. © Cambridge University Press 2007.

noted that 'the ego-syntonic quality of symptoms can contribute to inaccuracy in self-report, avoidance of treatment, difficulties in establishing a therapeutic relationship, and high rates of attrition and relapse. Individuals with bulimia nervosa (BN) are typically more motivated to recover, but often ambivalent about forfeiting the ideal of slenderness and the protective functions of binge-purge behavior'. In their review they recommended that 'clinicians acquire a frame of reference that can help them understand the private experience of individuals with eating disorders, empathize with their distress at the prospect of weight gain, and acknowledge the difficulty of change'. This is especially true for patients with chronic medical complications. Although no organ system is spared the effects of dysfunctional weight control habits, there are targets that deserve special attention with respect to such complications. These include the heart, brain, gonads and skeleton.

Chronic medical complications

Heart

Although Gull (1874) noted bradycardia as a prominent chronic medical complication of the first reported cases of anorexia nervosa (AN), it was the research of Keys' group (1948) on young adult male volunteers undergoing 24 weeks of experimental protein-calorie malnutrition (PCM) that demonstrated the effects of starvation on the cardiovascular system. These individuals lost an average of 24% of body weight and experienced profound bradycardia – an average pulse of 37 beats/minute (bpm). Systolic and diastolic blood pressures both fell, as did stroke volume and all variables related to physical work of the heart decreased, by as much as 50%. Cyanosis of the nail-beds was also observed. These same changes occur in children and adolescents with chronic AN and are due to the malnutrition and not the eating disorder, per se. Furthermore, many cardiovascular changes found in eating disorders, such as sinus bradycardia, sinus arrhythmia and low blood pressure likewise are physiological adaptations to starvation; they do not represent 'complications' because they are evidence of inadequate nutrition, occur gradually, are not life-threatening and meet the diminished demands of tissue perfusion. They may be considered protective (Kreipe & Harris, 1992) insofar as a lower heart rate conserves caloric expenditure and the reduced afterload associated with lower blood pressure reduces ventricular wall forces required to eject blood during systole. Without such downregulation, then higher energy expenditures and higher forces than required would persist. In contrast, primary cardiovascular abnormalities such as prolonged corrected QT interval (QT_c), ventricular dysrhythmias or reduced myocardial contractility are abnormal complications that reflect myocardial impairment, occur more quickly, can be lethal and may interfere with tissue perfusion sufficient to meet metabolic demands.

Intermediate between these two extremes are the orthostatic pulse changes seen with weight loss. Our group (Kreipe *et al.*, 1994) found that pulse variability is related to hypothalamic autonomic imbalance (excessive para-sympathetic and inadequate sympathetic output) often associated with supine pulse < 50 bpm. On standing, the parasympathetic tone does not decrease as it normally should and the sympathetic tone is excessive, often resulting in an increase in pulse of > 30 bpm. Shamim *et al.* (2003) studied orthostatic pulse changes in 36 adolescent females with chronic restrictive AN during inpatient refeeding and found that pulse on admission averaged 54 bpm, which slowly increased to 70 by day 12 of hospitalization. Orthostatic changes from supine to standing of > 20 bpm decreased from a peak of 85% to a nadir of 15% of patients. Positional variation in pulse is a more sensitive indicator of haemo-dynamic instability than orthostatic blood pressure changes and takes longer to resolve. Thus, orthostatic pulse differential, which is reversible, is a reliable measure of cardiovascular stability in chronic AN.

Although various nonspecific changes most commonly associated with electrolyte imbalance can be observed, systematic investigations have not found a significant risk of life-threatening arrhythmias in adolescents with chronic eating disorders. Prolonged QT_c has been reported in some series, but the majority of reports do not demonstrate an increased incidence. A review of ECG changes in 47 subjects with AN found prolonged QT_c in only one, associated with hypokalaemia (Vanderdonckt *et al.*, 2001). However, young adults who have had AN for several years may be at greater risk for fatal arrhythmias (Isner *et al.*, 1985) and deserve special attention. Especially im-portant in this respect are patients who use ipecac to induce vomiting. Although this is seen less commonly now that its availability is more restricted, chronic ipecac use does result in a reversible myopathy affecting striated muscles, including the heart (Palmer & Guay, 1985). Patients who are found to have prolonged QT_c deserve ECG monitoring and cardiac evaluation, since fatal ventricular tachyarrhythmias, including torsade de pointes, have been observed as the cause of death in these circumstances.

Loss of ventricular mass is proportionately greater than the loss of body weight in AN (St. John Sutton *et al.*, 1985), suggesting that left ventricular mass reduction is related to decreased left ventricular after-load, possibly linked to the blunted heart rate and blood pressure responses mediated by reduced α-adrenergic receptor activity. The fall in left ventricular mass was associated with major left ventricular remodelling such that wall stresses remained normal, chamber shape and architecture remained normal, and chamber function and stress-shortening relationships remained normal. These variables remained normal during refeeding, when heart size returned to normal. Thus, left ventricular mass decrease during chronic starvation and subsequent increase during refeeding may be due to physiological adaptation of downregulation and upregulation, respectively.

The treatment of the chronic cardiovascular complications of EDs remains nutritional rehabilitation and weight gain. With respect to the prevention of potentially fatal dysrhythmias, electrolyte imbalances should be corrected, and medication use reviewed. Roche *et al.* (2005) studied 10 adolescent and young adult females with AN and found that QT dynamicity and RR intervals both could be restored with weight gain. Adolescents with chronic AN are often interested in continuing to exercise vigorously, even when severely underweight. Rowland *et al.* (2003) studied eight adolescent females with chronic AN undergoing exercise testing. As would be expected given their reduced lean body mass, subjects had resting and maximal heart rates and maximal oxygen uptakes that were significantly lower than controls. However, there was a normal pattern of response to progressive exercise in maximal stroke index, and peak aortic velocity and mean acceleration of flow were similar in the two groups when adjusted for heart rate, providing no evidence of abnormal myocardial performance during maximal exercise testing. Therefore, as long as the chronically ill patient is demonstrating weight gain and improvement in nutritional status and does not have prolonged QT_c or hypokalaemia, there is no cardiac contraindication to a progressive aerobic exercise programme. We encourage a programme that is developed in partnership with a physical therapist or trainer knowledgeable about EDs.

Brain

The brain has been studied extensively in adults chronically ill with an ED, initially with computerized tomography, then with magnetic resonance imaging (MRI) and most recently with functional MRI and positron emission tomography (PET) scanning. Only recently have studies focused on younger patients. Kerem & Katzman (2003) have summarized the changes in brain structure and function in adolescents with AN, noting that although structural changes improve with weight recovery, it is uncertain if they are completely reversible. For example, Katzman *et al.* (1997) found persistent grey but no longer white-matter deficits following almost 3 years of weight recovery in adolescents with AN. Total grey-matter volume correlated positively with lowest body weight and negatively with urinary cortisol levels, suggesting that grey-matter volume loss may be related to degree of weight loss and cortisol elevation. Although these researchers found statistically lower grey-matter volume in weight-recovered subjects, only half of them had resumed menses and there was significant overlap with controls, raising the possibility of continued return toward normal. Similar to Kohn *et al.* (1997), they found that increased ventricular volumes rapidly normalized with nutritional rehabilitation and weight gain.

Gordon *et al.* (2001) reported elevated medial temporal lobe cerebral blood flow on PET similar to that found in psychotic patients, suggesting that these changes may be related to body image distortion. Furthermore, visualizing high-calorie foods was associated with exaggerated responses in visual association cortex, similar to that seen in patients with specific phobias. Searching for a similar biological substrate for the unusual behaviours exhibited by patients with EDs, another research group (Gordon *et al.*, 1997) using single-photon emission computerized tomography (SPECT) found that 13 of 15 adolescents had unilateral temporal lobe hypoperfusion, eight on the left side and five on the right, and that abnormalities persisted in all three girls who had a follow-up scan after weight restoration. Although these authors propose that their findings suggest an underlying primary functional abnormality, further studies are needed to determine whether such alterations in brain function contribute to the development of the ED or are the result of it.

Several researchers have proposed that EDs are primarily brain disorders. With respect to chronic medical complications, however, the cumulative evidence is that structural abnormalities are reversible with weight restoration to normal, with dramatic improvements being noted with as little as 10% gain in body weight. Residual functional changes are of unknown significance and should deter neither the patient nor the practitioner from attempting to work toward normal weight and eating habits. From a clinical standpoint, the primary area of the brain affected by EDs, especially with weight loss, is the hypothalamus, with important influence on the endocrine regulatory function. Thermoregulation, satiety, sleep, as well as reduced gonadal activity and excessive adrenal cortex activity, can all be traced back to hypothalamic dysfunction, evidenced as acute medical complications. Even heart rate regulation is affected by weight loss. Fortunately, these central regulatory functions of the brain all appear to be reversible, with weight restoration.

Gonads and reproductive system

Because gonadotropin releasing hormone (GnRH) from the hypothalamus is decreased in both males and females with AN, both the testes and ovaries have reduced output of male and female sex steroids. However, because the overwhelming preponderance of patients are females and amenorrhoea is a core clinical finding in AN, testicular function has not been widely studied. Although menstrual function tends to be more normal in patients with bulimia nervosa (BN), they also exhibit dysfunction. For example, Ramacciotti et al. (1997) compared purging with nonpurging subjects with BN and found, even in the absence of overt menstrual disturbances, an altered LH secretion elicited by pulsatile stimulation of endogenous GnRH, with a more severe impairment in purging than in nonpurging subtype, possibly related to their greater psychopathological and physical burden.

Amenorrhea related to decreased hypothalamic function is one of the most clinically relevant chronic medical complications of EDs: it is a diagnostic feature of AN and is associated with both infertility and low levels of sex steroids. Our group studied adolescents a minimum of 4 years after treatment for AN and found that 80% of subjects had either resumed or initiated menses, at a mean of 90% average body weight (ABW) for height and age (Kreipe et al. 1989). In a similar study, Golden et al. (1997) also found that menses resumed at a weight approximately 90% of standard body weight; 86% of patients who achieved this goal resumed menses within 6 months. Measuring body composition, they found that menstrual return was not dependent on body fat content. Thus, a weight of 90% ABW or height is a reasonable target to expect menses to return. Swenne (2004) has suggested that weight Standard Deviation Scores (SDS) at the onset of amenorrhoea correlated more highly ($r^2 =$ 076; $P < 0.001$) with SDS on return of menses than other measures, including absolute weight, BMI or SDS for weight or BMI. Applying weight SDS is complicated in clinical practice, however, and it is important to note that there is large individual variation in the weight at which menses returns because menstruation is related to many factors in addition to weight. The weight to achieve menses may not be sufficient to achieve full reproductive system function, however. Using trans-abdominal ultrasound to assess ovarian and uterine maturity based on standardized criteria, Key et al. (2002) proposed that 90% of average weight may be sufficient for menses, but not for reproductive maturity. They reported that even at 100% of expected weight for height (BMI 20), 12% of girls still had immature ovaries and uterus.

The first report of bulimia nervosa (BN) as a distinct entity (Russell, 1979) reported a higher prevalence of menstrual dysfunction than the general population, but amenorrhoea was relatively uncommon. This was supported by a report by Crow *et al.* (2002) reporting on the menstrual and reproductive function of 173 women with BN an average of 11 years after initial presentation. While menstrual irregularities were common, they tended to be associated with low weight. They also concluded that a history of BN appeared to have 'little impact' on later fertility. They noted that abnormal LH secretion may be related to current weight < 85% of the highest lifetime weight, rather than current low body weight per se. Thus, if a previously overweight patient with BN has menstrual disturbance, she may need to gain more weight than otherwise expected to return to normal function.

Assuming that patients gain sufficient weight to achieve full reproductive capacity and become pregnant, what is known about their fertility and neonatal outcomes? Our group (Shomento & Kreipe, 1994) found that all subjects who had tried to become pregnant (many were still in college or graduate school) were able to do so, resulting in 22 pregnancies, 14 deliveries, five abortions, no known miscarriages and three ongoing pregnancies. These findings are similar to Franko *et al.* (2001) who evaluated the outcome of 49 live births among women with an ED – about half of whom had active symptoms at the onset of pregnancy – and found that the majority had healthy babies: average birth weight of 3500 g after an average gestation of 38.9 weeks, with normal Apgar scores and no differences between subjects with AN or BN, or between those who had a history of an ED compared with those with active symptoms. More recently, Kouba *et al.* (2005) reported the outcomes of 49 subjects with a past or current ED. In sum, adolescents and young adults with EDs who have concerns about future fertility can be reassured that there is little evidence that EDs, per se, are causally linked with poor pregnancy outcomes. As long as they recover sufficiently to maintain a healthy weight and menstruate regularly, their ability to conceive and deliver a healthy baby is similar to the general population. Obviously, obstetricians need to be aware of the increased risk for symptom relapse, hyperemesis and postpartum depression should a future pregnancy occur.

As is true of all chronic medical complications, the primary focus of treatment for adolescent patients with EDs who experience menstrual irregularities and amenorrhoea should be weight recovery and normalization of eating habits. For amenorrhoeic patients who have achieved 90% ABW, a 'progesterone challenge' has both diagnostic and therapeutic purposes. If any withdrawal vaginal bleeding occurs after taking 10 mg of medroxyprogesterone daily for 10 days, the hypothalamic-pituitary-gonadal-endometrial axis is intact, any proliferated endometrium will be shed, and nothing further needs to be done, although further weight gain may be needed for ovulation to occur. It is important to note that this manoeuvre does not 'kick start' the menstrual cycle, since menses begin at the level of the hypothalamus. Progestins are only effective in transforming a proliferated endometrium into a secretory one. Likewise, taking birth control pills regularly does cause a female to 'have her menstrual cycle'. Functioning at the level of the endometrium, oestrogen and progesterone cause endometrial proliferation and maturation, respectively. At the level of the hypothalamus, they provide *negative* feedback, resulting in suppression of the LH surge and ovulation. Moreover, patients taking birth-control pills often report feeling 'fat', like they need to lose weight, or because they are 'menstruating' no longer need to gain weight. Therefore, unless they are being prescribed for contraception, their use can actually be countertherapeutic to the long-term goals of treatment. Some providers prescribe sex hormones in the form of birth-control pills because of the desired effect on bone metabolism. However, as will be demonstrated next, there are no data to suggest a positive effect on bone mineral density.

Skeletal

Because inadequate nutrition in eating disorders may result in reduced insulin-like growth factor-I (IGF-I) levels, there is reduced hypothalamic negative feedback that may result in elevated levels of growth hormone (GH). Anorexia nervosa represents an acquired GH insensitivity related to low IGF-I production (Grottoli *et al.*, 2003). This is especially important for young patients who have not yet achieved their adult height. In general, studies have shown that children and early pubertal adolescents have the potential for catch-up growth if they improve their nutritional status, but it appears as if they might not reach their adult height potential, based on mid-parental height predictions. Modan-Moses *et al.* (2003) studied 12 male adolescents with AN, of whom 11 had growth retardation. Weight restoration resulted in accelerated linear growth (up to 2 cm/mo) in all patients and was strongly positively correlated with rate of weight gain. Boys who gained at least 1 kg/year gained an average of 7 cm/year, while those who gained < 1 kg/year averaged less than 3 cm/year height increment. Complete catch-up growth was only achieved in 25% of boys, however. Interestingly, in some cases the growth retardation preceded the detection of the ED. A similar finding of catch-up growth lacking the achievement of full expected adult height for girls was reported (Lantzouni *et al.*, 2002). Therefore, the most appropriate treatment is adequate caloric intake. For boys the focus of treatment may be more effectively placed on gaining stature, rather than weight. Although gains in height may be slow, we have found that measuring height with a stadiometer on outpatient visits can provide valuable feedback to patients to motivate them to change. GH-related deficiencies of IGF-I may also impair bone formation.

If there is any irreversible chronic medical complication for adolescents and young adults with eating disorders, it is decreased bone mineral density (BMD) that can lead to osteoporosis. Multiple factors predispose an adolescent to bone loss: (1) low body weight, (2) low calcium and vitamin D intake, (3) ineffective impact loading exercise, (4) low IGF-I levels, (5) high cortisol levels and for females (6) low oestrogen levels. Because of the remarkable positive effect that sex hormone replacement therapy (HRT) has on the bone density of postmenopausal women, birth-control pills are often prescribed with the dual purpose of improving bone density and resuming menstrual periods.

Recognized as a complication of chronic AN among adults, osteoporosis among patients as young as 12 years old was described in 1990 (Bachrach *et al.*, 1990). Newman & Halmi (1989) noted that among adults, high cortisol levels correlated better with low BMD than did low oestrogen levels, a suggestion echoed by Misra *et al.* (2004). Nonetheless, HRT dominated treatment studies of adolescents and young adults with osteoporosis or osteopenia for more than 10 years. This was due to amenorrhoea being both a diagnostic feature of AN and predictive of low oestrogen levels, known to be linked to low bone formation and high bone resorption. However, because of a remarkable concordance of findings from studies between 1993 and 2003 that HRT was of little benefit with respect to bone health in either adolescents or adults with EDs, newer treatment approaches have been studied.

Our group (Kreipe *et al.*, 1993) found that bone mineral accretion was related more to weight than to HRT, with subjects weighing less than 80% ABW and taking HRT losing BMD, while amenorrhoeic subjects averaging almost 90% of average weight gained BMD. Klibanski *et al.* (1995) performed the definitive randomized placebo-controlled trial of HRT in AN and concluded that: (1) oestrogen replacement generally does not prevent progressive osteopenia; (2) only subjects < 70% ABW taking HRT improved their BMD compared to controls and (3) recovery from AN is associated with significantly improved BMD. Although the difference in BMD compared to controls was better for patients on HRT if their weight was < 70% ABW, if their weight was > 70% ABW, they had only half the increase in BMD found in controls. Moreover, only 15% of those on HRT had recovered, whereas 40% of those on placebo had recovered over the 18 months of the trial. Patients who recovered from their eating disorder and were taking HRT had an increase in BMD of only 7.5%, compared with 19.3% in the placebo group who recovered. Translated into practical terms, 70% of average body weight for a 14-year-old girl 63 inches tall is only 82 pounds (approximately 1.60 metres, 37.3 kg), severely emaciated. Other researchers have had similar findings, leading Mehler (2003) to conclude: In contrast to the many other medical complications of anorexia, osteoporosis and its sequelae of fractures, kyphosis, and pain may persist regardless of the overall treatment outcome . . . Traditional well-proven therapies for postmenopausal osteoporosis are not as effective against osteoporosis in AN. Therefore, clinicians who treat these patients must become increasingly vigilant about osteoporosis in regards to preventive, diagnostic, and treatment strategies. Gordon & Nelson (2003) noted that adolescents with amenorrhoea who diet, but who do not meet diagnostic criteria for AN, such as the 'female athlete triad' (osteoporosis, disordered eating and menstrual disturbance), are also at risk for low bone density. Likewise, Turner's group (2001) found that dieting and amenorrhoea, without clinically evident eating pathology, was associated with decreased BMD. Although some reports still suggest the use of HRT (Birch, 2005), there is no evidence that there is any benefit to bone health in low-weight athletes (Kazis & Iglesias, 2003).

Potentially useful in the treatment of osteoporosis in EDs are IGF-I, either alone or in combination with HRT (Grinspoon *et al.* 2002) and newer, shorter-acting bisphosphonates (Miller *et al.* 2004). Although the early results using risedronate in older adults have been encouraging, not only because there was a dramatic increase in BMD in a brief period of time, but also because these changes were not weight dependent, bisphosphonates should be used with great caution. They are incorporated into the bone and their effect on the fetus if a patient were later to become pregnant is unknown. Current evidence-based practice regarding improving bone health in adolescents and young adults with osteopenia or osteoporosis associated with an ED is best summarized by Golden (2003): 'until more effective treatment regimens become available, the mainstay of treatment remains weight gain, nutritional rehabilitation, and spontaneous resumption of menses'.

Summary

Although chronic dysfunctional weight control habits practised by children and adolescents with eating disorders have recognized effects on all tissues, the primary foci with respect to chronic medical complications are the heart, brain, gonads and bones. Despite uncertainty regarding the completeness of recovery for the brain and bones, it is reasonable to expect recovery in each of these tissues with weight restoration and normalization of nutrition – targets themselves sometimes difficult to achieve. This requires persistence and motivation by both patient and their providers.

REFERENCES

Bachrach, L. K., Guido, D., Katzman, D. & Litt, I. F. (1990). Decreased bone density in adolescent girls with anorexia nervosa. *Pediatrics*, **86**, 440–7.

Birch, K. (2005). Female athlete triad. *British Medical Journal*, **330**, 244–6.

Crow, S. J., Thuras, P., Keel, P. K. & Mitchell, J. E. (2002). Long-term menstrual and reproductive function in patients with bulimia nervosa. *American Journal of Psychiatry*, **159**, 1048–50.

Franko, D. L. & Rolfe, S. (1996). Counter-transference in the treatment of patients with eating disorders. *Psychiatry*, **59**, 108–16.

Franko, D. L., Blais, M. A., Becker, A. E. *et al.* (2001). Pregnancy complications and neonatal outcomes in women with eating disorders. *American Journal of Psychiatry*, **158**, 1461–6.

Golden, N. H., Jacobson, M. S., Schebendach, J. *et al.* (1997). Resumption of menses in anorexia nervosa. *Archives of Pediatrics and Adolescent Medicine*, **151**, 16–21.

Golden, N. H. (2003). Osteopenia and osteoporosis in anorexia nervosa. *Adolescent Medicine State of the Art Reviews*, **14**, 97–108.

Gordon, C. M., Dougherty, D. D., Fischman, A. J. *et al.* (2001). Neural substrates of anorexia nervosa: a behavioral challenge study with positron emission tomography. *Journal of Pediatrics*, **139**, 51–7.

Gordon, C. M. & Nelson, L. M. (2003). Amenorrhea and bone health in adolescents and young women. *Current Opinion in Obstetrics and Gynecology*, **15**, 377–84.

Gordon, I., Lask, B., Bryant-Waugh, R., Christie, D. & Timimi, S. (1997). Childhood-onset anorexia nervosa: towards identifying a biological substrate. *International Journal of Eating Disorders* **22**, 159–65.

Grinspoon, S., Thomas, L., Miller, K., Herzog, D. & Klibanski, A. (2002). Effects of recombinant human IGF-I and oral contraceptive administration on bone density in anorexia nervosa. *Journal of Clinical Endocrinology and Metabolism*, **87**, 2883–91.

Grottoli, S., Gasco, V., Ragazzoni, F. & Ghigo, E. (2003). Hormonal diagnosis of GH hypersecretory states. *Journal of Endocrinological Investigation*, **26** (10 Suppl), 27–35.

Gull, W. W. (1874). Anorexia nervosa. *Transactions of the Clinical Society of London*, **7**, 22–8.

Hasler, G., Delsignore, A., Milos, G., Buddeberg, C. & Schnyder, U. (2004). Application of Prochaska's transtheoretical model of change to patients with eating disorders. *Journal of Psychosomatic Research*, **57**, 67–72.

Isner, J. M., Roberts, W. C., Heymsfield, S. B. & Yager, J. (1985). Anorexia nervosa and sudden death. *Annals of Internal Medicine*, **102**, 49–52.

Katzman, D. K., Zipursky, R. B., Lambe, E. K. & Mikulis, D. J. (1997). A longitudinal magnetic resonance imaging study of brain changes in adolescents with anorexia nervosa. *Archives of Pediatrics and Adolescent Medicine*, **151**, 793–7.

Kazis, K. & Iglesias, E. (2003). The female athlete triad. *Adolescent Medicine State of the Art Reviews*, **14**, 87–95.

Kerem, N. C. & Katzman, D. K. (2003). Brain structure and function in adolescents with anorexia nervosa. *Adolescent Medicine State of the Art Reviews*, **14**, 109–18.

Key, A., Mason, H., Allan, R. & Lask, B. (2002). Restoration of ovarian and uterine maturity in adolescents with anorexia nervosa. *International Journal of Eating Disorders*, **32**, 319–25.

Keys, A. (1948). Cardiovascular effects of malnutrition and starvation. *Modern Concepts in Cardiovascular Disease*, **27**, 21.

Klibanski, A., Biller, B. M., Schoenfeld, D. A., Herzog, D. B. & Saxe, V. C. (1995). The effects of estrogen administration on trabecular bone loss in young women with anorexia nervosa. *Journal of Clinical Endocrinology and Metabolism*, **80**, 898–904.

Kohn, M. R., Ashtari, M., Golden, N. H. *et al.* (1997). Structural brain changes and malnutrition in anorexia nervosa. *Annals of the New York Academy of Sciences*, **817**, 398–9.

Kouba, S., Hallstrom, T., Lindholm, C. & Hirschberg, A. L. (2005). Pregnancy and neonatal outcomes in women with eating disorders. *Obstetrics and Gynecology*, **105**, 255–60.

Kreipe, R. E., Churchill, B. H. & Strauss, J. (1989). Long-term outcome of adolescents with anorexia nervosa. *American Journal of Diseases of Children*, **143**, 1322–7.

Kreipe, R. E. & Harris, J. P. (1992). Myocardial impairment resulting from eating disorders. *Pediatric Annals*, **21**, 760–8.

Kreipe, R. E., Hicks, D. G., Rosier, R. N. & Puzas, J. E. (1993). Preliminary findings on the effects of sex hormones on bone metabolism in anorexia nervosa. *Journal of Adolescent Health*, **14**, 319–24.

Kreipe, R. E., Goldstein, B., DeKing, D. E., Tipton, R. & Kempski, M. H. (1994). Heart rate power spectrum analysis of autonomic dysfunction in adolescents with anorexia nervosa. *International Journal of Eating Disorders*, **16**, 159–65.

Lantzouni, E., Frank, G. R., Golden, N. H. & Shenker, R. I. (2002). Reversibility of growth stunting in early onset anorexia nervosa: a prospective study. *Journal of Adolescent Health*, **31**, 162–5.

Mehler, P. S. (2003). Osteoporosis in anorexia nervosa: prevention and treatment. *International Journal of Eating Disorders*, **33**, 113–26.

Miller, K. K., Grieco, K. A., Mulder, J. *et al.* (2004). Effects of risedronate on bone density in anorexia nervosa. *Journal of Clinical Endocrinology and Metabolism*, **89**, 3903–6.

Misra, M., Miller, K. K., Almazan, C. *et al.* (2004). Alterations in cortisol secretory dynamics in adolescent girls with anorexia nervosa and effects on bone metabolism. *Journal of Clinical Endocrinology and Metabolism*, **89**, 4972–80.

Modan-Moses, D., Yaroslavsky, A., Novikov, I. *et al.* (2003). Stunting of growth as a major feature of anorexia nervosa in male adolescents. *Pediatrics*, **111**, 270–6.

Newman, M. M. & Halmi, K. A. (1989). Relationship of bone density to estradiol and cortisol in anorexia nervosa and bulimia. *Psychiatry Research*, **29**, 105–12.

Palmer, E. P. & Guay, A. T. (1985). Reversible myopathy secondary to abuse of ipecac in patients with major eating disorders. *New England Journal of Medicine*, **313**, 1457–9.

Ramacciotti, C. E., Guidi, L., Bondi, E. *et al.* (1997). Differential dynamic responses of luteinizing hormone to gonadotropin releasing hormone in patients affected by bulimia nervosa-purging versus non-purging type. *Eating and Weight Disorders: EWD*, **2**, 150–5.

Roche, F., Barthelemy, J. C., Mayaud, N. *et al.* (2005). Refeeding normalizes the QT rate dependence of female anorexic patients. *American Journal of Cardiology*, **95**, 277–80.

Rowland, T., Koenigs, L. & Miller, N. (2003). Myocardial performance during maximal exercise in adolescents with anorexia nervosa. *Journal of Sports Medicine and Physical Fitness*, **43**, 202–8.

Russell, G. F. M. (1979). Bulimia nervosa: an ominous variant of anorexia nervosa. *Psychological Medicine*, **9**, 429–48.

Shamim, T., Golden, N. H., Arden, M., Filiberto, L. & Shenker, I. R. (2003). Resolution of vital sign instability: an objective measure of medical stability in anorexia nervosa. *Journal of Adolescent Health*, **32**, 73–7.

Shomento, S. H. & Kreipe, R. E. (1994). Menstruation and fertility following anorexia nervosa. *Adolescent and Pediatric Gynecology*, **7**, 142–6.

St. John Sutton, M. G., Plappert, T., Crosby, L. *et al.* (1985). Effects of reduced left ventricular mass on chamber architecture, load and function: a study of anorexia nervosa. *Circulation*, **72**, 991–1000.

Strober, M. (2004). Managing the chronic, treatment-resistant patient with anorexia nervosa. *International Journal of Eating Disorders*, **36**, 245–55.

Swenne, I. (2004). Weight requirements for return of menstruations in teenage girls with eating disorders, weight loss and secondary amenorrhoea. *Acta Paediatrica*, **93**, 1449–55.

Turner, J. T. Bulsara, M. K., McDermott, B. M. *et al.* (2001). Predictors of low bone density in adolescents with anorexia nervosa and other dieting disorders. *International Journal of Eating Disorders*, **30**, 245–51.

Vanderdonckt, O., Lambert, M., Montero, M. C., Boland, B. & Brohet, C. (2001). The 12-lead electrocardiogram in anorexia nervosa: a report of 2 cases followed by a retrospective study. *Journal of Electrocardiology*, **34**, 233–42.

Vitousek, K., Watson, S. & Wilson, G. T. (1998). Enhancing motivation for change in treatment-resistant eating disorders. *Clinical Psychology Review*, **18**, 391–420.

Wilson, G. T. & Schlam, T. R. (2004). The transtheoretical model and motivational interviewing in the treatment of eating and weight disorders. *Clinical Psychology Review*, **24**, 361–78.

18

Individual psychotherapy

Phillipa P. J. Hay[1] and Brett McDermott[2]

[1]James Cook University, Townsville, Queensland, Australia
[2]Mater Child and Youth Mental Health Service, South Brisbane, Queensland, Australia

Introduction and overview

To therapists and clinicians treating children and adolescents with eating disorders, the title 'individual psychotherapy' may appear a misnomer. Children and the majority of adolescents do not present alone and it is important in management to also engage family members, and others such as school counsellors. Guidelines and position statements for the specific care of young people emphasize this (Kreipe, 1995; National Institute for Clinical Excellence (NICE), 2004). Individual psychotherapy in most instances, particularly with children, should occur following a thorough assessment of the patient's family and social context, and will often occur in conjunction with family and other therapies. In anorexia nervosa treatment necessarily must also address the restoration of physical health. With this caveat, this chapter describes individual therapies that have been applied in eating disorders, summarizes their evidence base, and concludes with a commentary on their appropriateness for children and adolescents. The discussion is limited to anorexia nervosa (AN), bulimia nervosa (BN) and Eating Disorders not Otherwise Specified (EDNOS). For an account of psychotherapeutic approaches in the management of binge eating in obese and overweight children the reader is referred to Braet (Chapter 15, this volume).

Individual psychotherapies

It is not known which treatment approaches are most commonly used worldwide in AN. While cognitive–behavioural therapy for BN is now endorsed by leading authorities (NICE, 2004), a range of individual therapies have been described and are used for people with this condition. It is likely that use is

Eating Disorders in Children and Adolescents, ed. Tony Jaffa and Brett McDermott. Published by Cambridge University Press. © Cambridge University Press 2007.

influenced by factors such as availability of training and ongoing supervision for therapists, and health resource issues for consumers and providers that are outside the scope of this review. Most individual therapy for BN and EDNOS sufferers is conducted on an outpatient basis. While evidence is yet insufficient to support outpatient versus inpatient programmes (Meads *et al.*, 1999), the focus of treatment of AN has also moved from long-term inpatient programmes with outpatient follow-up, to more commonly outpatient care, with hospital back-up (Garner & Needleman, 1997). Care is usually offered in individual or group sessions, and family therapy is more usual in child or adolescent settings. Detailed accounts are found in Garner & Garfinkel (1997). Family therapy is discussed by Lock and Couturier (Chapter 19, this volume).

Psychodynamic therapy

Psychodynamic therapies have the longest history in therapies for eating disorders. A key figure in the application of such therapies in AN was Bruch (1973). She described the core therapeutic elements to change as being through developing an understanding of the meaning of food for the patient, and helping them find alternatives to anorexic self-experience and self-expression. Self-psychology for eating disorders such as BN (Goodsitt, 1997) has developed out of the older psychodynamic traditions. This approaches BN as a specific case of the pathology of the self. The treated person cannot rely on people to fulfil their needs such as self-esteem. They rely instead on a substance, food, to fulfil personal needs. Therapy progresses when people move to rely on humans, starting with the therapist.

These therapies by their nature are long term and therapist time-intensive. They also require specific training that may often not be readily accessible or available. Dare and colleagues (Dare & Crowther, 1995) have developed focal psychoanalytic therapy (FPT) as a standardized form of time-limited psychoanalytic therapy that may be both more readily accessible and disseminated, and subject to empirical evaluation. The therapist takes a nondirective stance, gives no advice about the eating behaviours or other problems of symptom management, but addresses first the unconscious and conscious meanings of the symptom in terms of the patient's history and family experiences; second, the effects of the symptom and its influence on current interpersonal relationships; and third, the manifestation of those influences in the patient's relationship with the therapist. A nondirective stance however presents challenges in child and adolescent treatment settings given parental pressure for a 'cure' and the expectation of active interventions by referrers, general practitioners and paediatricians.

Cognitive–behaviour, cognitive and behaviour therapies

Cognitive–behaviour and cognitive therapy (CBT and CT) are time-limited manual-based therapies that address abnormal cognitions (beliefs) and behaviours thought to promote and maintain the disorder. They have a robust evidence base for the treatment of child and adolescent depression and anxiety disorders (Compton *et al.*, 2004) and in parent effectiveness training. Garner & Garfinkel (1997) describe CBT for AN as a therapy that addresses the patient's set of beliefs, attitudes and assumptions about the meaning of body weight. The cognitive–behavioural model holds thinness as the principal construct for self-worth and weight gain is therefore feared. Combinations of positive and negative reinforcers maintain the patient's behaviour and help explain the ego-syntonic nature of the illness. Strategies are proposed that challenge these beliefs, and behaviours to normalize eating patterns are promoted. More recently, Fairburn *et al.* (1999) have proposed that cognitive therapy in AN should focus on the excessive need for self-control over weight and shape. Fairburn *et al.* (2003) have subsequently developed an extended CBT approach that addresses four key illness-maintaining factors, i.e. clinical perfectionism, low self-esteem, mood intolerance and interpersonal difficulties, and note this approach is not inconsistent with the involvement of the family 'in the treatment of young cases'.

A specific form of CBT has been developed for BN, termed CBT–BN (Fairburn *et al.*, 1993; NICE, 2004). This uses three overlapping phases. Phase one aims to educate the person about BN. People are helped to increase regularity of eating, and resist urge to binge or purge. Phase two introduces procedures to reduce dietary restraint (e.g. broadening food choices). In addition, cognitive procedures supplemented by behavioural experiments are used to identify and correct dysfunctional attitudes and beliefs, and avoidance behaviours. Phase three is the maintenance phase. Relapse prevention strategies are used to prepare for possible future set backs. The standard CBT-BN regime for adults is 19 sessions over 20 weeks (Fairburn *et al.*, 1993). A further variation, sometimes used as a comparison therapy, is behaviour therapy (BT), which applies behavioural strategies only, such as keeping a diary of eating patterns, exposure to 'normal' eating and techniques to help distract from extreme weight-control behaviours such as vomiting. The highly structured and manualized nature of CBT or BT render them amenable to empirical evaluation and dissemination. See Robin *et al.* (1998) for further discussion of applying adult psychotherapeutic techniques for use with children and adolescents.

A modification of the exposure and response prevention therapy developed for obsessive-compulsive disorder has been developed for adults with BN. It involves exposure to food and then psychological prevention strategies of weight-control behaviour, such as vomiting after eating, until the urge or compulsion to vomit has receded (Leitenberg *et al.*, 1988). It has been evaluated for efficacy in enhancing the effectiveness of CBT-BN (Agras *et al.*, 1989) but not in children or adolescents.

Griffiths *et al.* (1994) have developed hypnobehavioural psychotherapy for BN. It uses a combination of behavioural techniques, such as self-monitoring to change maladaptive eating disorders, and hypnotic techniques to reinforce and encourage behaviour change.

Multimodal therapies

Cognitive–analytic therapy (CAT) is a treatment that combines elements of CT and brief-focused psychodynamic therapy. Cognitive–analytic therapy integrates active symptom management, and has been recommended as a viable alternative to CBT (Garner & Needleman, 1997). People are helped to evolve a formal, mapped-out structure of the place of AN in their experience of themselves and their early and current relationships. This is drawn in diagrammatic form, and the figure may be modified over the course of the treatment (Treasure *et al.*, 1995). Treatment is conducted in 20 weekly sessions, with monthly 'booster' sessions over three months. Therapists require specific training and supervision.

Cognitive orientation theory aims to generate a systematic procedure for exploring the meaning of a behaviour around themes. For overeating, for example, the cognitive orientation refers to themes such as rejection or avoidance of overt expressions of hostility, which are thought to govern the overeating. Therapy for modifying eating disordered behaviour(s) focuses on systematically changing beliefs related to themes, such as aggression or avoidance, not beliefs referring directly to the eating behaviour. No attempt is made to persuade the people that their beliefs are incorrect or maladapative (Bachar *et al.*, 1999) but rather the therapist helps the patient to develop beliefs that are the opposite of the ones underlying the behaviours.

Finally, dialectical behaviour therapy is a type of behavioural therapy that views emotional dysregulation as the core problem in BN, with binge eating and purging understood as attempts to influence, change or control painful emotional states. Patients are taught a repertoire of skills to replace dysfunctional behaviours (Safer et al., 2001). In addition, there is a strong theme on acceptance of the person as they are, combined with the expectation that current behaviours need to change. The tension that arises between this need for both acceptance and change is the 'dialectical' tension. These three treatments have been developed more for adults than adolescents or children, but dialectical behaviour therapy has been applied in young people with borderline personality structure and young female offenders (Trupin et al., 2002).

Feminist therapy

Feminist therapy rests on the proposition that cultural constructions of gender are central to the understanding and treatment of eating disorders. Katzman & Lee (1997), Striegel-Moore (1995) and Wooley (1995) are key figures in the integration of feminist and transcultural approaches to eating disorders. Other descriptions are found in Dolan & Gitzinger (1994). Potentially this therapy could be applied and/or adapted for use in young people. There are no randomized controlled trials evaluating its approach but addressing feminist issues in therapy has 'face validity' for a disorder in which 90% of sufferers are women with body image concerns.

Interpersonal psychotherapy

Interpersonal psychotherapy (IPT) was first developed for treatment of depression including with adolescents (Mufson et al., 1999), and later modified for treatment of BN (Fairburn et al., 1991). Like CBT, it is a manual-based therapy and thus readily amenable to empirical evaluation. In BN it uses three overlapping phases. The first phase analyses the interpersonal context of the eating disorder leading to a formulation of the person's problem area(s) which form the focus of the second phase. The third phase aims at monitoring progress in making interpersonal changes and exploring ways to cope with further interpersonal difficulties. In BN, but not necessarily in AN, attention is not paid to eating patterns or body attitudes. Specific training is required, and it is unclear how common its use by therapists has become.

Motivational enhancement therapy

Vitousek et al. (1998) and Ward et al. (1996) have developed motivational enhancement therapies (METs) in eating disorders. These treatments target the ego-syntonic nature of the illness and are based on a model of change with focus on stages of change. Stages of change represent constellations of intentions and behaviours through which individuals pass as they move from having a problem to doing something to resolve it. People in 'pre-contemplation' do not acknowledge that there is a problem and show no intention to change. People in 'contemplation' acknowledge they have, or may have, a problem and are thinking about change, but have not yet made a commitment. People in the third 'action' stage are actively engaged in overcoming their problem while those in 'maintenance' work to prevent relapse. The aim of MET is to help patients move from earlier stages into 'action', utilizing cognitive and emotional strategies. For example pre-contemplators are invited to consider whether their thoughts, feelings and behaviours are normal or whether they are consistent with a diagnosis, for instance, of AN and then the pros and cons of doing something about it (namely, they are invited to contemplate the possibility that they have an eating disorder, and the possibility of change being a good idea). Open-ended questions are used to elicit client expression, and reflective paraphrase is used to reinforce key points of motivation. During a session following structured assessment, most of the time is devoted to explaining feedback to the client. Therapy then progresses to developing and consolidating a change plan. (See: Prochaska *et al.* (1992) and http://www.dualdiagnosis.org/library/nida_00_4151/9.html for more general references.) This is a widely used approach in psychiatry and psychology, has established applications with substance-using adolescents (Tevyaw & Monti, 2004) and has applicability in AN where there is often strong resistance to change. As an approach, it would arguably be a useful adjunct to other specific therapies, but is as yet unsupported by evidence.

Self-help therapy

Self-help therapy is a modified form of cognitive–behavioural therapy, in which a treatment manual is provided for people to proceed with treatment on their own, or with support from a nonprofessional. Guided self-help usually implies that the support person may or may not have some professional training, but is usually not a specialist in eating disorders. A good discussion of the development and types of self-help can be found in Williams (2000).

Evidence for treatments

As a source for trials evaluating individual psychotherapy in eating disorders, four systematic reviews were identified with search dates November 2002 (AN participants; RANZCP, 2004); December 2003 (AN participants; Treasure & Schmidt, 2004), June 2004 (BN and binge-eating participants; Hay & Bacaltchuk, 2004, update submitted August 2004), and 2004 (Eating Disorder participants; NICE, 2004). An additional search of MEDLINE was done by the authors for more recent publications (dated December 2004) using the terms 'psychotherapy' and 'eating disorders or anorexia or bulimia'. This generated 92 papers of which one new systematic review was identified (Gowers & Bryant-Waugh, 2004) and five new RCTs (Pike et al., 2003; Schmidt et al., 2004; Grilo & Masheb, 2005; Grilo et al., 2005; McIntosh et al., 2005).

Anorexia nervosa trials

In AN treatment we identified six randomized controlled trials evaluating an individual psychotherapy compared to a control therapy or wait-list group and two trials comparing individual therapy to family therapy (Russell et al., 1987; Robin et al., 1999). Only three trials (Russell et al., 1987; Bachar et al., 1999; Robin et al., 1999) included children or adolescents. Bachar et al. (1999) reported a comparison of self-psychology treatment and cognitive–orientation treatment (COT) for 25 participants with BN and eight late adolescent (mean age 18.1 years, SD 2.4) AN patients. All AN patients had nutritional counselling in addition to the specific psychotherapy. Five of the six treated with self-psychology remitted (BMI > 17.5 and menses resumed) and neither of the two treated with cognitive–orientation therapy remitted after 6 months of therapy. Robin et al.'s (1999) trial comparing a psychodynamically orientated individual therapy with family therapy was inconclusive. However, Russell et al. (1987) found a significant advantage for posthospitalization family therapy over psychodynamically orientated individual therapy in a subgroup of adolescents with short duration of illness. Significant differences persisted at 5-years follow-up (Eisler et al., 1997).

In the adult trials specific psychotherapies, CAT or FPT, and in one trial also family therapy (Dare et al., 2001) were favoured over treatment as usual or a similar therapy (Treasure et al., 1995; Dare et al., 2001). However, in Dare et al. (2001) only 21 of the 65 (32%) allocated to a specific therapy (family therapy, FPT or CAT) met Morgan and Russell criteria for weight recovery, and 24 of the 65 (37%) did not complete treatment. One study (McIntosh et al., 2005) differed from the others in that it favoured a nonspecific approach over a specific psychotherapy. In one study, CBT appeared more acceptable than dietary advice alone, the latter having a 100% noncompletion rate (Serfaty et al., 1999). There was little difference between cognitive–behavioural therapy

(CBT) and behavioural therapy (BT) in Channon *et al.* (1989). However, subjects were reported to be more compliant with the CBT as they had missed significantly fewer treatment sessions. Pike *et al.* (2003) found strong support for greater efficacy for CBT versus nutritional counselling in relapse prevention following hospitalization in 33 women. However, seven of the eight women receiving CBT who had a good outcome were taking an antidepressant during the course of the trial, suggesting a medication effect for CBT (but this was not found for nutritional counselling).

In these AN trials acceptability of treatments, as reflected in noncompletion rates, varied widely and may have been influenced as much by specific type of therapy as by vicarious participant, therapist's style and other effects. In the two (Channon *et al.*, 1989: Serfaty *et al.*, 1989) studies with end-of-treatment and follow-up data, reported effects were maintained at 12 months.

All systematic reviews we identified (Gowers & Bryant-Waugh, 2004; NICE, 2004; RANZCP, 2004; Treasure & Schmidt, 2004) concluded that evidence from randomized controlled trials is insufficient to make treatment recommendations. Trials are few and no trial directly replicates another, although two were closely similar in treatments evaluated – namely the CAT in Dare *et al.* (2001) was similar to the CAT in Treasure *et al.* (1995), and EBT (Treasure *et al.*, 1995) was similar to 'treatment as usual' in Dare *et al.* (2001). In addition quality, particularly adequate power, is lacking. Overall most trials reported that some subjects showed improvement after treatment but the numbers of those having a good outcome was either variably defined, or not defined at all. In the largest trial (Dare *et al.*, 2001) over half (62%) of participants had a poor outcome. Trials also differed on when therapy was provided, e.g. at onset of care or post-hospitalization (e.g. Pike *et al.*, 2003).

Bulimia nervosa

The evidence base for psychotherapy in BN, is much stronger than that of AN, and all systematic reviews (Gowers & Bryant-Waugh, 2004; Hay & Bacaltchuk, 2004; NICE, 2004; Treasure & Schmidt, 2004) concurred in supporting CBT–BN from results of randomized controlled trials (RCTs) where it was compared with wait-list or a control therapy. IPT has been found to be of similar efficacy to CBT–BN at one year follow-up in two studies (Fairburn *et al.*, 1991, 1993; Agras *et al.*, 2000) but effects were delayed compared with CBT–BN. One RCT supported the efficacy of hypnobehavioural therapy over a waiting list control group. One RCT supported group based IPT over a wait-list control group. One RCT partially supported IPT over behaviour therapy alone. One small RCT reported efficacy of dialectical behaviour therapy (DBT) over a waiting list control group. Evidence for other psychotherapies was inconclusive.

Evidence for self-help therapy is more equivocal. One RCT has found no support for efficacy of pure self-help-CBT versus wait-list. One RCT provided limited support for guided self-help over pure self-help. One RCT did not support specific CBT pure self-help versus nonspecific self-help and one RCT found no benefits compared with fluoxetine. One RCT provided support for guided self-help CBT reducing bulimia and depressive symptoms to a similar degree as specialist care.

Notwithstanding these findings, no study was identified of individual psychotherapy in children or adolescents with BN although three studies did include some adolescents: Thackwray et al. (1993) had age range 15–62 years but the mean age was 31.3, SD 10.4 and median 30 years; and Wilson et al. (1986, 1991) included 13 of 17 and 14 of 22 participants of 'college' age with mean ages between 19.2 and 21.9 years.

Eating disorder not otherwise specified (EDNOS)

Cognitive–behavioural therapy and IPT have been found to be effective in reviews that have included trials of EDNOS or binge-eating disorder (Hay & Bacaltchuk, 2004; NICE, 2004) and one review supported the efficacy of a guided self-help CBT compared with behavioural weight control in rates of remission from binge eating in people with binge-eating disorder (BED; NICE, 2004; Grilo & Masheb, 2005). However, no study was identified of individual psychotherapy in children or adolescents with BED or EDNOS.

Commentary and conclusions

It is evident that while much has been written about theoretical models for these and other therapies, empirical evaluation of these treatments in children and adolescents is severely limited. Studies of adult therapy in AN in addition are few, of small size, and not necessarily of the most widely used or accessible therapies. There are a number of difficulties extrapolating from adult studies as discussed by Gowers & Bryant-Waugh (2004). These include the problem that EDNOS is more common in younger people, there is almost no evidence base for treatment of EDNOS and irrespective of aetiological issues parents are necessarily involved at some level. There are also specific psychological issues related to stages of development, such as psychological adjustment to normal body morphology changes at puberty, and peer beliefs about dieting and ideal body image that would not be addressed in a prescriptive adult therapy such as CBT–BN.

At present the limited evidence base for AN interventions suggests family therapy is the treatment of choice (see Lock and Couturier, Chapter 19, this volume). However, family therapy is not the treatment of choice across all child and adolescent mental health presentations. As previously mentioned individual CBT approaches are effective for anxiety and depressive conditions, individual therapies are also effective for common childhood difficulties such as low self-esteem and social difficulties. More individual therapy treatment research is required prior to accepting exclusivity of family therapy interventions for child and adolescent ED patients. Research should broaden outcome domains to include not only diagnostic case status and ED psychopathology, but also typical comorbid psychopathology and peer, school and family impairment. It may prove that one treatment modality may assist in restoration of normal eating patterns and weight, while other specific individual therapies may more effectively target and ameliorate other presenting challenges.

REFERENCES

Agras, W. S., Schneider, J. A., Arnow, B., Raeburn, S. D. & Telch, C. F. (1989). Cognitive-behavioral and response-prevention treatments for bulimia nervosa. *Journal of Consulting Clinical Psychology*, **57**, 215–21.

Agras, W. S., Walsh, B. T., Fairburn, C. G., Wilson, C. T. & Kraemer, H. C. (2000). A multicenter comparison of cognitive-behavioral therapy and interpersonal psychotherapy for bulimia nervosa. *Archives of General Psychiatry*, **54**, 459–65.

Bachar, E., Eytan, B., Yael, L., Shulamit, K. & Berry, E. M. (1999). Empirical comparison of two psychological therapies. Self psychology and cognitive orientation in the treatment of anorexia and bulimia. *Journal of Psychotherapy Practice and Research*, **2**, 115–28.

Bruch, H. (1973). *Eating Disorders: Obesity, Anorexia Nervosa and the Person Within*. New York: Basic Books.

Channon, S., de Silva, P., Hemsley, D. & Perkins, R. (1989). A controlled trial of cognitive-behavioural and behavioural treatment of anorexia nervosa. *Behavioral Research and Therapy*, **27**, 529–35.

Compton, S. N., March, J. S., Brent, D. *et al.* (2004). *Journal of the American Academy of Child and Adolescent Psychiatry*, **43**, 930–59.

Dare, C. & Crowther, C. (1995). Living dangerously: psychoanalytic psychotherapy of anorexia nervosa. In *Handbook of Eating Disorders: Theory, Treatment and Research*, ed. Szmulker, G., Dare, C. & Treasure, J. Chichester: John Wiley & Sons, pp. 125–39.

Dare, C., Eisler, I., Russell, G., Treasure, J. & Dodge, L. (2001). Psychological therapies for adults with anorexia nervosa. *British Journal of Psychiatry*, **178**, 216–21.

Dolan, B. & Gitzinger, I. (1994). *Why Women? Gender Issues and Eating Disorders*. London: The Athlone Press.

Eisler, I., Dare, C., Russell, G. F. *et al.* (1997). Family and individual therapy in anorexia nervosa; A 5-year follow-up. *Archives of General Psychiatry*, **54**, 1025–30.

Fairburn, C. G., Jones, R., Peveler, R. C. *et al.* (1991). Three psychological treatments for bulimia nervosa: a comparative trial. *Archives of General Psychiatry*, **48**, 463–9.

Fairburn, C. G., Jones, R., Peveler, R. C., Hope, R. A. & O'Connor, M. (1993). Psychotherapy and bulimia nervosa: longer-term effects of interpersonal psychotherapy, behaviour therapy and cognitive behaviour therapy. *Archives of General Psychiatry*, **50**, 419–28.

Fairburn, C. G., Shafran, R. & Cooper, Z. (1999). A cognitive behavioural theory of anorexia nervosa. *Behavioral Research Therapy*, **37**, 1–13.

Fairburn, C. G., Cooper, Z. & Shafran, R. (2003). Cognitive behaviour therapy for eating disorders: a ' transdiagnostic' theory and treatment. *Behavioral Research Therapy*, **41**, 509–28.

Garner, D. M. & Garfinkel, P. E. (ed.) (1997). *Handbook of Treatments for Eating Disorders*, 2nd edition. New York: Guilford Press.

Garner, D. M. & Needleman, L. D. (1997). Sequencing and integration of treatments. In *Handbook of Treatment for Eating Disorders*, 2nd edition, ed. Garner, D. M. & Garfinkel, P. E. New York: Guilford Press, pp. 50–66.

Garner, D. M., Vitousek, K. M. & Pike, K. M. (1997). Cognitive-behavioural therapy for anorexia nervosa. In *Handbook of Treatments for Eating Disorders*, 2nd edition, ed. Garner, D. M. & Garfinkel, P. E. New York: Guilford Press, pp. 67–93.

Goodsitt, A. (1997). Eating disorders: a self-psychological perspective. In *Handbook of Treatments for Eating Disorders*, 2nd edition, ed. Garner, D. M. & Garfinkel, P. E. New York: Guilford Press, pp. 205–28.

Gowers, S. & Bryant-Waugh, R. (2004). Management of child and adolescent eating disorders: the current evidence base and future directions. *Journal of Child Psychology and Psychiatry*, **45**, 63–83.

Griffiths, R. A., Hadzi-Pavlovic, D. & Channon-Little, L. (1994). A controlled evaluation of hypnobehavioural treatment for bulimia nervosa: immediate pre-post treatment effects. *European Eating Disorders Review*, **2**, 202–20.

Grilo, C. M. & Masheb, R. M. (2005). A randomized controlled comparison of guided self-help cognitive behavioural therapy and behavioural weight loss for binge eating disorder. *Behavior Research and Therapy*, **43**, 1509–25.

Grilo, C. M., Masheb, R. M. & Wilson, G. T. (2005). Efficacy of cognitive behavioral therapy and fluoxetine for the treatment of binge eating disorder: a randomized double-blind placebo-controlled comparison. *Biological Psychiatry*, **57**, 301–9.

Katzman, M. A. & Lee, S. (1997). Beyond body image: the integration of feminist and transcultural theories in the understanding of self-starvation. *International Journal of Eating Disorders*, **22**, 385–94.

Kreipe, R. E., Golden, N. H., Katzman, D. K. *et al.* (1995). Eating disorders in adolescents. A position paper of the Society for Adolescent Medicine. *Journal of Adolescent Health*, **16**, 476–9.

Hay, P. J. & Bacaltchuk, J. (2004). Psychotherapy for bulimia nervosa and binge eating. Cochrane Database Systematic Reviews, **3**, CD000562.

Leitenberg, H., Rosen, J., Gross, J., Nudelman, S. & Vara, L. S. (1988). Exposure plus response-prevention treatment of bulimia nervosa. *Journal of Consulting Clinical Psychology*, **56**, 535–41.

McIntosh, V. V. W., Jordan, J., Carter, F. *et al.* (2005). Three psychotherapies for anorexia nervosa: a randomized controlled trial. *American Journal of Psychiatry*, **162**, 741–7.

Meads, C., Gold, L., Burls, A. & Jobanputra, P. (1999). *In-patient versus Out-patient Care for Eating Disorders*. DPHE Report no. 17. University of Birmingham.

Mufson, L., Weissman, M. M., Moreau, D. & Garfinkel, R. (1999). Efficacy of interpersonal psychotherapy for depressed adolescents. *Archives of General Psychiatry*, **56**, 573–9.

National Institute for Clinical Excellence (2004). Eating Disorders: Core interventions in the treatment and management of anorexia nervosa, bulimia nervosa and related disorders. London: National Institute for Clinical Excellence (NICE), p. 35.

Pike, K. M., Walsh, B. T., Vitousek, K., Wilson, G. T. & Bauer, J. (2003). Cognitive behavior therapy in the posthospitalisation treatment of anorexia nervosa. *American Journal of Psychiatry*, **160**, 2046–9.

Prochaska, J. O., DiClemente, C. C. & Norcross, J. C. (1992). In search of how people change: applications to addictive behaviors. *American Psychologist*, **47**, 1102–14.

RANZCP: Royal Australian and New Zealand College of Psychiatrists Clinical Practice Guidelines Team for Anorexia Nervosa (2004). Australian and New Zealand clinical practice guidelines for the treatment of anorexia nervosa. *Australia and New Zealand Journal of Psychiatry*, **38**, 659–70.

Robin, A. L., Gilroy, M. & Dennis, A. B. (1998). Treatment of eating disorders in children and adolescents. *Clinical Psychology Reviews*, **18**, 421–46.

Robin, A. L., Siegel, P. T., Moye, A. W. *et al.* (1999). A controlled comparison of family versus individual therapy for adolescents with anorexia nervosa. *Journal of the American Academy of Child and Adolescent Psychiatry*, **38**, 1482–9.

Russell, G. F., Szmukler, G. I., Dare, C. & Eisler, I. (1987). An evaluation of family therapy in anorexia nervosa and bulimia nervosa. *Archives of General Psychiatry*, **44**, 1047–56.

Safer, D. L., Telch, C. F. & Agras, W. S. (2001). Dialectical behavior therapy for bulimia nervosa. *American Journal of Psychiatry*, **158**, 632–4.

Serfaty, M. A., Turkington, D., Heap, M., Ledsham, L. & Jolley, E. (1999). Cognitive therapy versus dietary counselling in the outpatient treatment of anorexia nervosa: effect of the treatment phase. *European Eating Disorders Review*, **7**, 334–50.

Schmidt, U., Cooper, P. J., Hans, E. *et al.* (2004). Fluvoxamine and graded psychotherapy in the treatment of bulimia nervosa. A randomized, double-blind, placebo-controlled, multi-centre study of short and long term pharmacotherapy. *Journal of Clinical Psychopharmacology*, **24**, 549–52 (letter).

Striegel-Moore, R. H. (1995). A feminist perspective on the etiology of eating disorders. In *Eating Disorder and Obesity. A Comprehensive Handbook*, ed. Brownell, K. D. & Fairburn, C. G. New York: Guilford Press, pp. 224–9.

Tevyaw, T. O. & Monti, P. M. (2004). Motivational enhancement and other brief interventions for adolescent substance abuse: foundations, applications and evaluations. *Addiction*, **99** (Suppl 2), 63–75.

Thackwray, D. E., Smith, M. C., Bodfish, J. W. & Meyers, A. W. (1993). A comparison of behavioral and cognitive-behavioral interventions for bulimia nervosa. *Journal of Consulting Clinical Psychology*, **61**, 639–45.

Treasure, J. & Schmidt, U. (2004). Anorexia nervosa. *Clinical Evidence*, **12**, 1–3.

Treasure, J., Todd, G., Brolly, M. *et al.* (1995). A pilot study of a randomized trial of cognitive analytical therapy vs educational behavioural therapy for adult anorexia nervosa. *Behavioral Research and Therapy*, **33**, 363–7.

Trupin, E. W., Stewart, G., Beach, B. & Boesky, L. (2002). Effectiveness of a dialectical behaviour therapy program for incarcerated female juvenile offenders. *Child and Adolescent Mental Health*, **7**, 121–7.

Vitousek, K. M., Watson, S. & Wilson, G. T. (1998). Enhancing motivation for change in treatment resistant eating disorders. *Clinical Psychology Reviews*, **18**, 391–420.

Ward, A., Troop, N., Todd, G. & Treasure, J. (1996). To change or not to change – 'How' is the question? *British Journal of Medical Psychology*, **69**, 139–46.

Williams, C. (2000). New technologies in self-help: another effective way to get better? *European Eating Disorders Review*, **11**, 170–82.

Wilson, G. T., Rossiter, E., Kleifield, E. I. & Lindholm, L. (1986). Cognitive-behavioural treatment of bulimia nervosa: a controlled evaluation. *Behavioral Research Therapy*, **24**, 277–88.

Wilson, G. T., Eldredge, K. L., Smith, D. & Niles, B. (1991). Cognitive behavioral treatment with and without response prevention for bulimia. *Behavioral Research and Therapy*, **29**, 575–83.

Wooley, S. C. (1995). Feminist influences on the treatment of eating disorders. In *Eating Disorders and Obesity: A Comprehensive Handbook*, ed. Brownell, K. D. & Fairburn, C. G. New York: Guilford Press, pp. 294–8.

19

Evidence-based family psychotherapy interventions

James Lock[1] and Jennifer Couturier[2]

[1]Stanford University School, Stanford, CA, USA
[2]University of Western Ontario, London, ON, Canada

The role of families in treating this disorder was debated by the two individuals who first described anorexia nervosa (AN), William Gull in England and E. C. Lasègue in France. Gull suggested that families were the 'worst attendants' for their children with AN (Gull, 1874), whereas Lasègue believed the family to be essential to recovery and recommended their involvement (Lasègue, 1883). Specific family interventions for eating disorders started with Salvador Minuchin (Minuchin et al., 1975) and Mara Selvini–Palazzoli (Selvini, 1974). Hilde Bruch also provided a theory to support the use of family-based interventions, proposing that as a child, insufficient and inaccurate feedback was given by the mother, resulting in a distorted perception of self, a pervasive sense of ineffectiveness and poorly developed interoceptive awareness (Bruch, 1973; Dare & Eisler, 2002). More recently, family-based interventions have been gaining in popularity due to a growing evidence base.

Currently, there are many different views on the families of patients with eating disorders. Some believe that dysfunctional family systems are the cause of eating pathology, whereas others believe that the eating disorder brings about family dysfunction. Perhaps partly due to the success of early family therapists (e.g. Minuchin and Palazzoli) it appeared that AN originated in family disturbances that could be treated by targeting these supposed causative factors in family therapy. However, there have been no longitudinal studies that have investigated whether family dysfunction precedes or follows the onset of eating disorders. In fact, cross-sectional comparisons between the structure and functioning of families of patients with eating disorders and control groups suggest that these patterns are associated with more severe and more chronic illness rather than as aetiological factors (Dare & Eisler, 2002). Interestingly, while it remains unclear whether families have an

Eating Disorders in Children and Adolescents, ed. Tony Jaffa and Brett McDermott. Published by Cambridge University Press. © Cambridge University Press 2007.

aetiological role in the development of eating disorders in their children, the evidence supporting the involvement of the family in treatment is increasing.

This chapter will first review different models of family therapy for eating disorders, then review and synthesize the evidence from uncontrolled trials and randomized controlled trials. Although more studies have been completed on adolescent AN, the evidence for family treatment for individuals with bulimia nervosa (BN) will also be discussed.

Evolving models of family therapy for eating disorders

Structural family therapy for the treatment of AN began with Minuchin and his colleagues in Philadelphia, USA, in the 1970s. This model has not only been applied to AN, but is used in family therapy in general. The approach is based on the premise that the family of an individual with AN is a 'psychosomatic family', having the characteristics of enmeshment, overprotectiveness, rigidity and lack of conflict resolution along with a physiologically vulnerable child (Minuchin *et al.*, 1975; Minuchin, 1978). The child plays a key role in the family's general avoidance of conflict which, in turn, perpetuates the symptoms. The goal of this therapy is to alter the overall structural organization of the family through limiting pathological patterns of family interaction, by challenging alliances between parents and children that limit parental effectiveness, by encouraging development of stronger sibling subsystems and by encouraging more open communication. An important component of this therapy includes a family meal in which parents are encouraged to take control, thereby strengthening the parental dyad, and their confidence in their ability to refeed their child.

Strategic family models diverge from structural ones in their 'agnostic' view of the causes of psychological disorders. Haley was a strong proponent of this view, proposing a lack of speculation about the causes of the disorder (Haley, 1973). The interventions are focused on limiting the impact of the symptom on the individual and family. Typically, strategic interventions attack the role of the symptom, through powerful techniques that evoke change. One of these techniques is prescribing behaviours with paradoxical intentions. An example of this type of intervention would be to recommend that the patient eat in order to have the strength to fight against her parents.

The Milan systems group shares many characteristics with the strategic model, but Selvini–Palazzoli added the central idea that the family was a more rigidly organized system which was resistant to change from the outside

(Selvini, 1974). The eating disorder symptoms are seen as key to maintaining this system. In support of this observation, one defining characteristic of this model is that the therapist remains neutral towards the family, and towards the idea that change should occur. This stance avoids provoking the powerful homeostatic mechanisms within the family that resist change. Instead, the therapist encourages the family to be self-observers and challengers of their own process.

Feminist theory about authority and hierarchy has helped to refine some family therapy approaches. Feminist theory emphasizes the need for partnership and shared control of the therapeutic process rather than the hierarchical nature of the therapist–family relationship in which the therapist is the powerful expert (e.g. Minuchin). Also, in the case of young women, it focuses on the inequitable position of women in society and the role this plays in development and maintenance of eating disorders.

A different approach to family work in adolescent eating disorders that incorporates several aspects of each of these models of family intervention was developed at the Maudsley Hospital (Dare & Eisler, 1997). From the structural model, a family meal is used to enhance parental confidence. The importance of the parental dyad in maintaining control is emphasized, while sibling subsystems are strengthened. From the strategic approach, an agnostic view of the illness is held, along with the prescription of behaviours of paradoxical intentions. For example, asking a child to resist parental efforts at refeeding during the family meal in order to prevent premature compliance to parental authority (Lock et al., 2001). This family-based treatment (FBT) recognizes the adolescent's need to resist efforts at refeeding, while supporting parental efforts. From the Milan systems model, the family is encouraged to find solutions that work for them rather than relying on the therapist to provide answers, while from feminist approaches, the therapist is seen as a consultant rather than an expert, always holding the family in a noncritical and positive regard.

FBT includes three phases over approximately 20 sessions. The first phase involves a strong focus on parents regaining control of weight gain and of refeeding their child, and includes a family meal in the second session. The first phase includes weekly sessions, and lasts between 3 and 5 months. In the second phase, control over eating is gradually handed over to the child. This phase involves biweekly sessions for a period of about 3 months. And, in the third phase, components of normal adolescent development that were interrupted by the eating disorder are addressed as well as termination issues. This final phase typically consists of monthly sessions for a period of about 3 months (Lock et al., 2001).

Uncontrolled trials of family interventions in adolescent AN

There are few controlled trials of treatments for AN (Le Grange & Lock, 2005); therefore a brief review of case series studies of family treatment is warranted. Minuchin and his colleagues conducted the first and highly influential family therapy study of patients with AN using his structural model (Minuchin *et al.*, 1975; Minuchin, 1978). Their follow-up study of 53 patients with AN concluded that 86% had recovered (all but three patients were adolescents).

There have been two other similar studies examining structural approaches. Martin studied 25 adolescents with AN in Toronto, Canada, and found significant improvements at the end of treatment (Martin, 1985). Only 23% met the Morgan–Russell criteria (Morgan & Hayward, 1988) for good outcome at the end of treatment. However, at 5-year follow-up, 80% were classified as having a good outcome. As in the Minuchin study, patients in this study had a short duration of illness (about 8 months) and primarily received family therapy along with inpatient and individual treatments. In Buenos Aires, 30 adolescents were treated by a paediatrician and family therapist, and at 4–8.6 years later 60% were found to have a good outcome using Morgan–Russell criteria (Herscovici & Bay, 1996).

With respect to FBT, four studies (Dare, 1983; Mayer, 1994; Lock & Le Grange, 2001; Le Grange *et al.*, 2005) have examined FBT in an uncontrolled fashion, wherein adolescent subjects with short duration of AN appeared to respond well to FBT. Treatment outcomes in this group of studies suggest that about two-thirds of subjects did well. These studies have supported the development of controlled studies of FBT to be discussed below.

Randomized controlled family interventions in AN

There are five published randomized controlled trials (RCT) of family therapy that focused on adolescents with AN (Russell *et al.*, 1987; Le Grange *et al.*, 1992; Robin *et al.*, 1999; Eisler *et al.*, 2000; Lock *et al.*, 2005), and no RCTs involving adolescents with BN. Two of these studies compared FBT to individual therapy (Russell *et al.*, 1987; Robin *et al.*, 1999), and the others compared conjoint to separated FBT (Le Grange *et al.*, 1992; Eisler *et al.*, 2000), or dose-levels of FBT (Lock *et al.*, 2005).

The seminal study by Russell *et al.* (1987), from the Maudsley Hospital, involved 80 patients, 57 of these had AN and 23 had BN. The subjects with AN were first divided into three subgroups based on age and chronicity and then randomized to individual or FBT as described above. The individual therapy was 'supportive, educational, and problem-centered', and was designed to be a 'placebo' rather than active therapy. Although the sample size was small, they found that for those patients who had a duration of illness less than 3 years, and an onset of illness prior to age 18, FBT was superior to individual treatment, with 60% (6/10) of the adolescents having a good outcome (using Morgan–Russell criteria) in the family treatment, compared to 9% (1/11) in the individual therapy at the end of treatment (Russell *et al.*, 1987). At 5-year follow-up, 90% (9/10) of these adolescents in family treatment had good outcomes, compared with 36% (4/11) of those in individual treatment (Eisler *et al.*, 1997). It is important to note that the adult and more chronic subgroups did not differ in their response to the two treatments. The lack of robust response to FBT in the adult population was confirmed in a large study of adults with AN (Dare *et al.*, 2001).

In the other RCT to date comparing individual to family treatment, Robin *et al.* (1999) randomized 37 adolescent females to Behavioural Family Systems Therapy (BFST) or to a psychodynamic individual therapy called Ego-Oriented Individual Therapy (EOIT). BFST is similar to FBT, but has some differences. Like FBT, BFST encourages parents to take charge of their child's eating and weight gain in the first phase of treatment (Robin *et al.*, 1999). In the second phase, the therapist shifts the focus to cognitive distortions and family structure. Cognitive restructuring and strategic interventions are used respectively in this phase to tackle these two issues (Robin *et al.*, 1999). In the third phase, the therapist guides the parents in returning control over eating back to the adolescent, similar to FBT (see also Robin, 2003). In contrast, EOIT focuses on improving ego strength, and coping skills, while addressing individuation from the nuclear family, confusion about identity, and other interpersonal issues. At the end of 1 year of treatment Robin *et al.* (1999) found that both groups had improved on body mass index (BMI), with the BFST group having a significantly greater increase in BMI and increased rate of menstrual return. At 1 year follow-up, although patients continued to be improved, there were no longer any significant differences between the groups. These results suggest that family treatment is overall superior because of its more rapid effects. However, given the small sample size this finding remains tentative.

With the evidence growing for family therapy in adolescent AN, Eisler *et al.* (2000) compared conjoint (all family members present) FBT to separated (parents seen separately) FBT for AN drawing on a previous pilot study by le Grange *et al.* (1992) who found that high levels of maternal criticism were associated with a poor outcome and that this effect was stronger in the conjoint family therapy group than in the separated family therapy group. Eisler *et al.* (2000) randomized 40 patients and stratified the treatment allocation according to maternal criticism. Overall, 37.5% of the adolescents had a good outcome, 25% had an intermediate outcome and 37.5% had a poor outcome using Morgan–Russell criteria. For those families with high levels of maternal criticism, separated FBT was superior to conjoint FBT (Eisler *et al.*, 2000). The authors conclude that when treating families in which parents express high levels of criticism it is important to continue to include the parents, but to see them separately from the adolescent.

In order to better understand how much FBT was needed to produce good outcomes, Lock *et al.* (2005) used manualized FBT (Lock *et al.*, 2001) with 86 adolescents with AN, comparing 6 months (10 sessions) of FBT to 12 months (20 sessions) of FBT with random treatment allocation. The group receiving 6 months of FBT was followed for an additional 6 months, and outcomes between the two groups were compared at the 1-year point. In this adequately powered study, both groups improved significantly in terms of weight gain and Eating Disorder Examination (EDE) score, and there were no differences between the groups at the end of 1 year. The average amount of weight gained among the 86 subjects was 15 lbs (6.8 kg). At the 1-year point, 96% of the whole group (n = 86) no longer met the DSM–IV weight criteria for AN, and 65% had a good outcome according to Morgan–Russell criteria. There were two moderators of treatment effect in this study: eating-related obsessive-compulsive symptoms, and family status. When BMI was used as the outcome of interest, those with more severe eating-related obsessions and compulsions did better in 12-month treatment. And when EDE score was the outcome of interest, those with non-intact families did better in the 12-month treatment (Lock *et al.*, 2005). In addition to providing a large database generally supportive of the effectiveness of FBT for AN in adolescents, this study concluded that for most patients, a relatively brief course of FBT is as effective as a longer course.

It should be noted that the majority of these studies, though supportive of FBT for adolescent AN, suffer from significant methodological limitations (Le Grange & Lock, 2005). Most are very small in size (average cell size of 15 subjects), do not employ reliably replicable treatments (i.e. they did not use manuals) and outcome measures used were varied and often not the ideal (only one used the EDE, for example). Further the adolescent subjects studied were mostly patients with a relatively good prognosis having a short duration of AN (less than 1 year) (Russell *et al.*, 1987).

New applications of family treatments for adolescent eating disorders

Although a significant amount of research has been done in the area of adults with BN, very little research attention has been paid to adolescents with BN. In fact, there are no published treatment studies focused on adolescents with BN. Although there have not been any rigorous family therapy studies done to date with adolescents suffering from BN, Dodge *et al.* (1995) reported a small case series of eight adolescents with BN who received family therapy and had significant improvements. Good or intermediate outcomes using Morgan–Russell criteria were achieved by six out of eight patients (Dodge *et al.*, 1995). However, adults with BN treated with FBT did not appear to have a robust response to this intervention (Russell *et al.*, 1987).

Recently, work has been done on adapting FBT for adolescents with BN (Le Grange *et al.*, 2003). Whereas in AN the focus of treatment is on empowerment of the parents to refeed their starving adolescent, in the BN adaptation the focus is on helping the parents to assist their adolescent in regaining control over his/her eating and to prevent binge eating and purging (le Grange *et al.*, 2003). This adaptation has three phases. The first focuses on regulating food intake and preventing purging, and involves a family meal designed to provide an opportunity to prevent binge eating. The second phase, as in AN family-based treatment, focuses on assisting the adolescent to achieve full independent control over eating. The third phase addresses adolescent issues (autonomy, peers, independence) and termination. Studies examining the efficacy of FBT in BN are currently underway. Preliminary results suggest that significant reductions in binge and purge frequency, as well as improvements on EDE subscale scores are achieved with FBT for BN (Le Grange, 2004).

As involvement of family members appears to be important when treating adolescents with BN, cognitive–behavioural therapy (CBT) for BN (Fairburn *et al.*, 1993) has recently been modified for this age group. Parents can facilitate this treatment by altering their adolescent's environment, promoting engagement, motivation and stress management, and help compensate for different levels of cognitive abilities. Most importantly, they can learn how to best support their adolescent in order to encourage change (Lock & Le Grange, 2005). In CBT for BN, this might appear as parents assisting their adolescent to normalize eating patterns, and complete food logs, while discouraging binge eating and purging episodes (Lock, 2002). These modifications make it more likely that CBT will be acceptable and successful with adolescents (Lock, 2002). Preliminary results using a family-facilitated CBT approach with adolescent

BN are encouraging. In a small sample of 16 adolescents with BN, episodes of binge eating and purging declined from an average of 5.4 episodes per week to 1.2 episodes per week post-treatment, representing a reduction of 77%. Sixty-three per cent of these subjects were abstinent from binge eating and purging following treatment (Lock, 2002).

Intervention for eating disorders involving several families at the same time (multi-family group or MFG) is a relatively new approach that has most commonly been seen in the psychiatric literature in the area of schizophrenia (Chien & Chan, 2004). It is currently in an early stage of development, but two studies are ongoing in London, UK, and in Dresden, Germany (Dare & Eisler, 2000; Scholz & Asen, 2001). This treatment is delivered in a day treatment setting with families participating for 4 full days at the outset, followed by 4–6 one-day follow-ups spaced 1, 2, then several weeks later. As in FBT, MFG aims to help families by enhancing their own resources in order to help their son or daughter recover (Eisler et al., 2003). It has been used both in families with an adolescent with AN and families with an adolescent with BN. There appears to be a high level of patient and parent acceptability, with a very low drop-out rate of 2–3% (Scholz & Asen, 2001; Eisler et al., 2003). In Dresden, reduction in hospital admission rates has been seen, along with reductions in the length of stay, and in readmission rates (Scholz & Asen, 2001; Eisler et al., 2003). However, no systematic follow-up data examining symptomatology are available.

Summary

Family therapy has a long history in the field of eating disorder treatment. From its roots in structural, strategic, Milan and feminist theories, and the Maudsley approach, FBT has evolved and demonstrated effectiveness in adolescent patients with AN in several randomized controlled clinical trials. At this time, FBT is the treatment with the largest empirical evidence base for adolescents with AN, although large controlled studies are still urgently needed. In contrast, adolescent BN has received relatively little attention, which is surprising given the extensive literature base of psychotherapies for adult BN. The importance of families in treatments for adolescent eating disorders must be underscored. Future research might focus on differentiating family treatments from individual ones in AN, developing sorely needed family treatments for BN, along with determining the effectiveness of multifamily interventions in AN and BN.

REFERENCES

Bruch, H. (1973). *Eating Disorders: Obesity, Anorexia Nervosa, and the Person Within*. New York: Basic Books.

Chien, W. T. & Chan, S. W. (2004). One-year follow-up of a multiple-family-group intervention for Chinese families of patients with schizophrenia. *Psychiatric Services*, **55**, 1276–84.

Dare, C. (1983). *Family Therapy for Families Containing an Anorectic Youngster*. Columbus, OH: Ross Laboratories.

Dare, C. & Eisler, I. (1997). *Handbook of Treatment for Eating Disorders*, 2nd edition. New York: Guilford Press.

Dare, C. & Eisler, I. (2000). A multi-family group day treatment programme for adolescent eating disorder. *European Eating Disorders Review*, **8**, 4–18.

Dare, C. & Eisler, I. (2002). *Eating Disorders and Obesity: A Comprehensive Handbook*, 2nd edition. New York: Guilford Press.

Dare, C., Eisler, I., Russell, G., Treasure, J. & Dodge, L. (2001). Psychological therapies for adults with anorexia nervosa: randomised controlled trial of out-patient treatments. *British Journal of Psychiatry*, **178**, 216– 21.

Dodge, E., Hodes, M., Eisler, I. & Dare, C. (1995). Family therapy for bulimia nervosa in adolescents: an exploratory study. *Journal of Family Therapy*, **17**, 59–77.

Eisler, I., Dare, C., Hodes, M., Russell, G., Dodge, E. & Le Grange, D. (2000). Family therapy for adolescent anorexia nervosa: the results of a controlled comparison of two family interventions. *Journal of Child Psychology and Psychiatry*, **41**, 727–36.

Eisler, I., Dare, C., Russell, G. F., Szmukler, G., Le Grange, D. & Dodge, E. (1997). Family and individual therapy in anorexia nervosa. A 5-year follow-up. *Archives of General Psychiatry*, **54**, 1025–30.

Eisler, I., le Grange, D. & Asen, E. (2003). *Handbook of Eating Disorders*, 2nd edition. San Francisco, CA: John Wiley & Sons.

Fairburn, C. G., Marcus, M. D. & Wilson, G. T. (1993). Cognitive-behavioral therapy for binge eating and bulimia nervosa: a comprehensive treatment manual. In *Binge Eating: Nature, Assessment, and Treatment*, ed. Fairburn, C. G & Wilson, G. T. New York: Guilford Press, pp. 361–404.

Gull, W. (1874). Anorexia nervosa (apepsia hysterica, anorexia hysterica). *Transactions of the Clinical Society of London*, **7**, 222–8.

Haley, J. (1973). *Uncommon Therapy: The Psychiatric Techniques of Milton H. Erickson*. New York: Norton.

Herscovici, C. & Bay, L. (1996). Favourable outcome for anorexia nervosa patients treated in Argentina with a family approach. *Eating Disorders Journal of Treatment and Prevalence*, **4**, 59–66.

Lasègue, E. (1883). De l'anorexie hysterique. *Archives Generales De Medecine*, **21**, 384–403.

Le Grange, D. (2004). *Family-based treatment vs. individual psychotherapy for adolescent bulimia nervosa: What have we learned so far?* Paper presented at the Eating Disorders Research Society Annual Meeting, Amsterdam, The Netherlands.

Le Grange, D., Binford, R. & Loeb, K. L. (2005). Manualized family-based treatment for anorexia nervosa: a case series. *Journal of the American Academy of Child and Adolescent Psychiatry*, **44**, 41–6.

Le Grange, D., Eisler, I., Dare, C. & Russell, G. (1992). Evaluation of family treatments in adolescent anorexia nervosa: a pilot study. *International Journal of Eating Disorders*, **12**, 347–57.

Le Grange, D. & Lock, J. (2005). The dearth of psychological treatment studies for anorexia nervosa. *International Journal of Eating Disorders*, **37**, 79–91.

Le Grange, D., Lock, J. & Dymek, M. (2003). Family-based therapy for adolescents with bulimia nervosa. *American Journal of Psychotherapy*, **57**, 237–51.

Lock, J. (2002). Treating adolescents with eating disorders in the family context. Empirical and theoretical considerations. *Child and Adolescent Psychiatric Clinics of North America*, **11**, 331–42.

Lock, J., Agras, W. S., Bryson, S. & Kraemer, H. C. (2005). A comparison of short- and long-term family therapy for adolescent anorexia nervosa. *Journal of the American Academy of Child and Adolescent Psychiatry*, **44**, 632–9.

Lock, J. & Le Grange, D. (2001). Can family-based treatment of anorexia nervosa be manualized? *Journal of Psychotherapy and Practice Research*, **10**, 253–61.

Lock, J. & Le Grange, D. (2005). *Help Your Teenager Beat an Eating Disorder*. New York: Guilford Press.

Lock, J., Le Grange, D., Agras, S. & Dare, C. (2001). *Treatment Manual for Anorexia Nervosa: A Family-Based Approach*. New York: Guilford Press.

Martin, F. E. (1985). The treatment and outcome of anorexia nervosa in adolescents: a prospective study and five year follow-up. *Journal of Psychiatric Research*, **19**, 509–14.

Mayer, R. (1994). *Family treatment in the treatment of eating disorders in general practice*. Unpublished MSc Dissertation, Birkbeck College, University of London, London.

Minuchin, S. (1978). *Psychosomatic Families: Anorexia Nervosa in Context*. Cambridge, MA: Harvard University Press.

Minuchin, S., Baker, L., Rosman, B. L. *et al.* (1975). A conceptual model of psychosomatic illness in children. Family organization and family therapy. *Archives of General Psychiatry*, **32**, 1031–8.

Morgan, H. G. & Hayward, A. E. (1988). Clinical assessment of anorexia nervosa. The Morgan–Russell outcome assessment schedule. *British Journal of Psychiatry*, **152**, 367–71.

Robin, A. L. (2003). Behavioral family systems therapy for adolescents with anorexia nervosa. In *Evidence-Based Psychotherapies for Children and Adolescents*, ed. Kazdin, A. E. & Weiz, J. R. New York: Guilford Press, pp. 358–73.

Robin, A. L., Siegel, P. T., Moye, A. W. *et al.* (1999). A controlled comparison of family versus individual therapy for adolescents with anorexia nervosa. *Journal of the American Academy of Child and Adolescent Psychiatry*, **38**, 1482–9.

Russell, G. F., Szmukler, G. I., Dare, C. & Eisler, I. (1987). An evaluation of family therapy in anorexia nervosa and bulimia nervosa. *Archives of General Psychiatry*, **44**, 1047–56.

Scholz, M. & Asen, E. (2001). Multiple family therapy with eating disordered adolescents: concepts and preliminary findings. *European Eating Disorders Review*, **9**, 33–42.

Selvini, M. P. (1974). *Self Starvation: From the Intrapsychic to the Transpersonal Approach to Anorexia Nervosa*. London: Chaucer Publishing.

20

Models of service delivery

Simon Gowers and Lynne Green

University of Liverpool, Chester, UK

Introduction

Young people with eating disorders are treated in a range of service settings, but without, to date, good quality research evidence to determine which service configuration might benefit a particular patient at a particular time.

However, a number of recent clinical guidelines in the USA (APA, 2000), Australia and New Zealand (RANZCP, 2004), Finland (Ebeling *et al.*, 2003) and the UK (NCCMH, 2004) have exhaustively reviewed the treatment literature and made recommendations for good practice.

In the UK two further initiatives have offered the possibility of a more comprehensive approach to commissioning and developing services along evidence-based lines. First, the publication of the Children's National Service Framework (NSF) for mental health (Department of Health, 2004) set standards and defined service models for the promotion and treatment of mental health. It emphasized the need for age-appropriate services for children and young people requiring specialist intervention, whilst also acknowledging that in some adolescent cases where intensive, specialized treatment is required, contributions from services oriented to adults may be required. Second, an internet-based multidisciplinary special interest group of clinicians and academics, *EDNet,* was established to provide a forum for professionals, users and carers to review current knowledge and support service developments.

This chapter will review models of service delivery, the evidence to support them and the associated recommendations in clinical guidelines. Where evidence is lacking, priorities for further research are highlighted.

Eating Disorders in Children and Adolescents, ed. Tony Jaffa and Brett McDermott. Published by Cambridge University Press. © Cambridge University Press 2007.

Why this is an important area

Epidemiology

Epidemiological data are discussed at length by Nielsen (Chapter 7, this volume). The relative rarity of severe anorexia nervosa (an average community UK CAMHS team might be expected to see between 2 and 5 cases per year) suggests that specialist expertise and experience can not readily be obtained by generic community teams, nor can assembling a specialist team for a small population be justified if patient flows are small.

Range of severity

Although moderate eating concerns and associated dieting behaviours can be self-limiting, anorexia nervosa can be a very serious illness with the highest standardized mortality rate of any psychiatric disorder (Nielsen *et al.*, 1998). Medical and psychological comorbidity is very common and cases span a severity range from relatively mild to life threatening.

Meeting the needs of a diverse clinical group requires a range of provision from brief counselling delivered in primary care to long-term specialist provision. The latter can be extremely expensive, especially when lengthy inpatient care is undertaken; thus decision making has important economic as well as clinical considerations in a rationed health economy.

Dangers of treatment delay

The majority of eating disorder cases are treated on an outpatient basis and indeed less severe cases may be adequately managed in generic services, including primary care. Ensuring an effective system for the identification of high-risk cases with rapid referral to tertiary care is however important in order to avoid the development of secondary handicaps associated with chronicity. Any delay in initiating appropriate treatment also has important financial implications, as patients who may have been successfully treated in an outpatient service may end up being transferred as emergencies to specialist and more costly inpatient services.

A stepped care model in which patients move up from lower-level to higher-level care subject to locally agreed protocols (Fairburn & Peveler, 1990; Dalle Grave *et al.*, 2001) makes clinical sense, and this approach has been supported by the NICE guideline on the treatment of eating disorders (NCCMH, 2004). However, there is currently little evidence to guide clinical decision-making in this area and it is often difficult without the benefit of hindsight to know which cases in the early stages will require intensive treatment. In 1994, the Royal

College of Psychiatrists introduced a strategic approach to child and adolescent mental health services (CAMHS) based on tiers of service, subsequently adapted by the Health Advisory Service for the NHS (HAS, 1995).

Outpatient management

The phenomenology of eating disorders, comprising distorted cognitions about the value of weight and shape, coupled with maladaptive eating and compensatory behaviour, provides a theoretical basis for a cognitive–behavioural approach to treatment (Gowers, 2005). It is generally well accepted that cognitive–behavioural approaches favour treatment on an outpatient basis, to maximize personal responsibility for decision making (Vitousek et al., 1998) and a number of CBT approaches have been described in the eating disorder field (Fairburn et al., 1995). Alongside a behavioural programme designed to initiate weight restoration (where appropriate), individuals receive either group or individual psychotherapy (and usually both) to address underlying beliefs maintaining the eating disorder and to facilitate more adaptive ways of viewing the self and experimenting with new strategies for achieving their goals. Despite a growing amount of evidence for this approach for use with adults with bulimia nervosa, an absence of adequately powered trials means that there is little evidence for its effectiveness in cases of anorexia nervosa in general and with adolescents specifically (see Hay and McDermott, Chapter 18, this volume).

Family therapy approaches are often the treatment of choice for clinicians working with eating disorder patients in child and adolescent psychiatry, owing to their familiarity with systemic approaches and also a growing evidence base. The strongest evidence comes from the Maudsley Hospital in London (see Dare et al., 2001). Several small treatment studies have suggested the efficacy of family therapy, particularly in adolescent anorexia nervosa (see below).

Inpatient management

Although the majority of those with eating disorders are managed on an outpatient basis, there are potentially many benefits of admitting a severely ill patient to hospital. These include physical health monitoring, introduction of normal eating habits leading to weight restoration, intensive provision of psychological therapies and respite for the family. In addition to low levels of confidence and poor self-esteem, health-related quality-of-life studies have shown that eating disorder patients report more functional difficulties in daily living than do healthy controls (Keilen et al., 1994) and hospitalization may provide a welcome temporary escape. However, the extent to which such an admission improves these areas, particularly with more coercive treatments, where the emphasis is on the service taking control, has not been adequately studied. The personal costs of treatment to the patient, such as disruption of schooling and family life, as well as the additional problem of ensuring continuity of care postdischarge, when inpatient admission is at a distance from home, should be balanced against the benefits.

When inpatient admission is required, the choice of a medical or psychiatric facility should be carefully considered.

Inpatient medical units

Admission to a medical (paediatric) ward can be helpful or even life saving in stabilizing critically low-weight patients but such a benefit may be temporary, with subsequent inpatient admission to a comprehensive psychiatric service to address the eating disorder psychopathology usually being desirable.

In the absence of a psychiatric inpatient unit, management on a paediatric inpatient ward may be the best available for severely underweight patients requiring hospitalization. In such cases, appropriate communication with CAMHS staff and other agencies involved is vital.

Inpatient psychiatric units

Inpatient treatment programmes generally consist of a mixture of elements, usually involving a combination of nutritional and medical rehabilitation, psychotherapeutic treatment, psychosocial rehabilitation and often family interventions. There is usually a full-time teacher who provides daily education and maintains regular contact with the young person's own school. The multidisciplinary service at Great Ormond Street Hospital, London, has been described in detail (Lask & Bryant-Waugh, 2000).

Adaptations of the CBT model have been used in inpatient eating disorder units across the age range, and a CBT manual for use with adult and adolescent inpatients with eating disorders has recently been published in Italy (Dalle Grave, 2003). Essentially, the programme consists of 13 weeks of inpatient treatment, followed by 7 weeks of day patient treatment. The first 1-year follow-up data should be available early in 2006; interim results are promising, with 79.5% completing the programme and of those completers, significant reductions in eating-disordered behaviours (as measured using the Eating Disorders Examination) have been found (data presented at the European Association for Behavioural and Cognitive Therapy, Manchester, 2004).

There is a lack of consensus about the optimum length of stay in hospital as well as what should be achieved during that time. For example, from a CBT perspective, one might argue that once weight has stabilized, treatment should be continued in a less intensive facility where treatment gains can be more easily transferred to the natural environment. Others, particularly in Europe argue for a more lengthy admission with full weight restoration before discharge. Some of these variations in approach have been highlighted in a study investigating the range of service provision and treatment approaches in the treatment of adolescent anorexia nervosa in 12 European countries (Gowers et al., 2002). This survey found that the average length of stay varied at least four-fold between services and that the treatment style ranged from a strict behavioural approach to individually designed client-centred therapy.

Little agreement exists regarding the staffing of inpatient child and adolescent services in general and eating disorder services in particular, although anecdotal reports suggest that there is marked variation across services. The Eating Disorders Special Interest Group of the Royal College of Psychiatrists (2000) has made specific recommendations regarding staffing, based in part on previous recommendations by the Eating Disorders Association (EDA, 1994). This report suggests that in addition to a team of nonmedical, well-trained staff, including psychologists and nurses, the frequent occurrence of serious, life-threatening physical complications as well as psychiatric disorder in these patients would point to the need for a consultant psychiatrist with a specialist interest in eating disorders.

Day programmes

For those patients not requiring the intensity of inpatient treatment but requiring more than an outpatient programme, day hospital treatment may be considered. It may be helpful for patients who have not responded fully to outpatient treatment or as an intermediate (step down) treatment following an inpatient admission. It may also be used as a more cost-effective treatment for severe eating disorder cases. Birchall et al. (2002) costed the addition of an intensive day programme for the treatment of severe AN in a regional (adult) specialist service in the UK, finding that this reduced hospital costs per patient by about £1500.

Usually, day programmes run 4, 5 or 7 days weekly and consist of supervised meals, a variety of therapeutic groups and sometimes concurrent individual therapy (Olmsted, 2002). Additional family therapy and medical and pharmacological management are included as necessary. Specialized day patient treatments for anorexia nervosa have been described in various countries (Gerlinghoff et al., 1998; Birchall et al., 2002; Zipfel et al., 2002; Robinson, 2003) and seem to show short-term positive outcomes in older adolescents and adults. Without data from adequately powered RCTs, it is difficult to draw firm conclusions about the relative effectiveness of such programmes, but they may prove, in time, to be more cost-effective and developmentally appropriate than inpatient treatment.

A more intensive family-based intervention for adolescents with anorexia nervosa has recently been developed (Dare & Eisler, 2000; Scholz & Asen, 2001). This 'multi-family programme' is usually delivered within a day hospital facility and consists of a 4/5 day block of therapy followed by a limited number of day sessions. Whilst the treatment is at an early stage of evaluation, preliminary findings suggest promising outcomes, particularly regarding a reduced need for hospitalization (Scholz & Asen, 2001). (See Lock and Couturier, Chapter 19, this volume).

Specialist or general-purpose services?

Facilities for treating adolescent eating disorders vary greatly across and within countries, with some areas offering specialist eating disorder input and others providing a more generalized package of care, for example with medical and/ or psychiatric input but without specialist eating disorder expertise. The Eating Disorders Special Interest Group of the Royal College of Psychiatrists (2000) conducted a survey of all NHS and private services providing specialist treatments for patients with eating disorders in the UK. Services providing care for children and adolescents with eating disorders specifically were identified, in addition to a selection of general child and adolescent services. It was found that despite a willingness to treat young people with eating disorders in general units, in reality, relatively few patients were being treated as day or inpatients in them. Neither were many referred on to specialist units. The survey also showed that whilst at least one child-trained member of staff was present in 88% of the clinics, only 63% had a trained child psychiatrist on the staff, and only about half of the clinics had liaison with a paediatric team. It should be noted that these results were from a small sample of services across the UK (n = 24), and in the absence of a fully systematic survey, the shortage of provision is uncertain. Findings from a 1-day census of bed occupancy by diagnosis in child and adolescent psychiatric units in the UK revealed that more beds were occupied by young people with eating disorders than any other diagnostic group (O'Herlihy et al., 2003). This apparent discrepancy highlights the shortage of UK adolescent psychiatric beds overall and the high mean length of stay of those with eating disorders, thus a relatively small number of admissions occupy a large proportion of a limited inpatient provision.

The merits of specialist versus generalist care are being investigated in the TOuCAN trial – a randomized controlled treatment trial under way in the north of England. There would appear to be pros and cons to each approach. On the positive side, patients with eating disorders living in the same unit can be supportive of each other and share experiences. This can be the most positive aspect of the treatment experience for them. On the other hand, unhelpful competition between the young people can be counterproductive. In a general purpose unit, trying to treat people with eating disorders in the same unit as those with psychosis can sometimes limit the ability to meet individual treatment needs.

Research evidence for different treatment models

There are no comprehensive systematic reviews focusing on the child and adolescent age group (Treasure & Schmidt, 2003) and some extrapolation from the adult literature has been necessary (see Gowers & Bryant-Waugh, 2004, for a review of pros and cons of doing so). There is one systematic review summarizing the effectiveness of inpatient and outpatient care in the management of AN in the adult field (Meads et al., 2001). These authors concluded that outpatient treatment in a specialist eating disorder service was as effective as inpatient treatment in those not so severely ill as to warrant an emergency admission. Furthermore, they estimated the costs of outpatient treatment to be approximately one-tenth of the cost of inpatient treatment. However, it should be noted that the review included only one small RCT of service setting ('The St. George's Study', Crisp et al., 1991; Gowers et al., 1994).

Gowers et al. (2000) carried out a nonrandomized naturalistic comparison of outcome in adolescents with AN treated as inpatients and outpatients. They found that type of treatment received was strongly associated with outcome, with those treated as inpatients having a notably poorer outcome (despite initial weight restoration). However, the absence of a randomized design suggests some caution should be taken in interpreting these findings, for example those admitted to hospital were likely to have comprised some of the most severe cases.

CAMHS services in the northwest of England are currently undertaking an RCT (the TOuCAN trial), involving 35 child and adolescent mental health services covering a population of approximately 7 million. The study aims to assess the clinical and cost-effectiveness of inpatient versus outpatient treatment and generic versus specialist services for adolescents with anorexia nervosa. This trial hopes to make an important contribution to the evidence base in this area.

Evidence-based guidelines

The National Institute for Clinical Excellence (NCCMH, 2004)

The National Institute for Clinical Excellence (NICE) produces evidence-based guidelines for UK health commissioners, service providers and the general public. The Eating Disorders Guideline included an evaluation of the evidence for specific service delivery systems and service level interventions.

The recommendations for children and adolescents were limited by the paucity of good quality research evidence. NICE categorizes its recommendations hierarchically from A–C depending on the strength of evidence; category A being based on randomized controlled trials, B on findings from other research designs and C from consensus expert opinion.

In AN, the guideline made no category A recommendations and only one at level B, namely that family interventions that directly address the eating disorder should be offered; the remaining recommendations were all at category C.

When considering service recommendations, NICE recommended that the need for inpatient treatment to ensure weight restoration should be balanced against the educational and social needs of the young person. It also recommended that once a healthy weight is reached, the young person should maintain the necessary nutrients in their diet to support further growth and development and that carers should be included in any dietary education or meal planning.

The guideline refers to the importance of documenting the young person's consent or otherwise and the legal basis for embarking on treatment. If a young person refuses treatment that is deemed essential, consideration should be given to the use of the relevant Mental Health legislation. In the absence of research evidence NICE suggests adolescents with BN may be treated with CBT–BN adapted as needed to suit their age, circumstances and level of development and including the family as appropriate. Inpatient treatment is not recommended for bulimia nervosa in the absence of other indicators.

Throughout treatment, health professionals should remain alert to levels of risk to the patient's mental and physical health as well as any indicators of abuse. Health professionals are also advised to respect the young person's right to confidentiality as set out in national guidelines and local policies, and whether in- or outpatient treatment is proposed, children and adolescents should be offered individual appointments separate from their family or carer.

Consensus guidelines

In the absence of research trials addressing the effectiveness of service configurations in this area, a number of academic and professional bodies (Eating Disorders Association, 1994; the Society for Adolescent Medicine, Kreipe *et al.*, 1995; The American Psychiatric Association, 2000; Royal College of Psychiatrists, 2000; RANZCP, 2004) have published consensus guidelines to guide decision making. In practice, the recommendations are similar to the category C recommendations in the NICE guideline.

There is a general consensus that wherever possible, children and adolescents should be treated locally and in an age-appropriate manner. Assessment and ongoing management should be provided by a multidisciplinary team who have experience in the management of young people with eating disorders and who have knowledge about normal physical and psychological development. Transitions between services should be carefully planned and facilitated, for example in the case of older adolescents who may require ongoing treatment in an adult service.

Conclusions

Although the variation in services available for adolescents with eating disorders seems undesirable, this situation is to some extent the result of a lack of good quality evidence to guide decision making. It is unacceptable that the quality of a patient's treatment can depend largely on their home address and there is a clear need to standardize services and provide clear guidelines about how referrals are accepted and managed.

In choosing between different models of service, availability is a major consideration, with patients as well as referrers sometimes having to weigh up the advantages of a locally accessible service with those of a more comprehensive service at some geographical distance.

In many cases, a comprehensive outpatient CAMHS service will have the necessary skills to assess and initiate treatment with generic individual cognitive–behavioural therapy and family therapy where required. Each CAMHS service should have an established link with a paediatric medical facility to provide intensive/emergency inpatient treatment if required. Access to a specialist eating disorder service is desirable as part of the overall package of care (and particularly for severe cases), to provide second opinions, to offer more intensive or specialized management and to provide inpatient psychiatric management.

Whilst knowledge about the benefits of different service models and settings is largely anecdotal, decision making can be very difficult, particularly when faced with a young person who is poorly engaged and opposed to intensive treatment.

Guidelines such as those produced by NICE are useful in identifying gaps in knowledge and raising the profile of child and adolescent eating disorders. It is important that healthcare professionals are familiar with these guidelines in addition to local policies.

Most guidelines agree that whatever the type of service, the setting should be age-appropriate and take into account the young person's developmental, social and educational needs. Evidence-based treatment approaches should be provided where evidence is available. More training and support should be available for noneating-disorder specialists working in generic CAMHS services.

There is a clear need for further research investigating the effectiveness and cost-effectiveness of different service models (day patient, inpatient and outpatient) for young people with eating disorders.

Randomized Controlled Trials (RCTs) are required to improve the evidence base, for example in demonstrating the effectiveness of different and specialized models of care.

REFERENCES

American Psychiatric Association (2000). Practice guideline for the treatment of patients with eating disorders (revision). American Psychiatric Association Work Group on Eating Disorders. *American Journal of Psychiatry*, **157**, 1–39.

Birchall, H., Palmer, R., Waine, J., Gadsby, K. & Gatward, N. (2002). Intensive day programme treatment for severe anorexia nervosa – the Leicester experience. *Psychiatric Bulletin*, **26**, 334–6.

Crisp, A. H., Norton, K. W. R., Gowers, S. G. *et al.* (1991). A controlled study of the effect of therapies aimed at adolescent and family psychopathology in anorexia nervosa. *British Journal of Psychiatry*, **159**, 325–33.

Dalle Grave, R. (2003). *Terapia cognitivocomportamentale dei disturbi dell'alimentazione durante il ricovero*. Verona: Positive Press.

Dalle Grave, R., Ricca, V. & Todesco, T. (2001). The stepped care approach in anorexia nervosa and bulimia nervosa: progress and problems. *Eating and Weight Disorders*, **6**, 81–9.

Dare, C. & Eisler, I. (2000). A multi-family group day treatment programme for adolescent eating disorder. *European Eating Disorders Review*, **8**, 4–18.

Dare, C., Eisler, I., Russell, G. et al. (2001). Psychological therapies for adults with anorexia nervosa: randomised controlled trial of outpatient treatments. *British Journal of Psychiatry*, **178**, 216–21.

Department of Health (2004). The National Service Framework for Children. London: Department of Health.

Eating Disorders Association (1994). Eating Disorders: *A Guide to Purchasing and Providing Services*. Norwich: EDA.

Ebeling H., Tapanainen, P., Joutsenoja, A. et al. (2003). *Practice Guidelines for Treatment of Eating Disorders in Children and Adolescents*. Helsinki: Finnish Medical Association.

Eisler., I., Dare, C., Russell, G. F. M. et al. (1997). Family and individual therapy in anorexia nervosa. A 5 year follow up. *Archives of General Psychiatry*, **54**, 1025–30.

Fairburn, C. & Harrison, P. J. (2003). Eating disorders. *Lancet*, **361**, 407–16.

Fairburn, C. G., Norman, P. A., Welch, S. L. et al. (1995). A prospective study of outcome in bulimia nervosa and the long term effects of three psychological treatments. *Archives of General Psychiatry*, **52**, 304–12.

Fairburn, C. & Peveler, R. (1990). Bulimia nervosa and a stepped care approach to management. *Gut*, **31**, 1220–2.

Gerlinghoff, M., Backmund, H. & Franzen, U. (1998). Evaluation of a day treatment programme for eating disorders. *European Eating Disorders Review*, **6**, 96–106.

Gowers, S. G. (2005). Evidence based research in CBT with adolescent eating disorders. *Child and Adolescent Mental Health*, **10**, 1–4.

Gowers, S. G. & Bryant-Waugh, R. (2004). Management of child and adolescent eating disorders: the current evidence and future directions. *Journal of Child Psychology and Psychiatry*, **45**, 63–84.

Gowers, S. G., Norton, K., Halek, C. & Crisp, A. H. (1994). Outcome of outpatient psychotherapy in a random allocation treatment study of anorexia nervosa. *International Journal of Eating Disorders*, **15**, 165–77.

Gowers, S. G., Weetman, J., Shore, A., Hossain, F. & Elvins, R. (2000). The impact of hospitalisation on the outcome of adolescent anorexia nervosa. *British Journal of Psychiatry*, **176**, 138–41.

Gowers, S. G., Edwards, V. J., Fleminger, S. et al. (2002). Treatment aims and philosophy in the treatment of adolescent anorexia nervosa in Europe. *European Eating Disorders Review*, **10**, 271–80.

HAS (1995). Together we stand: The commissioning, role and management of Child and Adolescent Mental Health Services. London: HMSO.

Jaffa, T,. Lelliot, P., O'Herlihy, A. et al. (2004). The staffing of inpatient child and adolescent mental health services. *Child and Adolescent Mental Health*, **9**, 84–7.

Keilen, M., Treasure, T., Schmidt, U. & Treasure, J. (1994). Quality of life measurements in eating disorders, angina and transplant candidates – are they comparable? *Journal of the Royal Society of Medicine*, **87**, 441–4.

Kreipe, R. E., Golden, N. H., Katzman, D. K. et al. (1995). Eating disorders in adolescence. A position paper of the Society for Adolescent Medicine. *Journal of Adolescent Health*, **16**, 476–9.

Lask, B. & Bryant-Waugh, R. (ed.). (2000). *Anorexia Nervosa and Related Eating Disorders in Childhood and Adolescence*, (2nd edition). Hove: Psychology Press.

Lock, J., Le Grange, D., Agras, W. & Fairburn, C. (2001). *Treatment Manual for Anorexia Nervosa; A Family Based Approach*. New York: Guilford Press.

Meads, C., Gold, L. & Burls, A. (2001). How effective is outpatient care compared to inpatient care for treatment of anorexia nervosa? A systematic review. *European Eating Disorders Review*, **9**, 229–41.

Minuchin, S., Baker, L., Rosman, B. L. *et al.* (1975). A conceptual model of psychosomatic illness in childhood. *Archives of General Psychiatry*, **32**, 1031–8.

National Collaborating Centre for Mental Health (2004). *Eating Disorders: Core Interventions in the Treatment and Management of Anorexia Nervosa, Bulimia Nervosa and Related Eating Disorders; A National Clinical Practice Guideline*. London: National Institute for Clinical Excellence.

Nielsen, S., Moller-Madsen, S., Isager, T. *et al.* (1998). Standardised mortality in eating disorders – quantitative summary of previously published and new evidence. *Journal of Psychosomatic Research*, **44**, 412–13.

O'Herlihy, A., Worrall, A., Lelliott, P. *et al.* (2003). Distribution and characteristics of in-patient child and adolescent mental health services in England and Wales. *Clinical Child Psychology and Psychiatry*, **9**, 579–88.

Olmsted, M. (2002). Day hospital treatment of anorexia nervosa and bulimia nervosa. In *Eating Disorders and Obesity, a Comprehensive Handbook*, 2nd edition, ed. Fairburn, C. & Brownell, K. New York: Guilford Press, pp. 330–34.

RANZCP (2004). Australian and New Zealand clinical practice guidelines for the treatment of anorexia nervosa. *Australia and New Zealand Journal of Psychiatry*, **38**, 659–70.

Robinson, P. (2003). Day treatments. In *Handbook of Eating Disorders*, ed. Treasure, J., Schmidt, U. & Van Furth, E. Chichester: John Wiley & Sons, pp. 333–47.

Royal College of Psychiatrists (2000). Eating disorders in the UK: policies for service developments and training. *Council Report CR 87*. London: Royal College of Psychiatrists.

Scholtz, M. & Asen, E. (2001). Multiple family therapy with eating disordered adolescents. *European Eating Disorders Review*, **9**, 33–42.

Treasure, J. & Schmidt, U. (2003). Treament overview. In *Handbook of Eating Disorders*, 2nd edition, ed. Treasure, J., Schmidt, U. & Van Furth, E. Chichester: John Wiley & Sons, pp. 207–17.

Van Hoeken, D., Seidell. J. & Hoek, H. W. (2003). Epidemiology. In *Handbook of Eating Disorders*, 2nd edition, ed. Treasure, J., Schmidt, U. & van Furth, E. Chichester: John Wiley & Sons, pp. 11–34.

Vitousek, K., Watson, S. & Wilson, G. T. (1998). Enhancing motivation for change in treament-resistant eating disorders. *Clinical Psychology Review*, **18**, 391–420.

Zipfel, S., Reas, D. L., Thornton, C. *et al.* (2002). Day hospitalization programs for eating disorders: a systematic review of the literature. *International Journal of Eating Disorders*, **31**, 105–17.

21

Psychopharmacology and eating disorders

Kristine J. Steffen, James L. Roerig and James E. Mitchell

Neuropsychiatric Research Institute, Fargo, ND, USA

Introduction

Pharmacological options for the treatment of anorexia nervosa (AN) and bulimia nervosa (BN) are sequentially reviewed within this chapter. Randomized, controlled medication trials represent the primary focus of discussion. The majority of pharmacotherapy research in AN and BN has been conducted with adult patients. Owing to potential pathophysiological or pharmacokinetic differences, it is unclear how results derived from these trials translate into the treatment of paediatric or adolescent patients.

Psychotropic use in children

Particularly when treating younger children, the prescriber is left with the task of designing age-specific dosage regimens. Pharmacokinetic parameters change markedly with age, including absorption, metabolism, distribution and elimination. Further, although the literature on pharmacodynamics is sparse in paediatrics, it is generally assumed that developmental changes influence drug action and response. For a discussion on these paediatric pharmacology issues, the reader is referred to a review by Kearns et al. (2003).

Antidepressants

Underweight patients have an increased risk of arrhythmia with tricyclic antidepressants (TCAs) (Kotler & Walsh, 2000) and an association between certain TCAs and sudden death in children has been identified. A 2001 review describes eight cases of sudden death in paediatric or adolescent patients, six of which involved desipramine monotherapy and two of which involved imipramine in combination therapy (Varley, 2001). As discussed in this report, desipramine may be more specifically toxic compared with other TCAs, and

Eating Disorders in Children and Adolescents, ed. Tony Jaffa and Brett McDermott. Published by Cambridge University Press. © Cambridge University Press 2007.

imipramine may be implicated because it is metabolized to desipramine. Conversely, the absence of sudden death reports with other TCAs may be a result of a higher frequency of prescribing of desipramine and imipramine in paediatric patients. This reviewer concluded that the risk of sudden death may extend to other TCAs which have similar properties and are similarly lethal in overdose. Prescribing of TCAs in children requires close physician supervision and has been largely curtailed.

Compared with the TCAs, the selective serotonin reuptake inhibitors (SSRIs) are associated with a favourable adverse effect profile and reduced risk of cardiotoxicity (Table 21.2). Unfortunately, recent FDA reports have emerged suggesting that SSRIs appear to increase the risk of suicidality in children and adolescents. According to the FDA, pooled analyses of 24 short-term (4- to 16-week) placebo-controlled trials with nine antidepressant drugs in 4400 children and adolescents with a variety of psychiatric disorders have revealed a greater risk of suicidal thinking or suicidality during the first few months of treatment in those receiving antidepressants. The average risk of these events with drug treatment was reportedly 4%; comparatively, the placebo risk was 2%. No suicides occurred during these trials (FDA, 2004). The FDA has requested that all antidepressant manufacturers include a black-box warning at the beginning of each package insert regarding the increased risk of suicidal thinking and behaviour. The FDA states that the new warnings do not prohibit the use of antidepressants in children and adolescents, but rather encourages prescribers to weigh the suicidality risk against the clinical consequences of foregoing antidepressant treatment.

Antipsychotics

There are no controlled atypical antipsychotic trials published in AN. As conveyed in Table 21.2, however, several uncontrolled studies have included adolescent patients. Atypical antipsychotics have also been used successfully in other psychiatric disorders in children, and are considered 'first-line agents' in the treatment of psychotic symptoms associated with schizophrenia by the American Academy of Child and Adolescent Psychiatry (AACAP, 2005). The atypical antipsychotics offer several advantages over the conventional compounds, yet metabolic effects such as hyperinsulinaemia and hyperlipidaemia are a concern. The relative risk of adverse effects on glucose-insulin homeostasis and lipid levels appears highest for clozapine and olanzapine, moderate for quetiapine, rather low for risperidone and lowest for ziprasidone (Melkersson & Dahl, 2004). Upon request of the FDA, labelling of each atypical antipsychotic has been revised to contain a warning about the potential for hyperglycaemia, which can be extreme and has been reported to result in ketoacidosis or hyperosmolar coma or death in patients taking these drugs.

Anorexia nervosa

Pharmacotherapy literature

Anorexia nervosa is associated with the highest mortality rate of any psychiatric disorder (Sullivan, 1995), yet clinicians have a paucity of evidence-based treatment options available to offer these patients. The lack of clinical data in AN is partially attributable to the ill-defined aetiology of the illness. Other factors are also responsible, including the relative rarity of the illness, the severity of the condition and the consequent requirement for multiple interventions, and a patient population which is often adolescent and which frequently exhibits noncompliance resulting from a lack of appreciation for illness severity (Mitchell *et al.*, 2002).

Much of the existing clinical data have emerged from research protocols which have enrolled small subject numbers, lasted for a brief duration of time, or have used inadequate medication dosages (Kotler & Walsh, 2000). Several AN pharmacotherapy studies have been conducted with inpatients, the majority of whom receive simultaneous psychotherapy, dietary guidance, a refeeding programme and medical management, with resultant weight gain. Therefore, the superimposed benefit of pharmacotherapy may be inadequately appraised amid the myriad of other interventions these patients receive.

Pharmacotherapy objectives

In contrast to many historical outcome assessments, it is critically important that core psychological manifestations of AN, including fear of becoming fat, body image disturbance, perfectionism and obsessionality are assessed in tandem with measures of weight (Mitchell *et al.*, 2002). A recent review of AN pharmacotherapy generated a list of potential pharmacotherapy targets in AN, including weight gain, weight maintenance, obsessions and compulsions, cognitive deficits, anxiety symptoms (particularly phobic symptoms), depressive symptoms, psychotic symptoms including delusions and hallucinations, body image disturbances and impaired quality of life (Powers & Santana, 2004).

Antidepressants

It has been estimated that 50–75% of patients seeking treatment for AN in tertiary care centres present with comorbid major depression (MDD) or dysthymia. Further, the lifetime prevalence of obsessive–compulsive disorder

(OCD) in AN is about 25% (APA, 2005). For further discussion see Brewerton (Chapter 13, this volume).

Investigators originally looked toward the TCAs in search of a viable treatment strategy for AN. Propelling interest in these compounds was their documented propensity to cause dose-dependent weight gain, reported to be between 0.57 and 1.37 kg/month of treatment in depression studies (Garland et al., 1988). Three controlled trials have been conducted with TCAs in AN, a summary of which can be viewed in Table 21.1.

As a result of an improved adverse effect profile and demonstrated efficacy in conditions that include MDD and anxiety disorders, SSRIs largely supplanted TCAs in AN pharmacotherapy research. Similar to the majority of other medications, it appears that the role of the SSRIs is limited in the treatment of acutely ill, underweight AN patients. As summarized in Table 21.1, fluoxetine was not superior to placebo in a controlled treatment study in acute AN on weight gain or depressive symptom improvement (Attia et al., 1998).

Enduring negative mood, obsessionality, perfectionism and core eating disorder symptoms are frequently observed in recovered AN patients (Barbarich et al., 2003), thus providing therapeutic targets for SSRI maintenance therapy. SSRIs have been evaluated in a handful of uncontrolled trials in the maintenance treatment of AN which have produced variable results on weight gain and psychopathology. As summarized in Table 21.1, there are two controlled trial of fluoxetine in the maintenance treatment of AN (Kaye et al., 2001; Walsh et al., 2006). In the Kaye study, 10 out of 16 patients remained on fluoxetine for 1 year, compared with three of 19 given placebo. Subjects who remained on fluoxetine for 1 year displayed significantly increased weight, as well as decreased core eating-disorder symptoms, obsessive thoughts and depressed and anxious mood. Walsh et al. (2006) recently reported the results of a 52-week trial of fluoxetine versus placebo in 93 weight-restored outpatients with AN. This study did not find fluoxetine to be superior to placebo for preventing relapse. In the fluoxetine group, 26.5% of patients maintained a body mass index of at least 18.5 and remained in the study for 52 weeks, compared with 31.5% of the placebo group (P = 0.57). The groups did not differ in time to relapse. It is not entirely clear what accounts for the differing findings between these two studies.

Antipsychotics

It has been suggested that AN patients exhibit delusional thinking that is congruent with that of psychotic illness (Powers & Santana, 2004). Distorted or inaccurate perceptions about body shape and/or weight are commonly seen aberrations in thought (DSM–IV; APA, 1994). Several antipsychotic compounds are also potent weight-promoting agents. Thus, the typical antipsychotics were

Table 21.1. Controlled antidepressant trials in anorexia nervosa

Study reference	No. of inpatients/ outpatients	Duration	Mean baseline weight (kg)	Drug and dose	Outcome
Lacey & Crisp (1980)	16 inpatients	Until target weight reached	40.6 ($\pm$ 4.6) Clo 37.7 ($\pm$ 5.2) Plc	Clo 50 mg	No significant difference in weight gain or time to reach target weight.
Biederman et al. (1985)	38 inpatients and outpatients	5 weeks	38.2 ($\pm$ 4.2) Ami 35.5 ($\pm$ 5.8) Plc 35.8 ($\pm$ 6.7) Control	Ami Max 175 mg Mean 115 mg	Control group of drug-refusers who received psychosocial therapy only. No difference in weight gain; no decrease in depressive symptoms with Ami.
Halmi et al. (1986)	72 inpatients	4 weeks	—	Ami Max 160 mg Cyp Max 32 mg	Cyp increased treatment efficiency in nonbulimic subgroup. Antidepressant effect occurred with Cyp.
Attia et al. (1998)	33 inpatients	7 weeks	41.8 ($\pm$ 4.45)	Flu Max 60 mg Mean 56 mg	No difference in weight gain or mood symptoms between groups. Flu well tolerated.
Kaye et al. (2001)	39 outpatients	52 weeks	76–100% average body weight	Flu range of doses; 20 mg every other day to 60 mg/day	10/16 Flu subjects still on drug at 1 year, compared with 3/19 Plc subjects. Flu patients had higher weight and decreased core symptoms at 1 year.
Walsh et al. (2006)	93 outpatients	52 weeks	BMI: 20.16 ($\pm$ 0.48) Flu 20.45 ($\pm$ 0.51) Plc	Flu Mean 63.5 (15.8) mg/day Plc Mean equivalent 71.4 (13.2) mg/day	No advantage of Flu over placebo on relapse or completion rates

Ami, amitriptyline; Clo, clomipramine; Cyp, cyproheptadine; Flu, fluoxetine; Plc, placebo.

Table 21.2. Common or serious adverse effects with medications

Tricyclic antidepressants	Selective serotonin reuptake inhibitors (SSRIs)	Atypical antipsychotics
Anticholinergic	Headache	Sedation
Blurred vision	Insomnia/sleep disturbance	Dizziness
Constipation	Anxiety	Dry mouth
Delirium	Nausea, diarrhoea	Constipation
Dry mouth	Sexual dysfunction	Weight gain
Memory difficulties	Weight loss early in	Hyperglycaemia
Urinary retention	therapy, weight gain later	Extrapyramidal side effects (rarely)
Tachycardia	Diaphoresis	Parkinsonian effects
Dilated pupils	Discontinuation syndrome	Akathisia
Weight gain		Dystonic reactions
Sedation		Tardive dyskinesia (low risk)
Cardiovascular		Neuroleptic malignant syndrome
Orthostatic hypotension		Prolactin elevation
Prolonged cardiac conduction		Risperidone
Lower seizure threshold		Amisulpride
Switch to mania		
Lethal in overdose		
Arrhythmias, AV block		
CNS depression/coma		
Discontinuation syndrome		

initially studied in AN, where pimozide and sulpiride both failed to improve outcome (Vandereycken & Pierloot, 1982; Vandereycken, 1984). Coupling an improved side-effect profile to a propensity to stimulate weight gain that is virtually unrivalled by any other class of medications, the emergence of the atypical agents has renewed research enthusiasm in antipsychotic drugs in AN. A meta-analysis revealed that schizophrenic subjects gained 4–4.5 kg of weight at 10 weeks of treatment on clozapine, matched only by olanzapine. Risperidone is associated with approximately half the weight gain as olanzapine (Allison et al., 1999). At varying levels, these drugs are antagonistic at dopamine D1, D2 and D4 receptors, serotonin type 2, muscarinic and alpha-adrenergic receptors, and are thought to interact with GABA/glutamate neurotransmission (Allison & Casey, 2001). Along with quetiapine, olanzapine and risperidone have received preliminary study with promising results in AN, as summarized in Table 21.2.

Miscellaneous (Table 21.3)

By virtue of its weight gain and mood stabilization potential, lithium has been evaluated in a controlled study of AN but did not show substantial efficacy (Gross *et al.*, 1981). Further, the clinical use of lithium may be complicated by the fluid and electrolyte aberrations that frequently occur in AN, which may alter the pharmacokinetic parameters of the drug. Zinc supplementation has shown some benefit in a controlled study with adolescent AN patients with comorbid anxiety and depression, although weight gain was not superior to placebo (Katz *et al.*, 1987). Another controlled trial revealed a faster BMI increase with zinc compared with placebo, although this did not result in a shortened duration of treatment (Birmingham *et al.*, 1994). A variety of other drugs, including tetrahydrocannabinol, the opioid antagonist naltrexone, clonidine, recombinant human growth hormone, and the prokinetic agents metoclopramide, domperidone and cisapride have been demonstrated to either lack efficacy or result in adverse drug reactions (Pederson *et al.*, 2003).

Bulimia nervosa

Pharmacotherapy literature

Bulimia nervosa is a more prevalent condition than AN, affecting between 1% and 3% of adolescent and young adult females (DSM–IV; APA 1994). A more robust pharmacopoeia has been explored in BN, despite BN being characterized much later than AN. The antidepressant medication fluoxetine is currently FDA-approved for BN treatment, a designation that is still lacking for any drug in AN pharmacotherapy.

Pharmacotherapy objectives

In BN, subjects are characteristically of normal weight. Therefore, the focus of treatment shifts away from weight gain and toward a reduction in core symptoms of binge-eating (BE) episodes and associated inappropriate compensatory behaviours such as excessive exercise or purgation with laxatives or via vomiting. As with those afflicted with AN, patients with BN exhibit high rates of psychiatric comorbidity, including major depressive disorder (MDD), substance abuse/dependence and personality disorders (Agras, 2001). Symptoms associated with these conditions represent additional targets for pharmacotherapy.

Antidepressants

In BN, most of the controlled research trials to date have focused on antidepressant medications, as it is estimated that 50% or more of patients with

Table 21.3. Uncontrolled antipsychotic trials in anorexia nervosa

Study reference	No. of inpatients/ outpatients	Baseline weight/ BMI	Age (years)	Drug (daily dose)	Outcome/comments
Fisman et al. (1996)	1 inpatient	44.1 kg	13	RIS (1 mg)	Improvement in behaviour and paranoia. Weight gain of 2.3 kg maintained for 1 year.
Hansen (1999)	1 inpatient	31.2 kg	49	OLZ (5 mg)	Improved body image. Discharge weight 53.1 kg.
Jensen & Mejlhede (2000)	3 outpatient	BMI 13.8 BMI 15.8 BMI 18.5	50 30 34	OLZ (5 mg)	Patients gained weight and had decreased body image distortion.
La Via et al. (2000)	2 inpatient	16.9 kg	15	OLZ (10 mg)	Decrease in agitation and improvement in core eating-disorder behaviours. Gained 1.36 kg/week to 33.6 kg.
Newman-Toker (2000)	2 outpatient	48 kg 36.4 kg (BMI 14.6)	27 19	RIS (1.5 mg)	Gained 1.82 kg/week to 53.2 kg. Anxiety, food obsession and delusional thinking improved. Achieved and maintained normal body weight (49.5 kg). After drug discontinued, patient did well. QT$_c$ interval increased from 400–421 ms.
		37.7 kg (BMI 15.9)	12		Gained insight into illness and mood improved. Reached weight of 46.8 kg. (Randomized trial.)
Gaskill et al. (2001)	46 inpatient (open, non-randomized trial)			OLZ range 1.25–15 mg	No difference between OLZ group and nontreated group on weight gain.

Table 21.3. (*cont.*)

Study reference	No. of inpatients/ outpatients	Baseline weight/ BMI	Age (years)	Drug (daily dose)	Outcome/comments
Mehler *et al.* (2001)	5	30–39 kg	12–17	OLZ 5–12.5 mg	Decreased delusional thinking. Improved communication and social interaction. Weekly average weight gain unchanged with OLZ.
Ruggiero *et al.* (2001)	35 inpatients	37.61 kg (± 9.8) CLO 40.90 kg (± 6.9) FLU 38.41 kg (± 8.33) AMIS	23.69 (± 4.57) CLO 24.50 (± 5.06) FLU 24.33 (± 5.76) AMIS	CLO 57.7 mg FLU 28 mg AMIS 50 mg	Weight increase was not significantly different between groups. AMIS 11%, CLO 3.3%, FLU 4.5%.
Carver *et al.* (2002)	30 inpatients (retrospective chart review)	—	—	RIS 0.5–1.5 mg	Refractory AN patients. Weight gain (3.6 kg vs. 3.4) and caloric intake (1017 kcal vs. 943) slightly higher in RIS group.
Powers *et al.* (2002)	18 outpatients	BMI 16.4 (± 1.3)	26.8 (± 12.3)	OLZ 10 mg	10 of 14 completers gained average of 8.75 lb. Patients who gained weight had significant improvement on psychiatric rating scales by week 10.

Study	Sample	Baseline weight/BMI	Age	Drug/dose	Comments
Boachie et al. (2003)	3 inpatients	26 kg (BMI 13.6)	10	OLZ 2.5 mg	Comorbid OCD and MDD. Weight of 34.9 kg 3.5 mo after starting OLZ.
		27.4 kg (BMI 12.2)	12	OLZ 2.5 mg	Weight of 39.8 kg (BMI 17.8) at 10 weeks. Improved agitation and sleep, and improved relationships with family.
		23.8 kg (BMI 13.6)	10	OLZ 2.5 mg	Gained 5 kg during first four weeks of hospitalization and gained additional 2.4 kg over 3 weeks after OLZ was started to a weight of 31.3 kg (BMI 17.5). Patient was also on fluvoxamine 75 mg daily.
Barbarich et al. (2004)	17 inpatients	Proportion of IBW, %: 69 ± 10	20.5 ± 5.1 years	Mean 4.7 ± 1.6 mg (range 2.5–7.5 mg)	Some subjects also received SSRI. Significant decrease in depression, anxiety and core eating-disorder symptoms. Significant increase in weight to 81 ± 9% IBW ($P = 0.000$).
Powers et al. (2004)	20 outpatients	Mean BMI 16.5	14–48 (mean 26 years)	QTP (dose unknown)	10-week ongoing study. Mean weight gain for completers was 0.86 kg. Eight patients gained weight, 5 lost weight and 3 had no change. Significant decline in PANSS Positive Scale scores ($P = 0.047$) among those who gained weight.

AMIS, amisulpride; CLO, clomipramine; FLU, fluoxetine; IBW, Ideal body weight; mo., months; ms, milliseconds; OLZ, olanzapine; PANSS, Positive and Negative Syndrome Scale; QTP, quetiapine; RIS, risperidone; wks, weeks.

BN have a lifetime diagnosis of MDD (Agras, 2001). The majority of these trials have been conducted with adult subjects. Antidepressants have generally shown superiority over placebo in BN treatment, and no particular class of antidepressants has been substantially more efficacious than another (Roerig et al., 2002). Antidepressants appear to have efficacy not only on core BN symptoms of binge eating and vomiting, but also appear to improve mood and anxiety (Mitchell et al., 2002). As in AN pharmacotherapy, relapse prevention is a key point in BN treatment, an area where few trials have been conducted (Walsh et al., 1991; Fichter et al., 1996; Romano et al., 2002). Antidepressant trials in BN are numerous but not yet exhaustive, the sample sizes in the majority of the studies are modest and there is wide variability between placebo response rates (Mitchell et al., 2002).

Although the efficacy of the TCA compounds has been well established in BN, they are relegated primarily to historical interest and have been infrequently prescribed in this condition since agents with improved adverse effect profiles have become available.

Although it was not the only article to demonstrate the efficacy of fluoxetine in BN, the seminal work leading to its FDA approval in a dose of 60 mg/day was completed by the Fluoxetine Bulimia Nervosa Collaborative (FBNC) Study Group (1992). This was an 8-week, multicentre study that enrolled 387 BN subjects. Fluoxetine 60 mg/day was significantly better than placebo at reducing vomiting ($P < 0.001$) and BE ($P < 0.001$). Fluoxetine 20 mg/day separated from placebo only in terms of vomiting ($P = 0.040$), but not for BE ($P = 0.538$). The 60 mg/day fluoxetine dose was significantly superior to the 20 mg/day dose on reduction of vomiting as well as BE ($P = 0.014$ and 0.003, respectively).

Other studies have also supported the efficacy of SSRI medications in the treatment of BN (Goldstein et al., 1995, 1999; Romano et al., 2002). The treatment response to fluoxetine appears to be independent of pretreatment depression status, such that improvement in BN symptoms occurs irrespective of the presence or absence of depression (Goldstein et al., 1999). Antidepressant medications are not a cure for most BN patients. Agras found that on average, 25% of patients who began treatment and received an antidepressant recovered. With prolonged treatment, about one-third of those patients relapsed, revealing a sustained recovery rate of only 15% (Agras, 1997).

An 8-week, open-label trial of fluoxetine (titrated up to 60 mg/day) in adolescents was published in 2003 (Kotler et al., 2003). Subjects included females aged 12–18 years (average 16.2 ± 1.0 years) with BN or an eating disorder not otherwise specified (EDNOS). At baseline, all 10 subjects had depressive disorders and 4 of the 10 had an anxiety disorder. Average weekly binges decreased from 4.1 ± 3.8 to 0 ($P < 0.01$). Average weekly purges also decreased significantly from 6.4 ± 5.2 to 0.4 ± 0.9 (P < 0.005). Other clinical variables that decreased significantly included the Eating Disorder Inventory (Bulimia Subscale), Eating Attitudes Test and scores on the Self-Report for Childhood Anxiety Related Disorders (SCARED) test. No significant changes were seen on weight, body mass index or scores on the Beck Depression Inventory. It has been suggested that the optimum clinical approach to BN treatment involves psychotherapy, which medications can be used to augment, especially if the patient has comorbid anxiety or depression (Nakash-Eisikovits *et al.*, 2002). Generally, studies that have compared antidepressant therapy to psychotherapy have found a combination of the two superior to either treatment alone (Bacaltchuk *et al.*, 2003).

Miscellaneous

The antidepressant bupropion showed efficacy in a controlled BN study, but four out of 55 subjects experienced grand mal seizures, resulting in bupropion's contraindication in AN and BN patients (Horne *et al.*, 1988).

The anticonvulsant topiramate has been associated with weight loss and has shown potential promise in BN pharmacotherapy. Subjects aged 16–50 were randomized to 10 weeks of treatment with placebo or a titrated dose of topiramate (median dose, 100 mg/day, range 25–400 mg/day). Patients in the topiramate group exhibited a 44.8% reduction in mean weekly number of binge and/or purge days, whereas those in the placebo group demonstrated a 10.7% reduction (P = 0.004). Mean body weight for topiramate-treated patients decreased by 1.8 kg, whereas the placebo group had a mean increase of 0.2 kg (P = 0.004). Sixty-four subjects were included in the intent-to-treat analysis, with one topiramate-treated subject and two placebo-treated subjects withdrawing due to adverse events (Hoopes *et al.*, 2003).

The results of a recent controlled trial of adults with BN suggest that the androgen antagonist flutamide may be efficacious (Sundblad *et al.*, 2005). The selective norepinephrine reuptake inhibitor, reboxetine, has also shown promise in the preliminary study of BN (Fassino *et al.*, 2004). The anti-emetic, 5-HT3 antagonist, ondansetron appeared to have efficacy at reducing binge-purge episodes in a recent controlled paradigm (Faris *et al.*, 2000). Other drug modalities that have been explored include d-fenfluramine, lithium, phenytoin and naltrexone, none of which are clinically useful at this time (Pederson *et al.*, 2003).

Conclusion

The clinician is left with a lack of evidence-based pharmacological options to offer patients for the treatment of acute AN, and is required to make inferences to adolescent and paediatric treatment from data collected primarily with adult subjects. In maintenance AN therapy, one fluoxetine study has shown some benefit. While there is currently no pharmacological algorithm to guide the treatment of AN, anticipated atypical antipsychotic studies may yield new insight into the treatment of this disorder. In BN, pharmacotherapy is more advanced, although trials involving adolescent populations are scarce. Fluoxetine, 60 mg/day, is FDA-approved for BN treatment, and is frequently prescribed. Additional long-term antidepressant trials and further study into nonantidepressant compounds is indicated to enrich the pharmacotherapy of BN.

REFERENCES

Agras, W. S. (1997). Pharmacotherapy of bulimia nervosa and binge eating disorder: longer-term outcomes. *Psychopharmacology Bulletin*, **33**, 433–6.

Agras, W. S. (2001). The consequences and costs of the eating disorders. *Psychiatric Clinics of North America*, **24**, 371–9.

Allison, D. B., Mentore, J. L., Heo, M. *et al.* (1999). Antipsychotic-induced weight gain: a comprehensive research synthesis. *American Journal of Psychiatry*, **156**, 1686–96.

Allison, D. B. & Casey, D. E. (2001). Antipsychotic-induced weight gain: a review of the literature. *Journal of Clinical Psychiatry*, **62** (suppl. 7), 22–31.

American Academy of Child and Adolescent Psychiatry (AACAP) (2005). *Summary of the Practice Parameter for the Assessment and Treatment of Children and Adolescents with Schizophrenia.* www. aacap.org/clinical/schizo.htm.

American Psychiatric Association (1994). *Diagnostic and Statistical Manual of Mental Disorders*, 4th edition (DSM–N). Washington, DC: APA.

American Psychiatric Association (APA). *Practice Guideline for the Treatment of Patients With Eating Disorders*, 2nd edition. Accessed February 2005. http://www.psych.org/psych_pract/treatg/pg/eating_revisebook_index.cfm.

Attia, E., Haiman C., Walsh, B. T. & Flater, S. R. (1998). Does fluoxetine augment the inpatient treatment of anorexia nervosa? *American Journal of Psychiatry*, **155**, 548–51.

Bacaltchuk, J., Hay, P. & Trefiglior, R. (2003). Antidepressants versus psychological treatment and their combination for bulimia nervosa. In *The Cochrane Library*, *3*, Cochrane Review.

Barbarich, N. C., Kaye, W. H. & Jimerson, D. (2003). Neurotransmitter and imaging studies. In *Anorexia Nervosa: New Targets for Treatment. Current Drug Targets CNS Neurological Disorders*, **2**, 61–72.

Barbarich, N. C., McConaha, C. W., Gaskill, J. *et al.* (2004). An open trial of olanzapine in anorexia nervosa. *Journal of Clinical Psychiatry*, **65**, 1480–2.

Biederman, J., Herzog, D. B., Rivinus, T. M. *et al.* (1985). Amitriptyline in the treatment of anorexia nervosa: a double-blind, placebo-controlled study. *Journal of Clinical Psychopharmacology*, **5**, 10–16.

Birmingham, C. L., Goldner, E. M. & Bakan, R. (1994). Controlled trial of zinc supplementation in anorexia nervosa. *International Journal of Eating Disorders*, **15**, 251–5.

Boachie, A., Goldfield, G. S. & Spettique, W. (2003). Olanzapine use as an adjunctive treatment for hospitalized children with anorexia nervosa: case reports. *International Journal of Eating Disorders*, **33**, 98–103.

Carver, A. E., Miller, S., Hagman, J. & Sigel, E. (2002). *The Use of Risperidone for the Treatment of Anorexia Nervosa*. Academy of Eating Disorders Annual Meeting, Boston.

Faris, P. L., Kim, S. W., Meller, W. H. *et al.* (2000). Effect of decreasing afferent vagal activity with ondansetron on symptoms of bulimia nervosa; a randomized, double-blind trial. *Lancet*, **355**, 792–7.

Fassino, S., Daga, G. A., Boggio, S., Garzaro, L. & Piero, A. (2004). Use of reboxetine in bulimia nervosa: a pilot study. *Journal of Psychopharmacology*, **18**, 423–8.

US Food and Drug Administration (2004). *Labeling Change Request Letter for Antidepressant Medications*. www.fda.gov/cder/drug/antidepressants/SSRIlabelchange.html.

Fichter, M. M., Kruger, R., Rief, W., Holland, R. & Dohne, J. (1996). Fluvoxamine in prevention of relapse in bulimia nervosa: effects on eating-specific psychopathology. *Journal of Clinical Psychopharmacology*, **16**, 9–18.

Fisman, S., Steele, M., Short, J., Byrne, T. & Lavallee, C. (1996). Case study: anorexia nervosa and autistic disorder in an adolescent girl. *Journal of the American Academy of Child and Adolescent Psychiatry*, **35**, 937–40.

Fluoxetine Bulimia Nervosa Collaborative Study Group (1992). Fluoxetine in the treatment of bulimia nervosa. *Archives of General Psychiatry*, **49**, 139–47.

Garland, E. J., Remick, R. A. & Zis, A. P. (1988). Weight gain with antidepressants and lithium. *Journal of Psychopharmacology*, **8**, 323–30.

Gaskill, J. A., Treat, T. A., McCabe, E. B. & Marcus, M. D. (2001). Does olanzapine affect the rate of weight gain among inpatients with eating disorders? *Eating Disorders Review*, **12**, 1–2.

Goldstein, D. J., Wilson, M. G., Thompson, V. L. *et al.* (1995). Long-term fluoxetine treatment of bulimia nervosa. *British Journal of Psychiatry*, **166**, 660–6.

Goldstein, D. J., Wilson, M. G., Ascroft, R. C. & al-Banna, M. (1999). Effectiveness of fluoxetine therapy in bulimia nervosa regardless of comorbid depression. *International Journal of Eating Disorders*, **25**, 19–27.

Gross, H. A., Ebert, M. H., Faden, V. B. *et al.* (1981). A double-blind controlled trial of lithium carbonate primary anorexia nervosa. *Journal of Clinical Psychopharmacology*, **6**, 376–81.

Halmi, K. A., Eckert, E., Ladu, T. J. & Cohen, J. (1986). Anorexia nerovsa: treatment efficacy of cyproheptadine and amitriptyline. *Archives of General Psychiatry*, **43**, 177–81.

Hansen, L. (1999). Olanzapine in the treatment of anorexia nervosa. *British Journal of Psychiatry*, **175**, 592.

Hoopes, S. P., Reimherr, F. W., Hedges, D. W. *et al.* (2003). Treatment of bulimia nervosa with topiramate in a randomized, double-blind, placebo-controlled trial, Part 1: Improvement in binge and purge measures. *Journal of Clinical Psychiatry*, **64**, 1335–41.

Horne, R. L., Ferguson, J. M., Pope, H. G. *et al.* (1988). Treatment of bulimia with bupropion: a multicenter controlled trial. *Journal of Clinical Psychiatry*, **49**, 262–6.

Jensen, V. S. & Mejlhede, A. (2000). Anorexia nervosa: treatment with olanzapine. *British Journal of Psychiatry*, **177**, 187.

Katz, R. L., Keen, C. L., Litt, I. F. *et al.* (1987). Zinc deficiency in anorexia nervosa. *Journal of Adolescent Health Care*, **8**, 400–6.

Kaye, W. H., Nagata, R., Weltzin, T. E. *et al.* (2001). Double-blind placebo-controlled administration of fluoxetine in restricting and purging-type anorexia nervosa. *Biological Psychiatry*, **49**, 644–52.

Kearns, G., Abdel-Rahman, S., Alander, S. *et al.* (2003). Developmental pharmacology – drug disposition, action, and therapy in infants and children. *New England Journal of Medicine*, **349**, 1157–67.

Kotler, L. A. & Walsh, B. T. (2000). Eating disorders in children and adolescents: pharmacological therapies. *European Child and Adolescent Psychiatry*, **9**, I/108–16.

Kotler, L. A., Devlin, M. J., Davies, M. & Walsh, T. B. (2003). An open trial of fluoxetine for adolescents with bulimia nervosa. *Journal of Child and Adolescent Psychopharmacology*, **13**, 329–35.

Lacey, J. H. & Crisp, A. H. (1980). Hunger, food intake and weight: the impact of clomipramine on a refeeding anorexia nervosa population. *Postgraduate Medical Journal*, **56** (suppl. 1), 79–85.

La Via, M. C., Gray, L. & Kaye, W. H. (2000). Case reports of olanzapine treatment of anorexia nervosa. *International Journal of Eating Disorders*, **27**, 363–6.

Mehler, C., Wewetzer, C., Schulze, U. *et al.* (2001). Olanzapine in children and adolescents with chronic anorexia nervosa. A study of five cases. *European Child to Adolescent Psychiatry*, **10**, 151–7.

Melkersson, K. & Dahl, M. L. (2004). Adverse metabolic effects associated with atypical antipsychotics. *Drugs*, **64**, 701–23.

Mitchell, J. E., Crow, S., Myers, T. & Wonderich, S. (2002). The therapeutic armamentarium in eating disorders. In *Biological Psychiatry*, ed. D'haenen, H., den Boer, J. A. & Wilner, P. New York: John Wiley & Sons.

Nakash-Eisikovits, O., Dierberger, A. & Westen, D. (2002). A multidimensional meta-analysis of pharmacotherapy for bulimia nervosa: summarizing the range of outcomes in controlled clinical trials. *Harvard Review of Psychiatry*, **10**, 193–211.

Newman-Toker, J. (2000). Risperidone in anorexia nervosa. *Journal of the American Academy of Child and Adolescent Psychiatry*, **39**, 941–2.

Pederson, K. J., Roerig, J. L. & Mitchell, J. E. (2003). Towards the pharmacotherapy of eating disorders. *Expert Opinion on Pharmacotherapy*, **4**, 1659–78.

Powers, P. S., Santana, C. A. & Bannon, Y. S. (2002). Olanzapine in the treatment of anorexia nervosa: an open label trial. *International Journal of Eating Disorders*, **32**, 146–54.

Powers, P. S. & Santana, C. (2004). Available pharmacological treatments for anorexia nervosa. *Expert Opinion on Pharmacotherapy*, **5**, 2287–92.

Powers, P. S., Bannon, Y., Eubanks, R. & McCormick, T. (2004). *Anorexia Nervosa and Quetiapine: Effect on Weight and Psychopathology.* Poster presented at American Psychiatric Association meeting, New York, NY.

Roerig, J. L., Mitchell, J. E., Myers, T. C. & Glass, J. B. (2002). Pharmacotherapy and medical complications of eating disorders in children and adolescents. *Child and Adolescent Psychiatric Clinics of North America*, **11**, 365–85, xi.

Romano, S. J., Halmi, K. A., Sarkar, N. P., Koke, S. C. & Lee, J. S. (2002). A placebo-controlled study of fluoxetine in continued treatment of bulimia nervosa after successful acute fluoxetine treatment. *American Journal of Psychiatry*, **159**, 96–102.

Ruggiero, G. M., Laini, V., Mauri, M. C. (2001). A single blind comparison of amisulpride, fluoxetine and clomipramine in the treatment of restricting anorectics. *Progress in Neuro-Psychopharmacology and Biological Psychiatry*, **25**, 1049–59.

Sullivan, P.F. (1995). Mortality in anorexia nervosa. *American Journal of Psychiatry*, **152**, 1073–4.

Sundblad, C., Landen, M., Eriksson, T., Bergman, L. & Eriksson, E. (2005). Effects of the androgen antagonist flutamide and the serotonin reuptake inhibitor citalopram in bulimia nervosa. *Journal of Clinical Psychopharmacology*, **25**, 85–8.

Vandereycken, W. & Pierloot, R. (1982). Pimozide combined with behavior therapy in the short-term treatment of anorexia nervosa. *Acta Psychiatrica Scandinavica*, **66**, 445–50.

Vandereycken, W. (1984). Neuroleptics in the short-term treatment of anorexia nervosa: a double-blind placebo-controlled study with sulpiride. *British Journal of Psychiatry*, **144**, 288–92.

Varley, C. K. (2001). Sudden death related to selected tricyclic antidepressants in children: epidemiology, mechanisms, and clinical implications. *Paediatrics and Drugs*, **3**, 613–27.

Walsh, B. T., Hadigan, C. M., Devlin, M. J. *et al.* (1991). Long-term outcome of antidepressant treatment for bulimia nervosa. *American Journal of Psychiatry*, **148**, 1206–12.

Walsh, B. T., Kaplan, A. S., Attia, E. *et al.* (2006). Fluoxetine after weight restoration in anorexia nervosa: a randomized controlled trial. *Journal of the American Medical Association*, **295**, 2605–12.

Part V

Public health perspectives

22

Longitudinal perspectives, outcome and prognosis

Hans-Christoph Steinhausen

University of Zurich, Zurich, Switzerland

Given the limited understanding of the precise aetiology of eating disorders and the fact that there is no ultimate cure for these disorders, studies in the long-term development of the affected patients are of considerable interest. Along with the amazing increase in scientific studies of various facets of the eating disorders in the second half of the twentieth century, there have also been a notable number of outcome studies. In this chapter, separately for AN and BN, a review will be provided of the various studies on the outcome and prognosis of eating disorders.

Anorexia nervosa

Recently, the author has provided an exhaustive review of the outcome of AN in the twentieth century (Steinhausen, 2002). In this review, a total of 119 study series covering 5590 patients that were published in the English and German literature were analysed with regard to mortality, global outcome and other psychiatric disorders at follow-up.

The four major outcome parameters of mortality, recovery, improvement and chronicity and the other psychiatric disorders were analysed. Descriptive means and standard deviations were calculated as shown in Table 22.1. Given the rather wide standard deviations with extreme ranges across the studies and the varying sizes of the patient groups, the means in this table reflect only a central trend.

The mean crude mortality rate was 5.0%. In the surviving patients, on average, full recovery was found in only less than half (47%) of the patients, while a third improved and 20% developed a chronic course of the disorder. Outcome was slightly better for the core symptoms, with normalization of weight occurring in almost 60% of the patients, normalization of menstruation in 57% and normalization of eating behaviour in 47%. However, these

Eating Disorders in Children and Adolescents, ed. Tony Jaffa and Brett McDermott. Published by Cambridge University Press. © Cambridge University Press 2007.

Table 22.1. Outcome of anorexia nervosa based on 119 patient series (n = 5590)

Outcome variable	Group size	Rate of outcome (%)		
		Mean	SD	Range
Mortality	5,334	5.0	5.7	0–2
Recovery	4,575	46.9	19.7	0–92
Improvement	4,472	33.5	17.8	0–75
Chronicity	4,927	20.8	12.8	0–79
Symptom normalization				
Weight	2,245	59.6	15.3	15–92
Menstruation	2,719	57.0	17.2	25–96
Eating behaviour	1,980	46.8	19.6	0–97
Affective disorder	1,972	24.1	16.3	2–67
Neurotic or anxiety disorder	1.478	25.5	14.9	4–61
Obsessive-compulsive disorder	992	12.0	6.4	0–23
Schizophrenia	1,097	4.6	5.7	1–28
Personality disorder				
Unspecified or borderline	1,115	17.4	16.8	0–69
Histrionic	308	16.6	19.9	0–53
Obsessive-compulsive	202	31.4	25.1	0–76
Substance abuse disorder	627	14.6	10.4	2–38

Reprinted from Steinhausen, H.-C. (2002). *American Journal of Psychiatry*, **159**, 1284–93

slightly higher rates of normalization of the core symptoms, compared with the global outcome rating, may be largely due to different sample sizes. Nevertheless, this gap remained, even after adaptation for group size (when only the studies that reported both global outcomes ratings and normalization of the core symptoms were considered).

At follow-up a large proportion of anorectic patients suffered from additional psychiatric disorders. Frequent diagnoses at follow-up were neurotic disorders, including anxiety disorders and phobias, affective disorders, substance use disorders, obsessive-compulsive disorder (OCD) and unspecified personality disorders, including borderline states. A few studies reported a high rate of obsessive–compulsive personality disorder and a less pronounced rate of histrionic personality disorder. Schizophrenia was only rarely observed at follow-up.

In the analyses of the data only the four major outcome parameters and studies that reported these variables were considered for these analyses. It was possible to control for three major effect variables: duration of follow-up

($<$ 4 years, 4–10 years, $>$ 10 years), age at onset of the disorder (adolescence only vs. mixed samples with onset in adolescence and adulthood) and time period of study (1950–1979; 1980–1989; 1990–1999).

All four outcome parameters were significantly affected by duration of follow-up, and all four effect sizes were large. With increasing duration of follow-up, mortality rates also increased. In the surviving patients, there was a strong tendency toward recovery with increasing duration of follow-up. The rate of recovery increased while the rates of improvement and chronicity declined.

The comparison of the group of patients with adolescent onset and the group with a much wider age range at onset of illness revealed a significantly lower mortality rate in the group with the younger patients. The rates of recovery, improvement and chronicity were more favourable in the group with the younger patients. However, in each instance, in addition to duration of follow-up, the interactions between duration of follow-up and each outcome variable were significant, as shown in Figure 22.1. The interaction effects showed that the differences between the subgroups with different onsets of illness were wider or narrower or even inverted for the four outcome measures depending on the duration of follow-up. A comparison of the two effect sizes indicated that the effect of age at onset was stronger for mortality, whereas the effect of duration of follow-up was stronger for recovery, improvement and chronicity.

In the analyses of time trends, mortality showed a complex pattern and there were few differences between the studies for 1980–1989 and the studies for 1990–1999 on the other outcome measures – recovery, improvement and chronicity. For all four outcome measures, the effect sizes for duration of follow-up were markedly stronger than for time period.

Prognostic factors

A considerable number of outcome studies also provided some information on prognosis. However, there was a rather large variability as to the type and number of prognostic factors considered for analysis in the various studies. A summary of findings across all studies is given in Table 22.2.

As one can see from Table 22.2, the findings were considerably heterogeneous for the majority of the prognostic factors. Most obviously, this interpretation applies to the ambiguous findings regarding age at onset of illness. Furthermore, most studies indicated that a short duration of symptoms before treatment resulted in a favourable outcome. The impact of the duration of

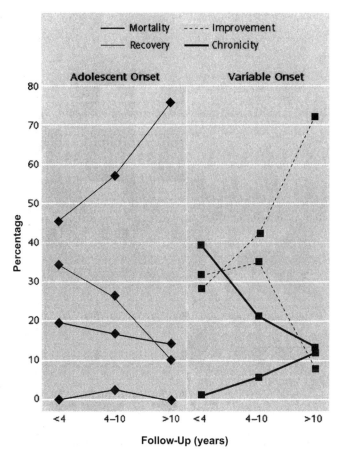

Figure 22.1. Outcome of anorexia nervosa in 119 patients series by duration of follow-up and age at onset. A total of 577 patients had less than 4 years of follow-up, 2132 had 4–10 years of follow-up and 438 had more than 10 years of follow-up.

Reprinted from Steinhausen, H.-C. (2002). *American Journal of Psychiatry*, **159**, 1284–93.

inpatient treatment is unclear because of ambiguous findings across the outcome studies. Similarly, no definite conclusions could be drawn as to whether greater weight loss at presentation had long-term effects on outcome.

In addition, it is quite clear that vomiting, bulimia and purgative abuse imply an unfavourable prognosis whereas hyperactivity and dieting as weight-reduction measures did not have any prognostic significance. A few studies also showed that premorbid developmental and clinical abnormalities, including eating disorders during childhood, carry the risk for a poor outcome of AN. In contrast, a good parent–child relationship may protect the patient from a poor outcome.

Table 22.2. Frequency of studies with identified prognostic factors of anorexia nervosa

Prognostic factor	Favourable prognosis N	Unfavourable prognosis N	Not significant N
Early age at onset of illness	13	2	14
Short duration of symptoms	14	0	7
Short duration of inpatient treatment	7	0	7
Heavy weight loss	0	8	8
Hyperactivity and dieting	1	0	7
Vomiting	0	9	2
Bulimia and purgative abuse	0	11	2
Premorbid developmental or clinical abnormalities	0	4	2
Good parent–child relationship	8	0	3
Chronicity	0	7	0
Hysterical personality	8	0	1
Obsessive–compulsive personality	0	6	1
High socio-economic status	6	0	8

Furthermore, the data clearly show that chronicity leads to poor outcome, a finding that implies that there are cases of AN in which treatment is refractory. A substantial number of studies provided evidence that the features of histrionic personality disorder indicate a favourable outcome. In addition, the features of coexisting obsessive–compulsive personality or compulsivity add to chronicity. Finally, no definite conclusions can be drawn from the outcome studies as to the relevance of socio-economic status.

Adolescent patients

So far, the reported findings from follow-up studies in AN have mostly included the full age range when these patients fell ill. When the adolescent age range at onset was considered separately it became clear that the course of these young patients might be different from those with later onset of the disorder. In fact, the smaller series of young patients in the author's review of follow-up studies (Steinhausen, 2002) showed a less serious outcome as compared with a mixed group of studies containing patients with either adolescent or later onset of AN. However, adolescent onset was not unequivocally supported as a favourable prognostic factor in all studies.

Within the International Collaborative Outcome Study of Eating Disorders in Adolescence (ICOSEDA), the author and his associates studied the clinical features, treatment and outcome in consecutive cohorts of adolescent patients at five sites in former West Berlin and East Berlin, Zurich, Sofia and Bucharest (Steinhausen *et al.*, 2003). All samples consisted of series of consecutively admitted patients who were initially seen in the 1980s and early 1990s. All patients fulfilled the ICD–10 criteria for the various forms of eating disorders. The samples were predominantly composed of anorectic patients, with only the Berlin sample and the Zurich sample having 10% each of patients suffering from either bulimia or atypical eating disorders. Almost all of the patients were female (between 90% and 100%).

The follow-up sample comprised a total of 241 patients that was re-assessed with semi-structured personal interviews at a mean age of 21.8 ($\pm$ 3.2 SD) years after a mean follow-up period of 6.4 ($\pm$ 3.0 SD) years. As one would expect with such diverse cultural sites and health systems, the provided treatment varied considerably both in terms of types of intervention and quantity of treatment. On average, the entire sample had spent 6% of the total follow-up period as inpatients and 23% as outpatients. Taken together, the total time spent in any form of treatment amounted to 30% of the entire follow-up period. Half of the sample required a second hospitalization, 25% a third, 10% a fourth and 5% a fifth hospitalization.

The average crude mortality rate in this rather young sample was only 2.9% and thus lower than calculated for the previously reported analysis of the literature which was 5% (Steinhausen, 2002). The outcome of the eating disorder itself was also more favourable. Around 80% of the sample had a normalization of the core symptoms weight, eating behaviour and menstruation at follow-up. On the diagnostic level, a total of 70% was free from any eating disorder whereas 10% still suffered from AN and another 20% had either BN or an atypical eating disorder.

ICOSEDA findings of follow-up psychosocial status and other psychiatric disorders based on a comparison of different outcome criteria are shown in Table 22.3. West Berlin data are missing in Table 22.3 because no other psychiatric disorder than the eating disorder was assessed in this patient group. Good or fair psychosocial outcome was seen in a similar mean proportion of 71%, with only a statistical trend for any differences across sites. Three-quarters of the entire sample did not have another psychiatric disorder at follow-up. The rate was significantly lower for the Zurich sample. The other psychiatric disorders in the sample were affective disorders (n = 25), obsessive–compulsive disorder (n = 8), anxiety disorder (n = 8), somatoform disorders

Table 22.3. Comparison of different outcome criteria in four samples of adolescent onset eating disorder (n = 191; data are percentages)

	East Berlin (n = 67)	Zurich (n = 36)	Sofia (n = 47)	Bucharest (n = 41)	Total (n = 191)
No eating disorder	79	64	81	54	70
Good or fair psychosocial outcome	82	67	64	64	71
No other psychiatric disorder	86	56	81	73	76
No eating disorder or other psychiatric disorder	67	44	68	42	55
No eating disorder, no other psychiatric disorder, and good or fair psychosocial outcome	62	42	57	34	51

(n = 9), substance abuse (n = 3), schizophrenia (n = 2) and other disorders (n = 21). Among those who had an eating disorder at follow-up, 40% also had an associated other psychiatric disorder.

From Table 22.3 one can also see that the outcome is worse if one combines the criteria. Only slightly more than half of the patients are free from both an eating disorder and any other psychiatric disorder, with the Zurich and the Bucharest patients having significantly lower rates than the two other groups. If one looks at the most complex outcome measure, i.e. the combination of being free from an eating disorder and any other psychiatric disorder and enjoying a good or fair psychosocial outcome, then only half of the sample fulfils this optimal criterion of mental health. The outcome regarding this most complex measure is significantly worse in the Zurich and in the Bucharest sample than in the two other samples.

Finally, prognostic factors were also analysed in the ICOSEDA. In contrast to previous studies, an exhaustive list of potential predictors of the outcome was tested and various outcome criteria were considered. Furthermore, multiple regression analyses were performed in order to control for an overlap of prognostic factors and to identify the essential associations. It was found that only a few out of 17 predictors were significant. The BMI at follow-up was predicted by the BMI at initial assessment and treatment adherence (in terms of a negative association with rejection or premature termination of treatment). An eating disorder score composed of five core symptoms (i.e. dieting, vomiting, bulimic episodes, laxative abuse and menstruation) was more abnormal with longer duration of outpatient treatment and rejections or premature termination of treatments. The same two variables and another psychiatric disorder than the eating disorder at follow-up jointly predicted also the total outcome score, which was composed of the eating disorder symptoms and five additional psychosocial items reflecting sexuality and the quality of social relationships.

Thus, in this rather young patient sample, the consideration of a large list of prognostic factors in rather parsimonious analytical models resulted only in very few significant predictors of the outcome. Irrespective of the outcome criterion, the most consistent finding was the unfavourable role that rejection or premature termination of treatment played for the long-term course of the eating disorders. Second, the findings point to a treatment-refractory subgroup because the outcome deteriorated with increasing duration of outpatient treatment. Both findings are indicative of the pivotal function that treatment variables have for the outcome of adolescent eating disorders.

Conclusions

Based on the analysis of a large body of follow-up studies across various age groups and the ICOSEDA addressing more specifically the age range of adolescence, various conclusions as to the long-term course of AN can be drawn.

A first, rather general conclusion has to state that AN is a mental illness with a serious course and outcome in many of the afflicted individuals. This conclusion is based on the high crude mortality rate that increases with length of follow-up and is corroborated by an analysis of an almost 18-fold increase in mortality in patients with AN including a high suicide rate (Nielsen et al., 1998). Further support for this conclusion comes from the high rate of chronic courses, which may be expected in approximately 20% of the cases across all ages at onset of the disorder and the fact that at follow-up more than half of the patients showed either a complete or a partial eating disorder in combination with another psychiatric disorder or another psychiatric disorder without an eating disorder. In the younger patients with an eating disorder at follow-up, a 40% probability of a comorbid mental disorder can be expected.

The second conclusion pertains to the mitigating factors of the outcome of AN. Two factors, namely age at onset of the disorder and duration of follow-up, stand out. Onset of the disorder during adolescence is associated with lower crude mortality rates and a better outcome of the eating disorder per se. There is less certainty whether or not other psychiatric disorders including comorbid disorder at follow-up occur at a lower rate than in patients who are older at onset of the disorder. Furthermore, it must also be kept in mind that onset of AN before puberty has a very poor outcome as shown in clinical reports (Russell, 1992). The other mitigating factor, namely duration of follow-up, shows a clear trend of an improved global outcome of AN with increasing course so that there is also substantial hope, even for some rather complicated cases.

The third conclusion has to deal with the very limited knowledge of how intervention actually affects the course of AN. There are some hints that an early intervention, short duration of inpatient treatment and adherence to the treatment programme are prognostically favourable. However, all these variables may only reflect more latent clinical factors in terms of severity of the disorder and patient characteristics. Clearly, the lack or scarcity of controlled intervention studies with a sufficient duration of follow-up represents a major obstacle in the field of outcome research in AN. A notable exception is the London family therapy study with its documentation that treatment effects were kept at a 5-year follow-up (Eisler & Dare, 1997).

The final major conclusion has to address the fact that our understanding of the prognosis of AN has serious limitations. Certainly, vomiting, bulimia and purgative abuse, chronicity and obsessive–compulsive features represent unfavourable prognostic factors, whereas hysterical personality features represent the only favourable prognostic factor that has been documented with very little conflicting evidence in the literature. However, the lack of replication of the factors in the ICOSEDA data set with adolescent onset patients and a rigorous control of overlapping effects of various prognostic factors asks for a more conservative interpretation. In the same way, the variability in findings on various other prognostic factors preclude any delineation of rules as to the individual prognosis in a patient suffering from AN.

Bulimia nervosa

In the recent past, several reviews of the course and outcome of BN have been published. Whereas the reviews by Keel & Mitchell (1997) and Steinhausen (1999) covered the outcome literature until 1997, the most recent review by Quadflieg & Fichter (2003) also included eight more recent studies that had been published between 1997 and 2002.

In the author's review (Steinhausen, 1999) 24 outcome studies covered a total of 1383 patients who were followed up at a mean of 31 months in 15 studies containing this information. The onset of the disorder had been at between 14 and 22 years. The patients had been predominantly treated on an outpatient basis including some sort of psychotherapy with additional drug treatment in six studies and psychopharmacotherapy alone in two studies.

In these 24 studies, crude mortality rates amounted to 0.7% (range 0–6) and were only slightly higher than those reported by Keel & Mitchell (1997), i.e. 0.3% (range 1–3). Quadflieg & Fichter (2003) in their review obtained crude death rates of 0–3.1% after varying follow-up periods of 2–11.5 years. So far, there are no studies reporting standardized mortality rates.

The major outcome parameter of BN based on the review of 24 outcome studies by Steinhausen (1999) were 47.5% (range 22–66) for recovery, 26% (range 0–67) for improvement and 26% (range 0–43) for chronicity. According to the review by Keel & Mitchell (1997), controlled treatment studies as compared with ordinary follow-up studies resulted in higher short-term recovery rates after 6 or 12 months (53 or 48 in contrast to 31%). However, this superiority was markedly lower after a follow-up interval of 5 years (54 vs. 48%).

Some more recent studies both converge with the average recovery rate around 48% (e.g. Fairburn et al., 2000) and some greatly exceed this figure. High recovery rates were obtained by Ben-Tovim et al. (2001), who included less impaired outpatients from secondary and tertiary services only and found a recovery rate of 77%, and in the follow-up study by Fichter & Quadflieg (1997) with a recovery rate of 55% after 2 years and 71% after 6 years, after intensive inpatient treatment in a primary service hospital.

In contrast to AN, there is no really strong association between recovery and duration of follow-up. Quadflieg & Fichter (2003) calculated a moderate Pearson correlation coefficient of 0.26 and concluded that, presumably, no stable recovery rate can be expected for the first 5–6 years after intake into a study on the long-term course of BN. After about 10 years a proportion of two-thirds to three-quarters of former patients with BN can be expected to show at least partial recovery.

The data on the chronicity and relapse rate are still far from being conclusive. The estimated relapse rate of 30% for BN in a time period of 6 months to 6 years by Keel & Mitchell (1997), and the average chronification of 26% by Steinhausen (1999), do not allow the differentiation between chronic cases with no remission at any point of the follow-up period and cases showing a relapse at the time of the follow-up assessment. Furthermore, the large variability of finding precludes any definite conclusion as to the association of duration of follow-up and poor outcome.

The crossover from BN to AN has been studied repeatedly. However, a lack of diagnostic accuracy and a lack of diagnostic hierarchy rules before DSM–IV may have led to an overestimation of figures. Recent studies indicate rather low frequencies of crossover to AN between 0.6 and 3.7% and varying for length of follow-up (Quadflieg & Fichter, 2003). In contrast, the crossover to eating disorders not otherwise specified (EDNOS) is much higher and amounts to figures between 1.6 and 26% in various studies and also depends on the duration of follow-up (Quadflieg & Fichter, 2003). These high rates may well reflect chronic cases of eating disorders.

Other psychiatric disorders than BN have been assessed only in a few follow-up studies. Thus, the figures calculated by Steinhausen (1999) may only be tentative. According to this review, 25% (range 9–37) of the patients had an affective disorder, 5% (range 2–18) a neurotic/anxiety disorder, 0.7% (range 3–5) a personality disorder and 10% (range 2–26) a substance-use disorder.

So far, the psychosocial outcome in BN has received very limited interest in follow-up studies. There is a trend that better social outcome matches re-covered and improved eating disorders outcome. However, taken as a whole, the patient groups at follow-up tend to function less well than community control samples. Furthermore, they tend to function better in terms of their social adjustment rather than their personal and sexual relationships (Quadflieg & Fichter, 2003).

Prognostic factors

Based on the reviews by Steinhausen (1999) and Quadflieg & Fichter (2003) prognostic factors are summarized in Table 22.4. Due to the smaller body of scientific studies, the overall prognostic picture in BN is even less clear than in AN. Studies indicating a favourable function of some prognostic factors like younger age at onset, short duration of illness prior to treatment, severity of the disorder or a positive history of alcohol abuse are clearly outbalanced by a similar or even higher number of studies with no significant findings. Among the unfavourable factors, borderline personality symptoms clearly stand out because of a replicated status in various studies. A few studies further indicate that comorbid psychiatric disorders like depression, anxiety disorder or alcohol abuse have a negative effect on outcome. The same is true also for low self-esteem whereas findings on impulsiveness are equivocal. All these findings on the prognostic function of comorbid disorder and personality features have to await further replication.

Table 22.4. Frequency of studies with identified prognostic factors in bulimia nervosa

Prognostic factors	Favourable	Unfavourable	Not significant
Younger age at onset	2	0	6
Short duration of illness prior to treatment	6	0	6
Severity of the disorder	4	0	3
Premorbid anorexia nervosa	0	0	6
Premorbid substance abuse	0	0	3
Premorbid obesity	0	0	1
Family history of alcohol abuse	1	1	1
Family history of depression	0	1	2
Coexistent borderline personalizing symptoms	0	6	1
Coexistent depression	0	2	3
Coexistent anxiety disorder	0	1	0
Coexistent alcohol abuse	0	1	0
Low self-esteem	0	2	0
Impulsiveness	0	1	1

Conclusion

The outcome of BN has only been studied since 1983 because the first description of the disorder was published only in 1979 (Russell, 1979). Consequently, the number of outcome studies and included patients is considerably smaller than in AN. However, some major conclusions can be drawn from these analyses and some comparisons can be made between the outcome of the two disorders.

There is clear evidence that treatment of BN is efficient in the short-term, whereas the longer-term outcome shows a similar though only slightly better result as compared to AN. The rates of relapse and chronicity of BN are still considerable. However, the rate of mortality is low. Diagnostic crossover from BN to AN or the more recently introduced binge-eating disorder is a rather rare phenomenon, whereas the high rates of EDNOS may explain a large proportion of chronic courses.

In the majority of the affected patients, social adjustment and the quality of personal relationships normalize. However, there is a substantial number of women who suffer not only from persistent bulimic symptoms but also from social and, most notably, from sexual impairment.

So far, the study of prognostic factors in BN does not allow any definite conclusions because the picture is diverse and partly also contradictory. Sampling bias (e.g. the inclusion of a high rate of chronic cases) and a lack of control for overlapping risk factors by use of adequate analytical models may have contributed to this limitation and have to be overcome in future research. As with AN, it would be most hazardous to delineate any conclusions from research to the prognosis of an individual patient.

Due to its more recent origin, studies on the course of BN have profited from prospective rather than retrospective samples which have been used in many follow-up studies of AN. However, there are also limitations as precisely addressed in the review by Quadflieg & Fichter (2003). The latter include the heterogeneity of the diagnostic definition reflecting the changes in psychiatric nosology in the recent past, and the variations in the definition of outcome measures, as is true also for outcome studies of AN. Also, further limitations pertain to outcome studies of both eating disorders, namely the lack of studies on the natural course without treatment and an insufficient focus on the process rather than the outcome of the disorder. Thus, it is not clear how long a given person suffered from the disorder, nor is there differentiation between relapse or chronic state of the disorder at follow-up. Finally, so far there are no data available on the outcome of BN in males.

Further studies will have to address these limitations, and with more systematic diagnostic categories, standardized assessment procedures, control of interventions, longer follow-up periods and a stronger focus on the process of change in the individual patients, certainly, a more refined picture of the outcome of BN will emerge.

REFERENCES

Ben-Tovim, D. I., Walker, K., Gilchrist, P. et al. (2001). Outcome in patients with eating disorders: a 5-year study. *Lancet*, **357**, 1254–7.

Eisler, I. & Dare, C. (1997). Family and individual therapy in anorexia nervosa. A 5-year follow-up. *Archives of General Psychiatry*, **54**, 1025–30.

Fairburn, C. G., Cooper, Z., Doll, H. A., Norman, P. & O'Connor, M. (2000). The natural course of bulimia nervosa and binge eating disorder in young women. *Archives of General Psychiatry*, **57**, 659–65.

Fichter, M. M. & Quadflieg, N. (1997). Six-year course of bulimia nervosa. *International Journal of Eating Disorders*, **22**, 361–84.

Keel, P. K. & Mitchell, J. E. (1997). Outcome in bulimia nervosa. *American Journal of Psychiatry*, **154**, 313–21.

Nielsen, S., Moller-Madsen, S., Isager, T. et al. (1998). Standardized mortality in eating disorders – a quantative summary of previously published and new evidence. *Journal of Psychosomatic Research*, **44**, 413–34.

Quadflieg, N. & Fichter, M.M. (2003). The course and outcome of bulimia nervosa. *European Child and Adolescent Psychatry,* **12** (Suppl. 1), 99–109.

Russell, G. (1979). Bulimia nervosa: an ominous variant of anorexia nervosa. *Psychological Medicine,* **9,** 429–49.

Russell, G. (1992). Anorexia nervosa of early onset and its impact on puberty. In *Feeding Problems and Eating Disorders in Children and Adolescents,* ed. Cooper, P.J. & Stein, A. Philadelphia, PA: Harwood Academic Publishers, pp. 85–112.

Steinhausen, H.-C. (1999). Eating disorders. In *Risks and Outcomes in Developmental Psychopathology,* ed. Steinhausen, H.-C. & Verhulst, F. Oxford: Oxford University Press, pp. 210–30.

Steinhausen, H.-C. (2002). The outcome of anorexia nervosa in the twentieth century. *American Journal of Psychiatry,* **159,** 1284–93.

Steinhausen, H.-C., Boyadijeva, S., Griogoroiu-Serbanescu, M. & Neumärker, K.J. (2003). The outcome of adolescent eating disorders. Findings from an international collaborative study. *European Child and Adolescent Psychiatry,* **12** (Suppl. 1), 91–8.

23

Primary prevention of eating disorders

Greta Noordenbos

Leiden University, Leiden, the Netherlands

Introduction

Given the serious physical, psychological, social and financial consequences of eating disorders (EDs) and the difficulties of treatment, successful prevention strategies would obviously be of paramount importance. Development of such strategies requires an understanding of risk factors and at-risk groups. Although there is growing evidence that EDs are increasing in African, Asian, Arab and Latin American women (Nasser *et al.*, 2001), the majority of EDs occur in young Caucasian women living in highly industrialized societies. Particularly high-risk groups include dancers, sportswomen and those whose peak performance depends on being slim (Sundgott-Börgen & Bahr, 1998) or who are categorized by weight division (Dale & Landers, 1998). In terms of risk factors the most important are low self-esteem, negative body image, internalized slimness ideal, fear of fat and extreme dieting (Jacobi *et al.*, 2004).

Optimum primary prevention strategies are those directed at the reduction of risk factors in higher risk groups. In this chapter several strategies for primary prevention interventions are described. The chapter will end with a discussion about the main results of primary prevention interventions and the implications for future initiatives.

Strategies for primary prevention
The slimming culture and the media

Because the slimming ideal can predispose women, especially those with low self-esteem and negative body image, to dieting behaviour, this idealization of the slim body has been a focus for ED prevention strategies. Media-activists have protested against the unhealthy ideals portrayed in advertisements and have advocated the use of models with more healthy body proportions (Levine

Eating Disorders in Children and Adolescents, ed. Tony Jaffa and Brett McDermott. Published by Cambridge University Press. © Cambridge University Press 2007.

et al., 1999). Pressure has also been brought to bear in relation to the 'heroine' look, diet pills and advertisements for rapid and unrealistically large amounts of weight loss. Such activism has at times proved effective, e.g. the termination of the chocolate advertisements featuring the slogan 'You can never be too rich or too thin' (Levine *et al.*, 1999). In Norway an advertising campaign which offered a year's free supply of a popular drink to whoever could achieve the highest weight loss was similarly stopped following student protest (Börreson-Gresko & Rosenvinge, 1998).

Since 1997 the Eating Disorders Awareness and Prevention Organization (EDAP) has campaigned against misleading advertisements in the USA. It has developed criteria for the media for 'Constructing Healthy Media Messages for Every Body' and has been relatively successful in its activities (Levine *et al.*, 1999).

Clearly, determined actions by pressure groups and members of the public can influence advertising strategies (Rosenvinge & Börreson, 1999). Positive media campaigns have included that of the Body Shop featuring an above-average weight Barbie doll, called Ruby, with the slogan: 'There are three billion women who do not look like super models, and only 8 women do'. A recent Unilever advertising campaign for Dove cosmetics utilized a diversity of women with different shapes and skin colours, with the message for women to celebrate their curves and that every skin should be taken care of. Most women have reacted positively to such campaigns. However, the effect of these on the prevention of eating disorders is yet to be evaluated.

Media literacy programs

In addition to challenging the cultural ideal of slimness in the media, it is also important to help young people to adopt a critical approach to the influence of the media. These media literacy strategies are probably particularly important in countries where young people watch television for many hours (Levine *et al.*, 1999). Media literacy programs aim to analyse, evaluate and discuss the messages of the media. They explain how advertisements are made, and how photographs are manipulated electronically to enhance the thinness of the models. 'Behind Closed Doors' is a video which documents the computerized development of a top model (Scholtz, 1997). Other films made to inform people about the construction of photographs include those produced by Jean Kilbourne entitled 'Slim Hopes: Advertising and the Obsession with Thinness' and 'Still Killing Us Softly' (Kilbourne, 1995). These movies criticize the construction of the ideal women as young, thin, beautiful, white and sexy.

Media literacy programmes promote critical questions such as: Do real women look like the women in the advertisements? Does buying the product help you to look like the women in the advertisements? Does being slim guarantee a happy and successful life? It is hoped that media literacy programmes can change the attitudes of young people who have not yet formed stable opinions or maybe even some of those who have (Steiner-Adair & Purcell Vorenberg, 1999). Media literacy programmes for high-school students have been evaluated, using post-test-only comparisons, as having a positive effect in increasing knowledge, and reducing the idealization of slimness and fear about weight compared with a control group (Irving et al., 1998). However, there were no significant differences between the groups in body dissatisfaction, anxiety about weight and shape, the desirability of looking like slender models, or positive expectations associated with being slender (Irving et al., 1998). This suggests that media literacy programmes alone are likely to be insufficient to prevent eating disorders.

Psycho-education

Eating-disorder preventative educational programmes have been developed for secondary schools and for the final year of primary schools as these are the age groups at highest risk for developing an ED. Most of these programmes focus on cultural, social and psychological risk factors for EDs, puberty and changes which happen to the body, the slimming culture, negative attitudes towards fat, excessive slimming behaviour, low self-esteem and negative body image. Information is also given about the characteristics of anorexia and bulimia nervosa and the physical, psychological and social consequences. As well as the material for universal distribution, teachers receive instructions on how to discuss eating disorders with pupils who they suspect may be at particularly high risk. Prevention programmes also tend to include information about treatment methods and how help can be accessed. Further reading and contact addresses are provided.

Most programmes are accompanied by a video about the slimming culture, dieting and the characteristics and consequences of EDs. These are intended to promote discussion between the students about dieting. In some school programmes ex-patients are invited to give talks about their experience of having an ED and to answer questions from the students. A limitation of psycho-educative prevention programmes in schools is the unevenness of their implementation, generally dependent on the degree of enthusiasm of individual teachers, mostly female. For those who do run these programmes the number of sessions may vary, generally in the range 1–8.

Evaluative studies have shown the main effect of these prevention programmes to be an increase in knowledge, with few students actually changing their attitude about fat and dieting. It is disappointing to note that almost no change in behaviour is observed (Rosenvinge & Börreson, 1999; Smolak, 1999; Dalle Grave, 2003; Pratt & Woolfenden, 2003; Stice & Shaw, 2004).

In addition to the modest results, there are also concerns regarding unexpected negative consequences of prevention programmes directed at the reduction of slimming behaviour. Carter *et al.* (1997) report on one such programme. The positive immediate effects had disappeared by 1 year and even more worryingly, there was an increase in anxieties about body size with associated increased dieting behaviour found within the 13–14-year-old cohort, raising the question as to whether the programme might have been counterproductive. Although the lack of a control group makes such interpretation speculative, it could be that the findings were due to the effects of the programme, an age effect over the course of the study period or some other factor operating at this time. It is of note that a replication of this study using an intervention group of 474 girls 13–14 years old, and a control group of 386 girls, did not demonstrate these negative effects (Stewart *et al.*, 2001). Positive effects of this programme were a slight reduction of slimming behaviour and a more positive attitude to body shape and weight.

Perhaps the somewhat disappointing results of the educative prevention programmes should not be a surprise. Most of the young people who received the programmes do not have significant problems with their body attitude or eating behaviour, and do not intend to embark on serious diets. While a successful programme may, therefore, improve their knowledge, it would not be expected that there would be such a significant shift in attitudes and behaviour.

Improving self-esteem and body image

The programmes described have a major focus on provision of information regarding eating disorders. There are, of course, other areas that could be targeted in an ED prevention programme. It is of note that few are directed at the reduction of social risk factors, such as teasing about bodily appearance, sexual abuse and other negative societal reactions to girls and women (Larkin *et al.*, 1999). Also little attention has been paid to psychological risk factors such as perfectionism and fear of failure. In contrast a greater focus for preventative programmes has been the low self-esteem and negative body image which are seen as the most general risk factors for EDs (Killen *et al.*, 1993; Stice, 2001). Allied to this have been attempts to teach young women how to become more assertive and how to handle conflict more successfully. An example is a programme directed at empowerment of young girls using discussion groups and role play to learn to express their own feelings, needs and opinions (Friedman, 1999). They also discuss social and cultural factors which produce negative feelings about themselves such as 'I feel stupid, fat, ugly' etc. The goals of these discussion groups are to improve the participants' self-esteem, to analyse the cause of their negative thoughts and to support each other in developing a positive self-image. The effect of this programme was that the girls became more assertive. However, this was not always evaluated as positive by their parents. Some schools were reluctant to introduce the programme due to these behaviour changes of students, and because they were afraid that the girls would learn to express all kinds of problems and negative experiences, which the teachers may find difficult to cope with (Friedman, 1999). To deliver the programme teachers needed special training, not only to lead the discussions but also to give professional advice in case the students express more severe problems.

A more recent programme directed at improving self-esteem and body image is the feminist prevention programme called 'Full of Ourselves: Advancing Girl Power, Health and Leadership' (Steiner-Adair *et al.*, 2002). The goal of this programme is empowerment of young girls and to make them less dependent on the opinion of others and cultural messages. Effects were measured using pre-, post- and follow-up tests after 6 months in the intervention and control group. This programme resulted in positive and maintained changes in knowledge and weight satisfaction for adolescent girls. However, eating-related behaviours such as dieting and skipping meals appeared unaffected.

An advantage of prevention programmes focusing on improvement of self-esteem and body image is that these are important for general health not just for eating disorders. As eating attitudes and behaviours are not the focus of such programmes there is less risk of the glamourization of EDs and making them more attractive to some girls (Carter *et al.*, 1997).

Prevention programmes for elementary schools and college students

Although the main risk group for EDs consists usually of girls attending secondary schools, it has recently been observed that young girls at the end of primary school are already afraid of becoming fat, have a negative body image and that some of them have already started to diet, sometimes resulting in an eating disorder (Ricciardelli & McCabe, 2001). This finding has motivated some researchers to start prevention programmes in elementary schools (Smolak, 1999). These aim to develop healthy attitudes to bodies and to healthy food intake. The programme 'Eating Smart, Eating for Me' is an example of such a programme focusing on learning about healthy food intake and healthy exercising, toleration of diversity in body sizes and development of a positive body attitude and reduction in slimming behaviour (Smolak, 1999). Evaluation showed that compared with a control group, the intervention group who did experience the programme demonstrated increased knowledge about food and the effects of slimming behaviour and increased knowledge about causes of overweight and obesity. However, although attitudes concerning fat people did improve, no change was seen in the attitude concerning their own bodies. Moreover, no changes were seen in eating behaviour, exercising and weight reduction. A reason might be that these young girls did not (yet) have a negative body attitude and had not (yet) started slimming behaviour. A negative consequence of this prevention programme, however, was that despite the finding of improved attitude to fat people, there was a slight increase in teasing of fat children, maybe because the children learned that healthy food and exercising can prevent overweight and obesity. Clearly, more research directed at the prevention of eating disorders in elementary schools is needed (Smolak, 1999).

A further target group for prevention programmes has been women of 18 years and above. An example of an initiative for college students is the 'Student Bodies Program' developed by Winzelberg et al. (2000). This is an interactive internet program for high-risk groups who have already a negative body image and who diet more or less severely. The program offers an 8-week intervention in which the slim ideal is discussed and healthy food and exercising are promoted. The intervention group (n = 31) and control group (n = 29) did not vary significantly directly after the intervention, but by 3 months the intervention group had a significantly more positive body image and a reduced need to slim. A problem however was a relatively high drop-out (n = 6). A comparable internet program called 'Student Bodies' was developed by Zabinski et al. (2001). They also showed a significantly more positive body attitude and reduction of pathological eating behaviour in the high-risk intervention group (n = 31) compared with a healthy control group (n = 31) at 3-month follow-up. It is likely that more sustained change requires ongoing support over longer periods though this is yet to be evaluated.

Interactive prevention programs

New technologies such as the internet and CD-ROMs have stimulated the development of interactive prevention programs. Winzelberg et al. (2000) and Zabinski et al. (2001) have developed interactive prevention programs for students focusing on body image, self-esteem, dieting behaviour, etc. Positive aspects of internet programs are the anonymity of the user, the easy distribution and the relative low costs of the program once it is developed. Limitations of this kind of intervention are the restriction of participation to those who have access to computers and the internet, and the social isolation involved in using such a program (Kraut et al., 1998). As social isolation is often one of the characteristics of eating disorder patients, this is a cause for concern. Both the student programmes cited here suffered from a lack of personal support and had high drop-out rates (Winzelberg et al., 2000; Zabinsky et al., 2001). Despite this clear limitation the initial results of internet-based prevention programs do seem sufficiently promising to justify further efforts.

Primary prevention programmes for parents

It might be expected that parents would be central to attempts to prevent EDs in their daughters. This would be through positive support and encouragement. Also, perhaps, through attention to parental risk factors in the development of EDs such as parental negative expressed emotion, dieting, ED or criticism of the body shape of their children (Jacobi et al., 2004). It is surprising, therefore, that only very few primary prevention programmes have been developed with parents as the main focus (Graber et al., 1999). One of the few programmes which involve parents is 'Eating Smart, Eating For Me' developed by Smolak (1999). In this programme parents received newsletters informing them about the goals of the prevention project. In addition, the children had tasks to complete with their parents and were required to communicate with them about food. Whether or not the specific incorporation of parental components contributed to the programme's effectiveness is yet unknown (Graber et al., 1999). It is assumed that parent–adolescent communication around eating attitudes and behaviours and related adolescent challenges can be improved by active participation of parents. A side effect might be more healthy food intake by parents. For example, programmes to prevent obesity showed that they were not only positive for daughters, but also for mothers (Fitzgibbon et al., 1995).

Evaluation of primary preventions

Stice & Shaw (2004) carried out a meta-analysis of the outcome of prevention programmes. Most prevention programmes were universal programmes for all adolescents (girls and boys) and some programmes were for selected high-risk girls. Included were studies about prevention trials that tested for intervention effects on eating pathology, as well as those that solely tested for intervention effects on risk factors that have been found to predict the onset of eating pathology. Only controlled trials were included in which participants were randomly assigned to an intervention or to a minimal-intervention, placebo, wait-list or assessment-only control condition, as well as trials in which some relevant comparison group was used (e.g. matched controls) in a quasi-experimental design.

In total 38 disorder prevention programmes were evaluated in 53 separate controlled trials. Stice & Shaw (2004) analysed whether these prevention programmes were effective in the areas of: (1) increasing knowledge, (2) reducing the thin-ideal internalization, (3) body dissatisfaction, (4) dieting, (5) negative affect, (6) eating pathology and (7) improving body mass.

Larger effects were found for selected (vs. universal), interactive (vs. didactic) and multisession (vs. single session) programmes; for programmes offered solely to females and to participants over age 15; for programmes without psycho-educational content; and for trials that used validated measures. This can be explained because targeted prevention programmes for high-risk groups of girls above 15 years old can show more effect than universal programmes for girls and boys. Risk factors and early signs of eating disorders are more commonly in evidence in girls of age 15 and above than in younger girls. For this reason they are often more motivated. Interactive programmes are more effective than more passive psycho-educational programmes. More sessions are needed to show any effect, and validated instruments are more sensitive to show any effects than nonvalidated instruments. Regarding the content of prevention programmes, it is clear that educative programmes which only warn against the negative effects of extreme dieting are less effective than programmes which focus on positive health promotion such as improving self-esteem, a positive body image, better coping strategies, healthy food intake, healthy exercising and a healthier weight (Piran, 1999; Börreson & Rosenvinge, 2002).

Discussion

Clearly, studies of prevention programmes raise a number of questions. Perhaps two of the most pressing relate to the optimum age to target and the effects that the programmes are designed to bring about.

It appears that there are conflicting opinions regarding at what age primary prevention interventions have the greatest effect. Some argue that primary preventions should be introduced before 15 years of age so as to intervene early in adolescents who are at risk of developing an ED (Smolak, 1999) and are easily accessible in the school environment. Moreover, it is assumed that it is easier to change knowledge about food and dieting, attitudes towards the body and the internalization of the thin-ideal at this relatively young age before maladaptive attitudes have had a chance to develop. Because EDs begin at a younger age, some prevention programmes have been developed for the final year of elementary schools, and the first year of secondary school when girls will experience substantial changes of their body, such as an increasing percentage of fat, the start of menstruation and the development of breasts. During puberty many girls are insecure about their bodies, have low self-esteem and a negative body image. They are also likely to become strongly influenced by cultural expectations about their bodies and gender role. This may create insecurity about their body, hence stimulating dieting behaviour. According to Smolak (1999) it is necessary to intervene at this stage before dieting has begun. The final year of the primary school and the first year of secondary school can be argued to be the most relevant period for primary prevention programmes.

Others, however, conclude that primary prevention directed at the whole population of young girls before 15 years of age would be neither successful nor cost-effective (Dalle Grave, 2003; Stice & Shaw, 2004). These authors argue that such a widespread intervention would not be effective as only a minority of female pupils are at risk to develop an ED. For this reason they conclude that the most effective period for primary prevention is after 15 years for a selective group of high-risk girls who already have a negative body image, have internalized the thin body ideal and are severely dieting. Such girls can learn to improve their self-esteem and their body image and to reduce their dieting behaviour (Stice & Shaw, 2004).

However, one of the problems with concentrating primary prevention on a selected group of high-risk girls over 15 years old is that only those who are motivated to change their dieting behaviour become involved in such prevention programmes, while those who deny their dieting would not be motivated to do so. Denial of severe dieting is characteristic of ED patients. The question remains as to whether primary prevention programmes before the start of dieting could have prevented the development of a negative body image and (extreme) dieting behaviour in such girls.

This brings us to the second question as to what kind of effects we wish to bring about. Should the goal of primary prevention be to reduce the occurrence of a negative body image, and decrease extreme dieting as suggested by Stice & Shaw (2004), or should it also aim to promote healthy attitudes towards diversity in physical shape, a more positive body image, better self-esteem and healthy food intake and exercising? Given the current epidemic of obesity, the question can also be raised as to whether prevention programmes for eating disorders should also be focused on this area (Neumark-Sztainer *et al.*, 2000).

One solution to these dilemmas may be to develop a two-step prevention programme. First, a general health promotion programme for all young girls and boys which promotes self-esteem, a positive body image, healthy food intake, healthy exercising and healthy weight (Börreson & Rosenvinge, 2002). The successful prevention programme described by Piran (1999) reminds us of the importance of involving the whole school management in this (Austin, 2000).

Second, for girls (and boys) who already have a negative body image and are already (severely) dieting, or who already demonstrate the first characteristics of an ED the next preventative step would be to target the thin idealization, negative self- and body-image, and severe dieting strategies of this high-risk group (Stice & Shaw, 2004). Also for those who are already overweight or obese a second step might be to improve healthy food intake and healthy exercising in order to develop a healthy weight. So far the question as to whether a two-stage prevention programme would prove effective is unanswered and further research in this area is much needed.

REFERENCES

Austin, S.B. (2000). Prevention research in eating disorders: theory and new directions. *Psychological Medicine*, **30**, 1249–62.

Börresen-Gresko, R. & Rosenvinge, J.H. (1998). The Norwegian school-based prevention model-development and evaluation. In *The Prevention of Eating Disorders*, ed. Vandereycken, W. & Noordenbos, G. London: Athlone Press, pp. 75–98.

Börreson, R. & Rosenvinge, J.H. (2002). From prevention to health promotion. In *Handbook of Eating Disorders*, 2nd edition, ed. Treasure, J., Schmidt, U. & van Furth, E. West Sussex: John Wiley & Sons, pp. 435–54.

Carter, J.C., Stewart, A., Dunn, V. & Fairburn, C.G. (1997). Primary prevention of eating disorders: might it do more harm than good? *International Journal of Eating Disorders*, **22**, 167–72.

Dale, K. & Landers, D.M. (1998). Weight control in wrestling: eating disorders or disordered eating? *Medicine and Science in Sports and Exercise*, **31**, 1382–9.

Dalle Grave, R. (2003). School-based prevention programs for eating disorders. Achievements and opportunities. *Disease Management and Clinical Outcomes*, **11**, 579–93.

Fitzgibbon, M.L., Stolly, M.R. & Kirschenbaum, D.S. (1995). An obesity prevention pilot program for African-American mothers and daughters. *Journal of Nutrition Education*, **27**, 93–9.

Friedman, S.S. (1999). Discussion groups for girls: decoding the language of fat. In *Preventing Eating Disorders. A Handbook of Interventions and Special Challenges*, ed. Piran, N., Levine, M.P. & Steiner-Adair, C. London: Brunner/Mazel, pp. 122–33.

Graber, J.A., Bastiani Archibald, A. & Brooks-Gunn, J. (1999). The role of parents in the emergence, maintenance, and prevention of eating problems and disorders. In *Preventing Eating Disorders. A Handbook of Interventions and Special Challenges* ed. Piran, N., Levine, M.P. & Steiner-Adair, C. London: Brunner/Mazel, pp. 44–62.

Irving, L.M., DuPen, J. & Berel, S. (1998). A media literacy program for high school females. *Eating Disorders: The Journal of Treatment and Prevention*, **6**, 119–31.

Jacobi, C., Hayward, C., de Zwaan, M., Kraemer, H.C. & Agras, W.S. (2004). Coming to terms with risk factors for eating disorders: application of risk terminology and suggestions for a general taxonomy. [Review] *Psychological Bulletin*, **130**, 19–65.

Kilbourne, J. (1995). *Slim Hopes: Advertising and the Obsession with Thinness* (video). (Available from the Media Education Foundation, 28 Center Street, Northampton, MA 01060; http://www.igc.apc.org/mef/mef.html).

Killen, J.D., Taylor, C.B., Hammer, L.D. *et al.* (1993). An attempt to modify unhealthful eating attitudes and weight regulation practices of young adolescent girls. *International Journal of Eating Disorders*, **13**, 369–84.

Kraut, R., Lundmark, V., Patterson, M. *et al.* (1998). Internet paradox: a social technology that reduces social involvement and psychological well-being? *American Psychologist*, **53**, 1017–31.

Larkin, J., Rice, C. & Russel, V. (1999). Sexual harassment and the prevention of eating disorders: educating young women. In *Preventing Eating Disorders. A Handbook of Interventions and Special Challenges*, ed. Piran, N., Levine, M.P. & Steiner-Adair, C. London: Brunner/Mazel, pp. 194–207.

Levine, M.P., Piran, N. & Stoddard, C. (1999). Mission more probable: media literacy, activism and advocacy as primary prevention. In *Preventing Eating Disorders. A Handbook of Interventions and Special Challenges*, ed. Piran, N., Levine, M.P. & Steiner-Adair, C. London: Brunner/Mazel, pp. 1–25.

Nasser, M., Katzman, M.A. & Gordon, R.A. (ed.). (2001). *Eating Disorders and Culture in Transition*. New York: Brunner.

Neumark-Sztainer, D., Martin, S.L. & Story, M. (2000). School-based programs for obesity prevention: what do adolescents recommend? *American Journal of Health Promotion*, **14**, 232–5.

Piran, N. (1999). The reduction of preoccupation with body weight and shape in schools: a feminist approach. In *Preventing Eating Disorders. A Handbook of Interventions and Special Challenges*, ed. Piran, N., Levine, M.P. & Steiner-Adair, C. London: Brunner/Mazel, pp. 148–59.

Pratt, B.M. & Woolfenden, S.R. (2003). Interventions for preventing eating disorders in children and adolescents (Cochrane Methodology Review). *In the Cochrane Library, Issue 4*. Chichester: John Wiley & Sons.

Ricciardelli, L.A. & McCabe, M.P. (2001). Children's body image concerns and eating disturbance: a review of the literature. *Clinical Psychopathology Reviews*, **21**, 325–44.

Rosenvinge, J.H. & Börresen, R. (1999). Preventing eating disorders: time to change programmes or paradigms? Current update and further recommendations. *European Eating Disorders Review*, **7**, 5–16.

Scholtz, E. (1997). *Behind Closed Doors*. Video. LMNO productions, Sherman Oaks, California. (For an update contact Eating Disorder Awareness & Prevention, Inc, 603 Stewart Suite 803, Seattle, WA 98101.)

Smolak, L. (1999). Elementary school curricula for the primary prevention of eating disorders. In *Preventing Eating Disorders. A Handbook of Interventions and Special Challenges*, ed. Piran, N., Levine, M.P. & Steiner-Adair, C. London: Brunner/Mazel, pp. 88–104.

Steiner-Adair, C. & Purcell Vorenberg, A. (1999). Resisting weightism: Media literacy for elementary-school children. In *Preventing Eating Disorders. A Handbook of Interventions and Special Challenges*, ed. Piran, N., Levine, M.P. & Steiner-Adair, C. London: Brunner/Mazel, pp. 105–21.

Steiner-Adair, C., Sjostrom, L., Franko, D.L. *et al.* (2002). Primary prevention of risk factors for eating disorders in adolescent girls: learning from practice. *International Journal of Eating Disorders*, **32**, 401–11.

Stewart, D.A., Carter, J.C., Drinkwater, J., Hainsworth, J. & Fairburn, C.G. (2001). Modification of eating attitudes and behavior in adolescent girls: a controlled study. *International Journal of Eating Disorders*, **29**, 107–18.

Stice, E. (2001). A prospective test of the dual pathway model of bulimic pathology. Mediating effects of dieting and negative affect. *Journal of Abnormal Psychology*, **110**, 124–35.

Stice, E. & Shaw, H. (2004). Eating disorder prevention programs: a meta-analytic review. *Psychological Bulletin*, **130**, 206–27.

Sundgott-Börgen, J. & Bahr, R. (1998). Eating disorders in athletes. In *Oxford Textbook of Sports Medicine*, ed. Harries, M. *et al.* Oxford: Oxford University Press, pp. 138–52.

Winzelberg, A.J., Eppstein, D., Eldridge, K.L. *et al.* (2000). Effectiveness of an Internet based program for reducing risk factors for eating disorders. *Journal of Consulting and Clinical Psychology*, **68**, 346–50.

Zabinski, M.F., Pung, M.A., Wilfey, D.E. *et al.* (2001). Reducing risk factors for eating disorders: Targeting at risk women with a computerized psycho-educational program. *International Journal of Eating Disorders*, **29**, 401–8.

24

Strategies for secondary prevention

Greta Noordenbos

Leiden University, Leiden, the Netherlands

Introduction

If those with anorexia nervosa (AN) or bulimia nervosa (BN) told their parents, teachers and general practitioners that they had an eating disorder and presented as motivated to change their eating behaviour, early detection would not be an issue. However, this is not the case. Most of those with eating disorders experience their slimming behaviour not as a problem but as a 'solution' for other problems such as having low self-esteem, a negative body image and feeling they are overweight. Their first success in losing weight generates higher self-esteem and a more positive attitude towards their body (Noordenbos, 1998). They are often very successful in hiding their eating disorder from others, sometimes even for years. This makes early detection by parents, teachers or general practitioners very difficult. The longer the duration of an ED, the more difficult it is to recover (Steinhausen *et al.*, 1991). For this reason early diagnosis and early intervention are seen as important. Because these strategies start when a person already has an ED, we speak about secondary prevention.

Secondary prevention is an early intervention approach to seek out emerging manifestations of EDs, and by early intervention to reduce the likelihood of disease progression. As so many cases are girls between 12 and 18 years old who live with their parents and are in education, parents, teachers, peers and general practitioners may all play pivotal roles in secondary prevention. This chapter will describe the major issues including effectiveness of secondary prevention.

Screening programmes for the detection of eating disorders

Screening programmes for risk factors and early signs of eating disorders have tended to focus on secondary schools and to be run in two stages. The first

Eating Disorders in Children and Adolescents, ed. Tony Jaffa and Brett McDermott. Published by Cambridge University Press. © Cambridge University Press 2007.

Table 24.1. Eating-disorder patients' ratings of who had been important in recognizing their problem and in facilitating them seeking help (n = 120)

Important for recognizing an eating disorder	%	Important for finding treatment	%
1. Mother	26%	1. Mother	56%
2. Friend	21%	2. General practitioner	43%
3. General practitioner	20%	3. Father	31%
4. Teacher	14%	4. Friend	19%
5. Father	11%	5. Teacher	18%
6. Classmate	8%	6. School doctor	2%
7. Lessons about ED	4%	7. Classmate	1%
8. School doctor	3%	8. Lessons about ED	0%
9. Lessons from ex-ED patient	1%	9. Lessons from ex-ED patient	0%

consists of a self-report questionnaire such as the Eating Attitudes Test (EAT) (Garner & Garfinkel, 1979). The second consists of interviewing those students with high scores on the questionnaire, often using the Eating Disorder Examination (EDE), a semi-structured interview developed by Fairburn & Cooper (1993). Evaluation of these screening strategies, however, suggests various problems. First, there are no risk factors highly predictive of the development of an ED. Second, students with early signs of an ED tend to deny having eating problems and may not fill in the questionnaire, may lie in their answers and are unlikely to attend the second stage interview. Third, those individuals who are detected by the screening instrument and who do come for interview have often already been diagnosed with an ED and are already in treatment (Rathner & Messner, 1993). It has therefore been argued that although intuitively attractive, screening programmes have limited effectiveness in the facilitation of early diagnosis and treatment of EDs (Schoemaker, 1998).

Who is important for secondary prevention?

It is usually only when dieting behaviour has become severe and the physical consequences visible that those with EDs consult a general practitioner (GP). Prior to this it tends to be family, friends and teachers who are in the best position to notice early symptoms of an ED and discuss them with the patient.

In recent research 120 young eating-disorder patients were asked who had been important in recognizing their ED, and helping them to realize they had an ED and to find treatment (Noordenbos & Vandereycken, 2005). Table 24.1 details the responses given to these questions.

It is of note that although parents are the most important source of help in early detection and in seeking intervention, very few programmes for secondary prevention are directed at assisting them in this. Most secondary prevention programmes are directed at schools and general practitioners who often recognize the eating disorder in a later stage.

Secondary prevention aimed at parents

In Table 24.1 we can see that many more mothers (26%) than fathers (11%) were the first to identify the change in eating behaviour of their daughter. Mothers often have more contact with their daughters than do fathers, and often buy the food and prepare the meals. Recent research by Van der Geest (2005) looking at possibilities of early identification of EDs by parents, in which 46 mothers and 12 fathers responded, found that the mean duration between the start of an ED and the arousal of suspicion in parents was 5 months. Partly because their daughters had developed strategies to hide the ED from their parents there was a mean delay of a further 7 months before the suspicions were confirmed either by the daughters accepting the nature of the problem or by professional diagnosis. The mean time between the start of the eating disorder and the first contact with professional help was 11 months (ranging from 0 to 48 months), with a further 3 months' delay before the treatment started (varying from 0–12 months). Parents reported that in order to be of help to their eating disordered child they needed better information about the early symptoms of EDs and the physical, psychological and social characteristics and consequences of EDs and about how to find professional treatment. Important questions for parents are: what is 'normal' dieting and what kind of dieting is a risk factor for an ED? Do I ask my daughter about her dieting behaviour or will she hide her dieting behaviour even more so that I lose contact with her? What kind of professional help is useful?

Secondary prevention aimed at peers and teachers

Most girls who develop an ED do so during their secondary school years. For this reason, teachers, friends and other pupils might be expected to have important roles in the detection of EDs. In Table 24.1 we can see that friends were seen as important in recognizing the eating disorder by 21% of those with EDs, and teachers and other pupils by 14% and 8%, respectively. Very few studies on secondary prevention have focused on how friends, teachers and other pupils can be more effective in the early recognition of eating disorders. This is clearly an area for further attention (Paxton, 1999).

Although it might be hoped that lessons about eating disorders may contribute to earlier recognition by eating disordered girls themselves, with consequent increased motivation to seek help, Table 24.1 suggests that this is not often the case. Only 4% of the ED patients realized that they had an ED after a lesson about EDs and only 1% after a lesson from a former ED patient. Whether this is because most of them did not get any prevention lessons about ED, or because the EDs lessons were ineffective or infrequent is not clear.

Secondary prevention aimed at school doctors and general practitioners

In Table 24.1 we can see that only 3% of the subjects mentioned the school doctor as the person who had recognized their eating disorder and only 2% felt that the school doctor had helped them to find treatment. By contrast, 20% of the ED subjects reported that their GP had diagnosed their ED and 43% reported that this had been the route to finding treatment. It should be noted that school doctors are by no means universally available and this varies considerably between countries.

The results of the considerable body of research carried out on secondary prevention in general practice are not very promising. Early diagnosis and treatment are hampered by a variety of factors such as patients' delay consulting their GP, communication problems within the consultation and GPs' problems in accessing specialist treatment.

Patients' delay consulting their general practitioner

Although more than 90% of ED patients consult their GP several times with complaints caused by their eating disorder, these patients are often in a late stage of the disorder (Noordenbos, 1998). It often takes several years before they are motivated to disclose their eating problems. Daaleman (1991) found a mean duration of 4 years between the onset of the ED and their first step to seek treatment for their ED. In a Dutch sample of 108 patients with AN and bulimia nervosa (BN) only 45% themselves took the initiative to see their GP, 23% were advised by others and 32% were sent by their parents (mostly mothers) (Noordenbos, 1998). Most patients fear that medical consultation will lead to them having to give up slimming and to gaining weight. Some fear hospitalization, particularly psychiatric hospitalization and being labelled as mentally ill. They may attempt to avoid such consequences by using water loading or weights to falsify their body weight. When they finally agree to visit their GP, it is often for secondary complications of their eating and slimming behaviour (Yanovski, 1991). Ogg et al. (1997) found that ED patients consult their general practitioner more frequently prior to the diagnosis with a variety of psychological, gynaecological and gastroenterological symptoms such as abdominal pain, bloating, constipation, cold intolerance, light headedness and amenorrhoea. Although these symptoms can be indicative of EDs, they often are very general and not specific enough to diagnose an ED.

Doctors' delay

General practitioners may struggle to identify EDs in an early stage (White-house *et al.*, 1992; Noordenbos, 1998). This is probably particularly the case when the diagnostic criteria are not all clearly met. Because women with BN often have normal weight, their diagnosis is missed even more often than the diagnosis of AN in which emaciation can become very visible. Hoek (1991) estimated that GPs may miss the diagnosis of more than 50% of patients with AN and nearly 90% of the patients with BN. The diagnosis is even more likely to be missed in those outside the main risk group i.e. in men, children below 12 years, women from ethnic minority groups and lower socio-economic classes.

One of the reasons for the difficulty in diagnosing EDs is that GPs often do not learn much about the characteristics of EDs in their medical education (Gurney & Halmi, 2001). A second reason is that given the low prevalence figures for EDs (Hoek, 1991) most GPs have limited exposure to these patients and do not become familiar with the conditions and the treatment needs (Burston *et al.*, 1996). King (1989) found that only 1.1% of the female and 0.5% of the male patients of GPs in the UK had an ED. More recent research of Noordenbos (1998) did not show a substantial change, although it was found that female GPs see more patients with eating disorders than do male GPs.

Diagnostic questions

For general practitioners the following symptoms can indicate an ED: weight loss, or weight swings, menstrual irregularities, loss of hair, fatigue, weakness and dizziness, dental problems, abdominal pain, constipation, cold intolerance, a sore throat, parotid swelling and dental enamel erosion (Pritts & Susman, 2003; see Birmingham, Chapter 16, this volume).

When a general practitioner suspects an ED it is very important that he or she approaches the issue very carefully and in a nonjudgemental fashion (Yanovski, 1991). Several brief ED questionnaires have been developed suitable for use by general practitioners. Perhaps the most useful of these is the SCOFF (Sick, Control, One Stone, Fat and Food) (Morgan *et al.*, 1999). The SCOFF questions are:

1.   Do you make yourself Sick (induce vomiting) because you feel uncomfortably full?
2.   Do you worry you have lost Control over how much you eat?
3.   Have you recently lost more than One stone (14 lb or 6.4 kg) in a 3-month period?
4.   Do you believe yourself to be Fat when others say you are thin?
5.   Would you say that Food dominates your life?
       (One point for every yes answer: a score $>=2$ indicates a likely case of anorexia nervosa or bulimia nervosa (sensitivity: 100%; specificity: 87.5%).

       Another instrument for adolescent women was developed by Anstine & Grinenko (2000). Their Rapid Screening Questionnaire (RSQ) for disordered eating in college-aged females in primary care consists of the following questions:

1.   How many diets have you been on in the past year?
2.   Do you think you should be dieting?
3.   Are you dissatisfied with your body size?
4.   Does your weight affect the way you think about yourself?

       A positive response to RSQ combined with positive clinical features should result either in management within primary care if not too complicated a condition and if the primary-care professional has relevant skills and interest, or otherwise in referral to an appropriate source of more specialist care. The GP may also ask about psychological risk factors for eating disorders such as low self-esteem, a negative body image, perfectionism and fear of failure (Kreipe & Birndorf, 2000). A problem is that the patient may be too ashamed to answer these questions honestly. It will often take more than one consultation before it is clear the patient has an ED (Noordenbos, 1998). It is essential to maintain a trusting relationship and to respect the feelings of fear and shame of the patient. In younger patients it is very important to include parents in the assessment and diagnostic process (Bryant-Waugh et al., 1992).

Communication problems between doctors and eating disorder patients

The diagnosis of an ED is not always accepted by the patients. In a Dutch study, 30 general practitioners reported that 27% of their ED patients completely denied their illness, 46% minimized their ED and were reluctant to be treated, 19% dropped out and only 8% had a positive attitude towards treatment (Noordenbos, 1998).

According to Vandereycken (1993) many GPs find it difficult to deal with the patient's denial of illness and their reluctance to be treated. 'Anorexics often evoke frustration and outrage in doctors who regard them as imposters because they do not have a "genuine illness", deliberately harm themselves, and refuse to cooperate in treatment, just like self-poisoners and addicts do' (Vandereycken, 1993, p. 13). Problems in the communication between patients and doctors can also be caused by gender differences (Dolan & Gitzinger, 1994). For female patients it is often more difficult to reveal their eating behaviour to male GPs, because they assume that male doctors do not understand why women are so concerned about becoming fat (Noordenbos, 1998). Male patients may be reluctant to tell their doctors about their ED, because they often feel ashamed to have a 'girl's disease'. Hence, EDs are often overlooked in males (Bryant-Waugh *et al.*, 1992).

Physical examination

In addition to a careful history an essential part of a general practitioner's assessment is the physical examination. This will include assessment for signs of purging and fluid restriction, and investigation of pulse rate, blood pressure, core temperature and a cardiovascular examination (Beumont *et al.*, 2003; Pritts & Susman, 2003; see Birmingham, Chapter 16, this volume). Laboratory investigations are not usually required and are often normal (NICE Guidelines, 2004). It is important, in this age group, not just to check weight and weight for height or BMI but to plot weight and height progression over time.

Management within general practice

Some doctors try to treat their ED patients themselves, especially those patients whose physical condition is not cause for serious concern. However, treatment by GPs is often not successful. Noordenbos (1998) found that of 93 ED patients who visited a GP, 68% were first unsuccessfully treated by their GP, before they were referred for more specialized treatment. The treatment administered by the GP consisted of medication (38%), prescription of a diet (16%) and talking about their problems more (14%) or less (32%) intensively. Recently GPs have increasingly prescribed fluoxetine, especially for patients with BN or binge-eating disorder (BED) or advised the use of self-help books (Loeb *et al.*, 2000; Carter *et al.*, 2003). Psychopharmacology interventions are discussed by Steffen, Roerig and Mitchell in Chapter 21, this volume.

Problems in referring patients for professional treatment

An important question for GPs is where to refer ED patients. Do they need a dietician, a self-help group, a psychologist, psychiatrist or medical specialist? Do they need out- or inpatient treatment? A wide variation of referrals of GPs in cases of eating disorders is found by Hugo *et al.* (2000).

Dutch studies showed that much has changed in the referral of ED patients by GPs (Noordenbos, 1998). A few decades ago 53% of ED patients were referred to a medical specialist because of the physical consequences of an ED, 19% were referred to a psychiatrist, 10% to a psychologist and 18% were treated by the GP. More recently, research carried out on 30 GPs showed an important change: 31% were referred to a community mental health centre, 23% to a psychologist, 23% to a psychiatrist and only 8% to a medical specialist. Moreover, the prescription of medication by GPs had fallen from 38% to 23%. To make a proper decision about the care which is needed, The American Psychiatric Association Work Group on Eating Disorders developed a practice guideline for treatment (APA, 2000). The levels of care vary from (1) outpatient, (2) intensive outpatient, (3) full-day outpatient, (4) residential treatment to (5) inpatient hospitalization.

Improvement of secondary prevention

Effective secondary prevention by GPs probably depends on improved educational material, enhanced diagnostic skills, good doctor–patient communication and optimized use of treatment strategies. Hoek *et al.* (1995) found that ED diagnostic skills of 58 GPs were improved by providing them with specialist training in this area. To improve early identification of EDs Gurney & Halmi (2001) developed a brief ED teaching programme for Primary Care focusing on identification of early signs, assessment and improving motivation and treatment within the primary care setting. It is probably helpful for GPs to have available, and to use, the recently developed nationally accepted guidelines for ED, such as the National Guidelines which are now developed in several countries: Australia, Canada, England, France, the Netherlands, New Zealand and the United States. The impact of these National Guidelines for improving secondary prevention of GPs is a question for new research.

Results of secondary prevention interventions

Effects of early diagnosis on anorexia nervosa

Is secondary prevention effective? Steinhausen *et al.* (1991) in their review of 67 follow-up studies between 1953 and 1989 found early diagnosis of AN to be an important predictor of earlier recovery. However, a more recent meta-analysis by Schoemaker (1997) presented a somewhat different picture.

He reviewed 33 articles on secondary prevention of AN and used the following nine criteria for inclusion in a meta-analysis: (1) a minimum of 15 patients; (2) who meet explicit diagnostic criteria for AN; (3) sufficient information on the age of onset, age of admission and duration of the illness; (4) no previous treatment for AN; (5) the period in which the patients were admitted into the study had to be less than 20 years; (6) a mean follow-up of at least 2 years after admission; (7) less than a 20-year range of follow-up; (8) 65% of the sample at admission should be included in the follow-up study and (9) use of multiple and well-defined criteria for the evaluation of the treatment outcome. Unfortunately 27 articles contained too many methodological problems and only six articles met the nine criteria for inclusion.

In four of these six the duration of the ED between the start and the first treatment was not related to recovery. In the other two a negative relationship was found between the duration of the ED and recovery, i.e. the longer the duration of the ED the poorer the results of the treatment.

Effects of early diagnosis of bulimia nervosa

In a meta-analysis Raes *et al.* (2001) found 24 articles which assessed secondary prevention of BN. However, only six articles met the same nine criteria for inclusion as mentioned for AN and were appropriate to answer the question of whether early diagnosis promoted early recovery of BN. Four studies demonstrated a negative relationship between the duration of the ED and recovery: the longer the ED the worse the outcome. Two other studies, however, showed that a longer duration of the BN was associated with a better outcome.

Summary and conclusion

Secondary prevention tries to achieve early diagnosis and early treatment. Early recognition of EDs is difficult because of the patients' delay (they do not see the seriousness of their eating behaviour or are too ashamed to talk about their ED) and the delay in recognizing an ED by parents, teachers, school doctors and GPs. Mothers are often the first to recognize the ED, followed by friends and GPs. Parents require more information if they are to be effective in secondary prevention. In case of strong suspicion of an ED parents can ask a GP for more information, or use a professional website for EDs.

Friends, teachers and schoolmates are the second group who may recognize an ED in an early stage, but they often lack the skills and instruments to make a diagnosis. They talk with the patient about her eating problems and can advise her to visit a school doctor or a GP. GPs, however, are often not well informed about EDs in their medical education and see only few ED patients, which makes it difficult for them to diagnose an ED. Recently better diagnostic instruments have been developed and many countries have national guidelines for the diagnosis and treatment of ED patients. New research is necessary to find out whether these new diagnostic instruments and national guidelines improve the diagnosis of an ED at an earlier stage.

Early recognition and diagnosis of the ED, however, does not yet guarantee early treatment and earlier recovery, as is shown by the AN meta studies of Schoemaker (1997) and the BN studies of Raes *et al.* (2001). After the diagnosis of an ED many problems can delay the process of recovery: (1) many ED patients are not motivated to change their eating behaviour and are very afraid of gaining weight; (2) patients often have to wait before they can start therapy; (3) not all treatments are effective and no treatments guarantee recovery; (4) many treatments focus only on improvement of eating behaviour, weight and menses, and full recovery in which improvement is also realized in psychological, emotional and social well-being is not always managed by the end of the treatment (Strober *et al.*, 1997).

To be effective secondary prevention has to be followed by prompt and effective treatment focusing not only on the motivation of ED patients to recover, the disordered eating behaviour and weight restoration, but also the psychological, emotional and social condition of the patient (Strober *et al.*, 1997; Fennig & Roe, 2002). Only when these conditions are fulfilled is it realistic to assume that early recognition might lead to early recovery. However, there is still a long way to go.

REFERENCES

Anstine, D. & Grinenko, D. (2000). Rapid screening for disordered eating in college-aged females in the primary care setting. *Journal of Adolescent Health*, **26**, 338–42.

American Psychiatric Association Work Group on Eating Disorders (2000). Practice guideline for the treatment of patients with eating disorders (revision). *American Journal of Psychiatry*, **157** (suppl. 1), 20.

Beumont, P.J.V., Hay, P. & Beumont, R.O. (2003). *Australian and New Zealand Clinical Practice Guideline for the Treatment of Anorexia Nervosa*. Royal Australian and New Zealand College of Psychiatrists.

Burston, M.S., Gabel, L.L., Brose, J.A., & Monk, J.S. (1996) Detecting and treating bulimia nervosa: How involved are family physicians? *Journal of American Board of Family Practitioners*, **9**, 241–8.

Bryant-Waugh, G.J., Lask, B.D., Shafran, R.L. & Fosson, A.R. (1992). Do doctors recognise eating disorders in children? *Archives of Diseases in Childhood*, **67**, 103–5.

Carter, J.C., Olmsted, M.P., Kaplan, A.S. *et al.* (2003). A: Self-help for bulimia nervosa: a randomised controlled trial. *American Journal of Psychiatry,* **160**, 973–8.

Daaleman, C.J. (1991). *More or less: Research on the prevalence of anorexia nervosa, bulimia nervosa, and obesity.* (In Dutch.) Warnsveld: Rigg Oost Gelderland.

Dolan, B. & Gitzinger, I. (ed.) (1994). *Why Women? Gender Issues and Eating Disorders.* London: Athlone Press.

Fairburn, C.G. & Cooper, Z. (1993). The Eating Disorders Examination (12th edn). In *Binge Eating: Nature, Assessment and Treatment,* ed. Fairburn, C. G & Wilson, G.T. New York: Guilford Press, pp. 317–60.

Fennig, S. & Roe, D. (2002). Physical recovery in anorexia nervosa: is this the sole purpose of a child and adolescent medical-psychiatric unit? *General Hospital Psychiatry,* **24**, 87–92.

Garner, D.M. & Garfinkel, P.E. (1979). The Eating Attitudes Test: an index of symptoms of anorexia nervosa. *Psychological Medicine,* **9**, 273–9.

Geest, M. van der (2005). Parents' capacities to recognise an eating disorder in an early stage. *Thesis.* Leiden University, Leiden.

Gurney, V.W. & Halmi, K.A. (2001). Developing an eating disorders curriculum for primary care providers. *Eating Disorders,* **9**, 97–107.

Hoek, H.W. (1991). The incidence and prevalence of anorexia nervosa and bulimia nervosa in primary care. *Psychological Medicine,* **21**, 455–60.

Hoek, H.W., Bartelds, A.I.M., Bosveld, J.J.F. *et al.* (1995). Impact of urbanization on detection rates of eating disorders. *American Journal of Psychiatry,* **152**, 1272–8.

Hugo, P., Kendrick, T., Reid, F., & Lacey, H. (2000). GP referral to an eating disorder service: why the wide variation? *British Journal of General Practice,* **50**, 380–3.

King, M.B. (1989). Eating disorders in a general practice population. Prevalence, characteristics and follow-up at 12–18 months. *Psychological Medicine,* Monograph Supplement 14.

Kreipe, R.E. & Birndorf, S.A. (2000). Eating disorders in adolescents and young adults. *Medical Clinics of North America,* **84**, 1027–49.

Loeb, K.L., Wilson, G.T., Gilbert, J.S. & Labouvie, E. (2000). Guided and un-guided self-help for binge eating. *Behaviour Research Therapy,* **38**, 259–72.

Morgan, J.F., Reid, F. & Lacey, J.H. (1999). The SCOFF questionnaire: assessment of a new screening tool for eating disorders. *British Medical Journal,* **319**, 1467–8.

NICE Guidelines (2004). *Core Interventions in the Treatment and Management of Anorexia Nervosa, Bulimia Nervosa and Related Eating Disorders.* Manchester: National Institute for Clinical Excellence.

Noordenbos, G. (1998). Eating disorders in primary care: early identification and intervention by general practitioners. In *The Prevention of Eating Disorders,* ed. Vandereycken, W. & Noordenbos, G. London: Athlone Press, pp. 214–29.

Noordenbos, G. & Vandereycken, W. (2005). *Prevention of Eating Disorders.* Mechelen: Kluwer.

Ogg, E.C., Millar, H.R., Pusztai, E.E. & Thom, A.S. (1997). General practice consultation patterns preceding diagnosis of eating disorders. *International Journal of Eating Disorders,* **22**, 89–93.

Paxton, S.J. (1999). Peer relations, body image, and disordered eating in adolescent girls; implications for prevention. In *Preventing Eating Disorders. A Handbook of Interventions and Special Challenges*, ed. Piran, N., Levine, M.P. & Steiner-Adair, C. London: Brunner/Mazel, pp. 134–47.

Pritts, S.D. & Susman, J. (2003). Diagnosis of eating disorders in primary care. *American Family Physician*, **67**, 297–304.

Raes, D.L., Schoemaker, C., Zipfel, S. & Williamson, D.A. (2001). Prognostic value of duration of illness and early intervention in bulimia nervosa: a systematic review of the outcome literature. *International Journal of Eating Disorders*, **30**, 1–10.

Rathner, G. & Messner, K. (1993). Detection of eating disorders in a small rural town: an epidemiological study. *Psychological Medicine*, **23**, 175–84.

Schoemaker, C. (1997). Does early intervention improve the prognosis in anorexia nervosa? A systematic review of the treatment-outcome literature. *International Journal of Eating Disorders*, **21**, 1–15.

Schoemaker, C. (1998). The principles of screening for eating disorders. In *The Prevention of Eating Disorders*, ed. Vandereycken, W. & Noordenbos, G. London: Athlone Press, pp. 187–213.

Steinhausen, H.C., Rauss-Masson, C. & Seidel, R. (1991). Follow-up studies of anorexia nervosa: a review of four decades of outcome research. *Psychological Medicine*, **21**, 447–54.

Strober, M., Freeman, R. & Morrell, W. (1997). The long-term course of severe AN in adolescents: survival analysis of recovery, relapse and outcome predictors over 10–15 years in a prospective study. *International Journal of Eating Disorders*, **22**, 339–60.

Vandereycken, W. (1993). Naughty girls and angry doctors: eating disorder patients and their therapists. *International Review of Psychiatry*, **5**, 13–18.

Whitehouse, A.M., Cooper, P.J., Vize, C.V., Hill, C. & Vogel, L. (1992). Prevalence of eating disorders in three Cambridge general practices: hidden and conspicuous morbidity. *British Journal of General Practice*, **42**, 57–60.

Yanovski, S.Z. (1991). Bulimia nervosa: the role of the family physician. *American Academy of Family Physicians*, **44**, 1231–8.

Index

In this index AN stands for anorexia nervosa, BN for bulimia nervosa and EDs for eating disorders. Note that only information specific to either AN or BN is indexed under those entry terms.